ASIAN BIOTECH

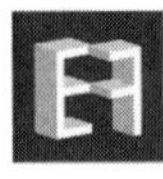

EXPERIMENTAL FUTURES

TECHNOLOGICAL LIVES, SCIENTIFIC ARTS, ANTHROPOLOGICAL VOICES

A series edited by Michael M. J. Fischer and Joseph Dumit

Edited by Aihwa Ong
and Nancy N. Chen

| ASIAN BIOTECH |

ETHICS AND COMMUNITIES OF FATE

| Duke University Press | Durham and London | 2010 |

Printed in the United States of America on acid-free paper ∞
Designed by Heather Hensley
Typeset in Chaparral Pro by Keystone Typesetting, Inc.
Library of Congress Cataloging-in-Publication Data appear on the last printed page of this book.

An earlier version of chapter 1, by Kaushik Sunder Rajan, was published as "Experimental Values: Indian Clinical Trials and Surplus Health," *New Left Review* 45 (2007): 67–88.

A different version of chapter 8, by Margaret Sleeboom-Faulkner, was published as "Debates on Human Embryonic Cells in Japan: Minority Voices and Their Political Amplifiers," *Science as Culture* 17, no. 1 (March 2008): 85–97.

Contents

Acknowledgments

The University of California Pacific Rim Research Program provided the funding for our workshop "Asian Biotech" that met in April 2006. The University of Hawaii John A. Burns School of Medicine generously offered conference facilities for the meeting, and we thank Lesley Sharp for her role as a discussant.

We are grateful to the workshop participants for their contributions, which make up this collection. Janelle Lamoreaux provided skillful assistance in preparing the final manuscript. Maura High's excellent copyediting is much appreciated. Finally, we thank the Abigail Reynolds Hodgen Publication Fund for defraying the costs involved in getting this book ready for publication.

INTRODUCTION **AIHWA ONG**

An Analytics of Biotechnology and Ethics at Multiple Scales

The dispersal of genetic science across the world raises questions about the interactions of biotechnologies and bioethics in diverse global locations. Yet the tendency has been to think in terms of general rules for governing the proliferation of scientific and commercial uses of biological resources. For instance, at the 2008 meeting of the World Economic Forum in Davos, a panel proposing "Rules for the Genomic Age" issued this statement:

> Genetic data about specific populations may soon be in the hands of a wide variety of interested players from pharmaceutical firms to insurance companies for scientifically and commercially valid reasons. How should access to, and the application of, this information be managed to both promote collaborative innovation and address societal concerns?"[1]

It is perhaps not surprising that meetings dominated by pharmaceutical interests do not list the nation-state as an interested player, nor is there any mention of resurgent nationalism and ethical debates in non-Western contexts as influences in the uses and effects of the biosciences. Even academic research has struggled to keep abreast of recent events that highlight the complex intersections of the life sciences and ethical dilemmas in Asia:

1. At the turn of the new century Singapore launched Biopolis, a biomedical research hub that seeks to combine researchers from the public and private sectors. The government boasted about the

"state-of-the-art infrastructure including shared resources and services catering to the full spectrum of R & D activities and graduate training." Stunning buildings with names like Genome, Matrix, Nanos, Centros, Helios, Proteos, Neuros, and Immunos house a spectrum of research institutes, many led by "world-class" (a favorite term) scientists from around the world. The complex has overcome initial global skepticism to win accolades such as "a high-tech heaven" and "Asia's biotech tiger," and to advertise itself in *Science* as "the Biopolis of Asia."[2]

2. Shortly after scientists on the Human Genome Project released a rough draft of their report in 2000, China was the only developing nation to contribute to ongoing sequencing. The Beijing Genomics Institute has since sequenced the genomes of the cucumber, the giant panda, an ancient human, and many microbes. Called "the sequence factory," the BGI is expected to surpass the total sequencing output of the United States.[3]
3. In early 2004, a scandal roiled the stem cells world, when the sensational claim of the South Korean scientist Dr. Hwang Woo-Suk, to be the first to clone a human embryo, was exposed as fraudulent. The research reported in two papers published by Dr. Hwang's team in *Science* was later revealed as fabricated. Not only was this scandal a major blow to South Korean science, it also raised ethical questions about lab practices surrounding the donation of human eggs.[4] The event cast an international spotlight on South Korea's quest to build a "world stem cell hub with new labs in California" and to influence global perception of "different ethical norms" for biomedical research in Asian sites.[5]
4. More recently, in 2007, stem cell research made a major advance in Asia. In Japan, Shinya Yamanaka successfully reprogrammed skin cells to produce stem cells, thereby expanding the toolkit beyond the use of human embryos in research. Although an American team also made a similar discovery at the University of Wisconsin, Yamanaka has single-handedly put Japan on the cutting edge of scientific research by developing an alternative technique to induce pluripotent stem cells.[6]

This book responds to the urgent need for examining the deployment of biotechnologies in economic growth, biosecurity, and ethical configurations in contemporary Asia. Its chapters present ethnographic studies of biotech projects in Asian countries, but also identify their convergence in practices of ethical reasoning. Some of the contributions to the volume report a trend in state entrepreneurialism that makes biotechnological innovations the new model for cutting-edge capitalism. At the same time, contributors frequently link biotechnologies in Asian contexts to issues of national security and management of a risky future.

There are growing efforts to make connections between the new tradability of "bio" in the bioeconomy and the securitization of "bio" in biopolitics. Crucially, for Asian states, biotechnologies are not merely about the transformation of nature into market shares, but also biosecurity mechanisms aligned with nationalist projects. For instance, as a region of postcolonial emergence, of "uncanny surplus" in population and pandemics, and ascendant nations and megastates, Asian countries treat their populations as a political artifact of risk and opportunity, as well as a fertile source of potential material and ethical values. The new biotechnologies, moreover, enable the materialization of an expanding national field of power that articulates nonmaterial values such as collective imaginings and affective mappings of identities.

While specific biotech policies and styles vary by the Asian countries considered here, there is a convergence of political thinking and of uses of the life sciences that articulate regimes of risk management and thus reinforce feelings and convictions about the collective fate—productivity, wealth, health, and security—of certain populations. By "communities of fate" I refer to three kinds of communalism that can be enhanced, invoked, and given new life through the deployment of biotechnologies, genomics, and molecular sciences. First, postcolonial nationalism in Asia is fundamentally about the regeneration of political and cultural communities on the global stage. As state-led enterprises, biotechnologies are allied to nationalist efforts to overcome past humiliations and to restore national identity and political ambition. The examples mentioned above all register a deep nationalist fervor in the race to be "number one" in cutting-edge sciences, with its promise of a lucrative science-driven economy.

Second, less obvious to outside observers are the social and symbolic effects of biotech innovations, the different ways biological anxieties get worked into biotech projects. Recent experiences of epidemics, new demands for biomedicine tailored to Asian populations, and an overriding sense of living with biological risks have instilled a need for greater biosecurity. Biotech enterprises are perceived to have the added value of enhancing human security and are thus legitimized as a necessity for emerging nations to combat certain biological vulnerabilities. Different kinds of biotechnology respond to national anxieties about food supplies, diseases, epidemics, and the still-unknown biological crises of the future.

Third, the assembling of databases and pharmacogenomics reinscribe traditional beliefs about ethnicity, nation, and even race, thus giving a molecular cast to collective fate at shifting and multiple scales. There are real differences among Asian situations, each shaped by a particular assemblage of technology, politics, and ethics.[7] In many cases, the articulation of biotechnologies and risk calculations stirs deep feelings about shared fate, and crystallizes new ethical configurations as "life" takes on new meanings, from ethnic inheritance to future present risk. But before I turn to a discussion of ethical practices thus mobilized, I will define the different forms of biotechnologies in question.

"Biotechnology" is defined in the *American Heritage Science Dictionary* as "the use of biological substances or techniques to engineer or manufacture a product or substance, as when cells that produce antibodies are cloned in order to study their effects on cancer cells."[8] To put it simply, "biotechnology" refers to technology that makes use of biology, as in the production of genetically modified (GM) foods and biofuels, and especially in the production of drugs and the engineering of therapies. Thus, biotechnology is involved in broad swaths of contemporary living. Biotechnology is also associated with biosecurity systems (such as surveillance tools and military capabilities), the efficiency of production systems, and consumer lifestyle choices in relation to food, energy, and medicine. Furthermore, today, the biological sciences have become digital and computer-intensive, and computational biologists are able to simulate experiments, predict outcomes, and design miniaturized devices and microorganisms for treating patients. The impact of computational biology for notions of what it means to be human is enormous, but the geopolitical context of technodecision and technoimplementation shapes the broader implications of such experimentations.

The biotech innovations in the above examples illustrate the interplay of nationalist security interests and scientific entrepreneurialism in many Asian sites, and the fraught outcomes of the specific ventures that ripple beyond the field of biosciences. The chapters that follow index developments in different biotech fields: genetically modified foods, clinical trials, stem cells research, drug consumerism and regenerative medical tourism, blood donation and banking, and pharmacogenomics and genetics research. These biotechnologies are investigated in complex evolving milieus, all already entangled with sovereign reason, neoliberal logic, and the logics of collectivist ethics. A major goal of the volume is to present recent ethnographic studies on specific contexts of claims about the ethical in and for Asian biotechnologies.

Although each chapter focuses on one kind of material technology or biotech field, in actuality different kinds of biotechnologies can be found in various combinations in the same country. The availability and uses of different forms of biotechnologies reflect state strategies in shaping biotech niches, but also divisive ethical practices that articulate different modes of bioeconomy. There are significant divergences in the extent of state involvement and the spillover effects of specific programs beyond the immediate experimental fields.

Nevertheless, despite political, programmatic, and social differences in each country's biotech revolution, this scientific turn articulates a transcendental notion of emerging Asia. The term "Asian biotech" captures some important points of convergence across this diversity in the biotech industry. First, the emerging combination of biotech expertise, national politics, and collective interests is constitutive of an "emerging technoscientific cosmopolitan world."[9] "Asian biotech" denotes a regional sphere of scientific imagination and endeavor. This is a historical moment when biotechnologies articulate powerful nationalist aspirations in newly affluent Asia. Indeed, Asian imaginations of "the West"[10] as the original source of biological sciences, and the negative Western judgments of Asian knowledges, shape the global context within which individual Asian countries position and project the life sciences in their own rise as modern nations. The biotech revolution represents a "Sputnik opportunity" for Asian states seeking to "catch up with" and potentially surpass "the West." By deploying a mix of neoliberal logics and molecular science, ambitious Asian states are reconfiguring the risks of surplus populations and surplus needs into biotech opportunities for growth and security.

Second, while global attention has focused on Asian commercialization of biological forms, biotech projects articulate biorisks that menace Asian futures, and are thus entangled with processes of ethical reasoning at many scales. In this diverse yet converging region of biotechnicity, the ethical reasoning surrounding science-driven politics, ethics, and sociality links moral subjects and collectives from kinship to nation and beyond. This collection of studies traces experiments with bioeconomies and tracks emerging ethical configurations that link regeneration, bioresponsibility, and biosecurity to the political constitution of subjects and communities of fate.

Finally, while biotech-related ethical processes are located in the specificity of contemporary Asia, I propose a generalizable analytics of ethics that can be divorced from particular Asian contexts and applied productively to other sites and moments of biotech and biopolitical governance.

Technology and Ethics

The yoking of bioeconomies and collective ethics may seem paradoxical, since many Marxists, sociologists, and social scientists tend to view technologies—in this case, political, neoliberal, and biotech—as forms of cold, instrumental materialism that cannot be aligned with ethical values. Indeed, as debates in the United States have shown, biotechnologies are widely viewed as a broad endangerment of ethical forms and human freedom, an overcoming of individual will by mechanic will to power. The Western liberal tradition of viewing machines as a threat to man, reinforced by George Orwell's *1984* and Aldous Huxley's *Brave New World*, is a specter that haunts modern Western consciousness.[11]

Such fears have influenced science and technology studies, which assume that nature/culture divides permeate epistemological and ontological claims of self, science, and beyond. The leading feminist scientist Donna Haraway has been both prescient and courageous in challenging science studies scholars and public activists on their beliefs in a fundamental nature/culture divide and taking a resolutely antitechnology stance. She argues that many of these scholarly and activist approaches make claims and arguments based on their own fear of recognizing the hybrid quality of human/nonhuman technology/bios. Because of culture's history of fiddling with nature, she argues, we are all entangled nature/culture subjects, or cyborgs.[12] Indeed, feminists and anthropologists have long viewed technology and ethics as mutually constitutive, and yet the exploration of ethics—a question of how to do the right thing in biosciences—beyond the clinic and the public has yet to engage nationalist and geopolitical issues.

In contrast to the skepticism and unease of the West, the embrace of Western technology by Asian countries seems overly determined by dual effects of Western imperialism and nation-building. For over two centuries, Western science and technologies were instrumental in facilitating European domination of Asia. To fend off Western encroachments, Japan became the first Asian nation to industrialize,[13] thus inspiring postcolonial countries to seek Western knowledge as a tool of national empowerment. A pragmatic and flexible approach to modern technology gave rise to the Asian tiger economies in the 1970s, first South Korea, Singapore, Hong Kong, and Taiwan, and in the 1980s, Malaysia, Thailand, Indonesia, and post-Mao China. Scientific gains in education, industry, and research gave concrete expression to the modern state's efforts in ensuring the future of their citizens. By 2010, China's accelerating economy had overtaken Japan's, becoming the engine that drives Asian (and global) economic activities.[14] Now as Asian nations shift beyond manufacturing to knowledge-based industries, they turn to biotechnologies for diagnostic tools and solutions to problems of life and national prowess. One should note that Asian attitudes toward modern technologies had not always been unambiguous. Deep tensions between Western rationalities and cultural values had long festered in China,[15] and not until the late twentieth century did the necessity of modern science for national empowerment largely silence lingering doubts. As in the West, there is recognition that modern technology endangers ethics, but ethics disarticulated from modern science does not appear to be a real option for the emerging world.

In truth, East Asian leaders are dazzled by the economic, social, and political gains that can stem from developing scientific expertise and knowledge. In science parks from Singapore to Shanghai, scientists are viewed as demigods and national heroes. Scientific work in converting nature into products is celebrated for its patriotic contribution to economic growth and for its ethical quest to treat diseases endemic in the region. For instance, the Singapore doctors who died in the course of dealing with the outbreak of severe acute respiratory syndrome, or

SARS, are honored as self-sacrificing patriots.[16] In a different example, before his fall from grace, Dr. Hwang Woo-Suk had a large fan club promoting Seoul as a world-class stem cell hub. Indeed, despite the devastating effects of accidents and pollution associated with rapid industrialization, and rigorous protests by public intellectuals, biotechnologies are not generally viewed in dystopian terms. Rather, there is a sense that biotechnologies are clean and innovative, flexible and versatile, bringing cutting-edge science to newly affluent populations. In South Asia, the populist dazzle is focused more on nuclear scientists than on clinicians; and while environmental movements led by charismatic environmentalists have caught international headlines (the movement against dams is one example), there is no mistaking the vital role of laboratory science in leveraging national prestige in the region.

Despite uneven achievements in biotech development across Asia, there is a common conviction that biotechnology is a necessary tool for defining and solving problems of national and collective interests. Biotech forms are not introduced in a purely technical context, but are always already enmeshed with preexisting social norms, cultural beliefs, and political goals. Their comingling crystallizes situated conditions for shaping life and its various implications for communities of fate mapped at different scales. The political tendency among the elites is not to question the compatibility of technologies and modern solidarity, but to deploy rational and materialist justifications for reinforcing the commitments of subjects, and for configuring a spirit of commonality and nationalist futures.

An Analytics of Ethics

While the ethical processes discussed in this book are located in the specificity of contemporary Asia, the studies taken together make the case for a more generalizable analytics of ethics beyond the region. Before enlarging on that ethics, I will briefly review different anthropological diagnoses of contemporary ethics associated with biotechnology and then propose the alternative analytics, which I call situated ethics.

ETHICS AS MORAL CRITICISM

A popular anthropological perspective has tended to find multiple examples of morally condemnable biotech conduct measured against a universalizing moral philosophy. In North America, bioethics tends to be narrowly focused on protecting the rights of individuals and of historically discriminated groups. For instance, besides the worry over the informed consent of patients and experimental subjects, debates have focused on customized drugs that target certain racial or ethnic groups. A report on "medical apartheid," for example, exposes the history of inhuman medical experimentation on African Americans.[17] New medical procedures and drugs stir fear that "misleading correlations of race, genetics, and behavior" will foster racist mistreatment at the hands of the law and penal system.[18]

The exposure of shocking misuses of research and biomedical practices has become a common anthropological project. Nancy Scheper Hughes has tracked black markets in organs that depend on kidnapping, trickery, and physicians' complicity to generate volunteers who wish to sell their body parts. She notes that even when regulations are in place, the lines between ethical donation and commercialized trading are becoming blurred because of the acceleration of the global traffic in organs.[19] Global pharmaceutical companies (collectively known as "Big Pharma") are also viewed as increasingly unreliable in protecting human bodies and as exercising a form of discriminatory "ethical variability" around the world. Noting the proliferation of opportunities for clinical trials in poor countries, Adriana Petryna and others have framed the ethical question as a matter of who gets treated and who doesn't; who is exploited for bioresources and who gains?[20] In such studies, the anthropologist is presented as a watchdog of ethical violations, or as a moral actor helping to forge ethical resolutions for more equitable distribution of value between donors and experimental subjects, on the one hand, and predatory commercial and medical entities, on the other.

Another related moral critical approach firmly situates biotechnologies as elements in contemporary capitalism, and thus allied to exploitative logics. Catherine Waldby and Robert Mitchell have argued that biotechnological forms and practices have become inseparable from the generation of "biovalue" that is produced when "the generative and transformative productivity of living entities can be instrumentalized along lines that make them useful for human projects—science, industry, medicine, agriculture or other arenas of technical culture."[21] The capture and use of human organs in a "tissue economy" maximizes their productivity through "circulation, leverage, diversification, and recuperation," thereby creating a hierarchy of values for these organs.[22] Kaushik Sunder Rajan more rigorously pursues the connection between markets and the life sciences, claiming that capitalism "overdetermines the emergence of new technoscience." He has identified a biotechnology-driven form of capitalism that has engendered novel forms of "alienation, expropriation, and divestiture" that go beyond Marx's formulation of exploitation.[23] Despite their critique of biocapitalism, Waldby and Mitchell, on the one hand, and Sunder Rajan, on the other, are also aware that global tissue and biotech networks have an effect on the politics of life and subject formation. Waldby and Mitchell note that the susceptibility of even altruistically donated tissues to global commercialization is nevertheless tempered by the flourishing of a tissue economy and alliances between commercial and civil society interests.[24] Sunder Rajan notes that the biotech-based markets shape new "individual and collective subjectivities and citizenships."[25]

This moral evaluation of commodified biotech systems becomes more nuanced in studies that see complex ethical possibilities associated with the use of transplant or reproductive technologies. Participation in intrusive surgery can involve a form of ethical self-validation. Charis Thompson has noted that biovalue produced by regenerative medicine exceeds market processes condemned by Marxist scholars. The "biopolitics of reproduction," she argues, captures forms of value intrinsic to life-giving potential. "Reproductive intrinsic value is self-validating and is not dependent on a community of experts and evaluation of skills." Furthermore, she notes, the productivity of stem cell research is not focused on immediate profit making, but is future-oriented with regard to "knowledge, technologies of life, and promise."[26] In this debate, there are interconnections between the production of biovalues and other kinds of ethical values beyond the strictly economic, including the symbolic value of life generation. Even at the molecular level, as Sarah Franklin has noted, genetic information is inherently inflected with specific aims and relationships that maintain social and political claims.[27]

When the viewpoint is enlarged beyond the laboratory, ethical decisions become negotiative practices with circles of significant others. Lawrence Cohen observes that the status of "operability" of poor Indians induces them to supply the growing market in kidneys. However, a decision to sell one's kidney for cash is often recognized as an act of sacrifice and love made within the moral economy of kinship. "Sellers usually sell to support loved ones, particularly in conditions of everyday or extraordinary debt."[28] Here is an important reminder that decisions surrounding the use of biotechnologies can have profound ethical implications that spill beyond the isolated patient or donor.

Thus, any mode of moral reasoning in a biotech setting articulates bioethics in the narrow ethical sense, and perhaps even more urgently in preexisting ethical scales beyond the clinical subject. An anthropological inquiry into ethical practices would examine how bioethical norms that regulate clinicians' practices and patients' choices unavoidably involve broader ethical considerations that spiral beyond the lab and the clinic. A new donor ethics in the United States is the "kidney daisy chain," whereby a donor whose kidney is not compatible with an intended recipient (usually a relative or friend) gives her organ to a more compatible patient. This anonymous gift triggers new donations by the loved ones of the recipient patient, thus generating a chain of donors and transplants.[29] The kidney daisy chain is a great example of how the bioethics of kidney donation (voluntary informed consent) articulates with an ethics of indirect reciprocity derived from kinship and altruism.

BIOMEDICAL LIBERALISM

Another approach ties contemporary biomedical practices largely to ethical expressions of liberal individualism. Following Foucault, scholars claim that individual choice, informed consent, and other forms of "nondirectness" express the very essence of "governmentality." Thus, contemporary techniques of governmentality exercised in the field of biomedicine represent an emergent form of governmentality that is free of state constraints.[30] Rose and Carlos Novas invoke the notion of "biological citizenship" to describe a process whereby patient groups in Britain both make claims for resources and challenge experts and authorities on health policies. They maintain that these medical consumers generate a kind of "public value" vis-à-vis the authorities.[31] Elsewhere, Rose asserts that the devolution of many responsibilities of the social state to quasi-autonomous bodies places increasing emphasis on self-management with a prudential focus on one's own future security.[32] This view of contemporary ethics follows Foucault's claim that liberal freedoms of self-constitution are autonomous of state power, leading to an eventual "'governmentalization' of the state."[33]

Ethnographic research in an array of settings, however, reveals a lacuna in the critique of ethics and the liberal individual perspectives, both of which ignore or reject ethical processes involving the state. The demands of self-managing subjects, after all, frequently involve claims on the state power and its capacity to respond to citizens' health demands. In her study of the Chernobyl meltdown, Adriana Petryna observes that victims were able to claim biomedical resources, social equities, and human rights from the state.[34] Her notion of biological citizenship allows for and addresses issues of sovereignty in a much more thorough way than Rose and Novas—who borrowed her concept—allow. As Mitchell Dean argues, biopolitical choices are claims on the appropriation and use of organized resources of the government, and also the political means "by which a settlement to a struggle can be forcibly imposed," adding that "what is at stake are often matters of life and death."[35]

SITUATED ETHICS

As an alternative to the perspectives described above, which make ethical judgments about particular ethnographic situations; seek to rectify them according to some universalizing ethical standard; or link biotech innovations to ethical possibilities of self-validation or enhancement of liberal subjectivity, I propose an analytics of situated ethics. Indeed, the anthropology of science and social medicine have long questioned the "coherence" model of philosophers, and anthropologists have variously posed relational and situational ethics as counters to the claims of universal systemic ethics.[36] This anthropological approach has focused on cultural (gender, ethnic, and racial) differences in ethical reasoning. But in contemporary conditions of heterogeneity, flux, and uncertainty, we cannot proceed from a position of stable or standardized props of culture. Rather, "ethics" become part of tentative experiments with heterogeneous elements that are amenable to control and valuation. Stephen J. Collier and Andrew Lakoff have suggested that an analytics of situated forms of moral reasoning ("regimes of living"), by resolving problems at hand, provides possible guides for ethical action. In contemporary times, this alternative vantage point would consider the rise of technology and biopolitics as "sources of dynamism that are critical to understanding how the constitution of ethical subjects, forms of ethical reasoning, and practices of living with respect to the good are at stake today."[37] My concept of situated ethics takes the emergent assemblage of diverse logics as the space and tension within which moral reasoning takes place, and is woven into overlapping contexts of technology and sociality. Several theoretical insights drawn from research on situated ethics in Asian biotech assemblages have greater applicability beyond the region. The following are not mutually exclusive but concern coexisting social phenomena.

First, an analytics of ethical practices dives below schematized descriptions of expropriation and alienation in biotech enterprises. Instead of proceeding from a position of moral certitude to make judgments about particular ethnographic situations or seek to remedy them according to a universal set of ethics, an anthropology of ethics is necessarily about locating ethical practices, that is, tracking ethical configurations where "ethicalizing" processes and decisions take place. Situated ethics happen at the intersection of competing logics of politics, technology, and culture. Overlaps and tensions between multiple ethical regimes are conditions within which moral decisions are made for solving a particular bioethical dilemma.

Second, moral reasoning, I maintain, is located not in the empirical individual, but in the space of convergence or contestation between shifting scales of ethical life. The classic question "What is the good life?" should be reposed as "What is the good life for my family, community, people, humanity at large?," depending on the context of broader engagement or consideration. "What ought I to do (in this moment of ethical decision making)?" takes into consideration how my action would affect these significant others, again at multiple scales of family, ethnicity, or community.

Third, in many unfolding situations, broader ethical scales can be invoked over that of the (presumed) isolated moral person. At various scales, questions about the "ethical decision" or "the good life" for the individual necessarily tack between individual, kinship, and large collectivities of ethnicity and nation.

The ethical critique approach is fixated on the moral subject as the locus of ethical formation, and from that isolated vantage point, makes large abstract claims about universal ethics. Another type of ethical scaling would merely displace a question from a scale we are familiar with to another one, for example, from self-management (e.g., as in the studies of Rose and Novas) to demands on the state for providing biosecurity (as in Petryna). In sharp distinction, an anthropology of situated practices captures novel forms of ethicalizing in the midst of an assemblage of interacting technical, political, and ethical possibilities. The notion of situated ethics offers a view that takes scale into account, yet cannot be reduced to any single scale, and holds that it is precisely the space between scales where ethical work takes place.

This diagnosis of ethicalization at multiples scales requires that we include state and nationalist collectivities in thinking through risk, biopolitics, and sovereignty. In a powerful and insoluble way, broader scales of ethical reasoning articulate geopolitical stakes of contemporary globalization. In an age of global risk, Ulrich Beck notes, "reflexive modernization" cannot transform uncertainty into issues of order, but has at its profound center calculations and risks in confronting uncertainty.[38] The essays in this volume indicate how each biotech-biosecurity assemblage crystallizes conditions for confronting ethical questions about life, risk, and security that cascade across multiple collectivities. Emerging Asian situations indicate that diverse biotechnologies are not necessarily divergent from ethical possibilities of welfare, security, and identity. Furthermore it remains an open question whether biomedical self-management undermines sovereign power, or whether it can also strengthen the sovereign power's control of technologies and provision of resources and services when the national interest is also at stake. Such broad ethicalizing processes become interwoven with everyday ethical decisions about biomedicine, biotechnology, and biosecurity, that is, ethicalizing practices at many levels of society that become constitutive of new communities of fate (as I will discuss in more detail below).

Subject and Sovereignty

Genomic science has unleashed infinite possibilities for reworking the "bio" in biopolitics, allowing a combination of different techniques to be exercised in the biotech management of life, and of the self. Foucault notes that biopolitics "is, finally . . . control over relations between the human race, or human beings in so far as they are a species, in so far as they are living beings, and the environment, the milieu in which they live. This includes the direct effects of the geographic, climatic, or hydrographic environment: the problem, for instance, of swamps, and of epidemics."[39] Biopolitics are simply the "security mechanisms . . . installed around the random element inherent in a population of living beings so as to optimize a state of life."[40] If, as Foucault argues, biopolitics is fundamentally an apparatus of security,[41] then how does the biopolitics of security change in an age of genomics and assertive Asian sovereignty?

Foucault himself is complicated and contradictory on the ways in which sovereignty and governmentality might coconstitute each other or at least exist simultaneously. For instance, he has cautioned against a "reductive view of the relative importance of the state" as expounded in Marxist ideas about the state as oppressor.[42] But elsewhere he notes that "in the second half of the eighteenth century, taking responsibility for the population will involve the development of, if not the sciences, then at least practices and types of intervention," such as social medicine, public hygiene, demography, and so on. Thereafter, "the population as a collection of subjects is replaced by the population as a set of natural phenomena," that is, as a constituted reality for which the state will have to be responsible.[43] The question is, how to explore Foucauldian ideas about biopolitics, on the one hand, and his assertions about the state role in shaping a biosocial milieu, on the other? An even more challenging task is to interrogate the complex entanglement of biotechniques of subjectivization and sovereign-inflected notions of the national subject. The challenge for analysts is to specify how biopolitics intersects political responsibility, and how the rights of individuals articulate the rights of states.

After Foucault, one may argue, the biopolitics of security must be situated in relation to the geopolitics of state security. For much of the twentieth century, "bio-regulation by the state"[44] was exercised through infrastructural systems, for instance, to protect domestic security against catastrophic threats such as nuclear attacks.[45] Gradually, health security has come to the fore, gaining its fullest realization yet in the new biotech mechanisms that configure new living forms, but such processes and materials increasingly circulate in an international context. Contrary to popular perceptions, the regulation of biotech flows is managed not only by pharmaceutical companies and global health agencies, but also by nationalist states that increasingly shape and patrol flows of human tissues and biotech products. In contrast to market-state systems, emergent players in the field of biotechnology and biomedicine are situated in political environments with robust sovereignty and paternalist rule. Having laid the foundation for capitalist development, Asian states are turning to biotechnologies as a mechanism of regeneration, not only of the economy and of the people, but also of national prestige.

Asian governments are called "authoritarian" for their explicit expression of a sovereign logic that stresses cultural paternalism and sovereign custody of the population in the space of the nation. "Sovereignist" thinking has been used in reference to those who hold the politico-juridical position that the United States Constitution or "American exceptionalism" takes precedence over certain international obligations.[46] "Asian exceptionalism," by contrast, identifies a rigorous sovereignty shaped by precolonial political culture and postcolonial regional influence. Contemporary sovereign thinking, especially in East and Southeast Asia, is inextricably linked to deep structures of feeling rooted in old civilizations. In the early modern era, this sense of cultural character vested in the history of kingdoms or empires was violently unsettled by encounters with European colonial powers. Benedict Anderson has emphasized the "imagined community" as a vital practice of contemporary nation building, and indeed, the moral act of imagining a nation into being draws on ancient glories that in contemporary time continue to be animated by master symbols (an Asian example is Tiananmen).[47] Especially for East Asian nations, the imagining has always been infused with biological notions of cultural commonality and political difference.

Sovereign logic in East Asia is therefore in excess of the politico-legal definition of sovereignty found in international law. It includes a robust sense of cultural identity that, however unevenly, invokes a former kingdom or empire. China is the preeminent civilization-state model of how sovereignty shapes a cultural notion of belonging, one that is given visceral force by colonial encroachments in modern times.[48] The political construction of racial and cultural categories as foundational truths reinforces a moral-visceral experience of nation and sovereignty. Cultural notions of the state as a father-protector of ordinary people persist—uncountable failures and betrayals notwithstanding—and governing is viewed as a form of collective caring from above that engenders a sense of national subjectivity and shared fate. In Southeast Asia, postcolonial nations have been characterized as "strong states,"[49] that is, authoritarian regimes that can maintain a moral order and foster market competition. Cultural authoritarianism from above and collectivist sentiments from below are perhaps more easily aligned in these countries than in Western contexts that celebrate unfettered individualism and participatory democracy. Given the enduring influence of historical and cultural factors of paternalism and dependency, modern East Asian nations emphasize national or state sovereignty over popular sovereignty.

In China's case, the ever-present memory of humiliations inflicted by the West reinforces the historical, moral, and visceral elements of its cultural exceptionalism rooted in its long continuous civilization and profound sense of cultural superiority. For thousands of years, Confucianism shaped a hierarchical ethical order of mutual responsibilities that instilled a unifying cultural identity among the predominantly Han population. In the twentieth century Confucianism was repeatedly subjected to violent repudiations, but since the era of market reforms, the communist state has resurrected Confucian thinking as a way to strengthen cohesion and support for authoritarian rule.[50] The resolute quest for modern sovereignty is most potent in the nationalist fervor to reunite with Taiwan, an island-nation that has tried to defend its political autonomy.[51] We shall see later this duel between the People's Republic of China and Taiwan expressed in the realm of DNA research. Furthermore, China's ascendancy as a world power intensifies its already vigorous sense of state sovereignty. For instance, Chinese foreign relations experts are using an index of "comprehensive national power" to measure the country's global profile.[52] In addition to the appeal of its gigantic economy, China competes for international influence under the labels of "peaceful rise" and "soft power" by exporting cultural ideas, legitimacy, and foreign aid from its multi-trillion-plus-dollar assets. A prime example of hypernationalism is the Beijing 2008 Olympics, a global coming-out event by which China sought to restore its claim to global stature. Sovereign power has been enhanced by shaping transnational relationships, not diluted by them. An unapologetic focus on national interest prevails not just in China but in much of Asia, despite the countries' differing political systems. In their different ways, Japan and India, for example, deflect Chinese power by forging alliances with the United States.

The Western legacy in India is markedly different from this legacy in other Asian nations. As Sunder Rajan has noted, the role of the Indian vanguard elite in leading the move against British rule was tempered from the start by the extensive constitutional mechanisms that were enshrined in the imagination of the independent India nation. The tension between a vanguard (rather than paternalistic) ruling elite and populist institutional mechanisms foster conditions for a more participatory democratic sensibility that is more akin to South Africa and Brazil.[53] South Asian states tend therefore to a more contested environment of political stewardship than do East Asian states; their embrace of biopolitical calculations is mainly a jingoistic rhetoric among the highest elites and is not widely disseminated across society.

Nevertheless, both China and India are sensitive about their national identity and political exceptionalism in the world. Whereas Indian sensitivity about its exclusivity is always in tension with its desire to be a "global player" by embracing global values of democracy and free trade, Chinese prickliness about its exceptionalism is more aloof, despite its extensive participation in global trade. These contrasting styles of sovereignty mean that in the area of biotech development, India positions itself as more closely aligned with global pharmaceutical practices and bioethical concerns, while China is more assertive about gaining state control over the knowledge of biotech companies and bioresources in relation to global research and trade. Other Asian nations considered in this volume are situated in the continuum between these two poles of assertive sovereignty. A logic of sovereign exception to pharmaceutical globalization is not so unexpected in an age of Asian emergence.

Sovereign thinking stresses cultural distinctiveness and national territoriality, but when species become the target of biopolitics, technologies of security shift from patrolling borders to controlling the circulation and futures of living bodies. Michael Dillon and Luis Lobos-Guerrero have noted that contemporary biotechnology is concerned not only with regenerative medicine, but exploits the fungibility of species life, that is, the "pluripotency" of stem cells allows a constant instigation of new life forms that can be used in tissue regeneration and the compression of mortality.[54] In recent decades, the coupling of political entrepreneurialism and the life sciences is extending security mechanisms for trading in and capitalizing on life forms in Asian milieus. As I argue below, genomic sciences allow the translation of a dynamic of surplus and risk into a synergy of fecundity and opportunity.

Biotechnologies unlock the potentialities of Asian bodies either as sites of experimental testing, as values to be harvested, or as consumers of security products. Does the production of biovalue and biotech-driven modes of subject formation challenge sovereign reason? Or do overlapping scales of ethical considerations articulate broad-level concerns about political security and risk? The governing and the governed are variously intertwined in emerging Asian biotech constellations, and no study can ignore their implications for national interest and the ethics of biopolitical belonging.

Communities of Fate

The promise of biotechnology in fostering a continual regeneration of life enhances the logic for ethicalization of the bioeconomy beyond the clinic, the laboratory, and the marketplace. In Asian milieus, biotech mechanisms are presented as ethical operations that link the immediate needs of the individual consumer or patient to the political generation of civic virtue, that is, appropriate conduct and social obligations to contribute to national prosperity and security. Especially in East Asian countries such as South Korea, Japan, Singapore, China, Taiwan, and Thailand, reciprocal relationships (sometimes patron-client ties, other times *guanxi*, or a web of personal connections) cut across public-private spheres. An implicit norm of reciprocity is embedded in the social contract between people and the state, a kind of social cohesion that is often misrecognized as corruption or authoritarian control. In such social contexts, our approach to ethics is not concerned with the repetition of universal norms of bioethics, but focuses on diverse moral reasoning that takes place in overlapping ethical spaces.

The phrase "communities of fate" has been used to denote communities bound by common fortunes and prospects beyond the state and national territory, that is, autonomous political networks of shared fate—represented by nongovernment organizations, environmental movements, human rights entities, and international law. Because of their interest in communities of fate as the building blocks of a "global civil society," theorists have written out the vital role of the state altogether in the formation of collective interests.[55]

In my use, "communities of fate" refers not to elements of a global civil society but to the network of collectivities that become connected as a result of diverse ethical decisions and feelings associated with technological innovations. Different forms of biotechnology can be used to manipulate corporeal and affective interests that reinforce a sense of community and shared fate, for instance by activating traditional values of family, ethnicity, and the nation in the course of ethical decision making. At another level, political authorities and venture capitalists variously participate in the ethical legitimation of biotech projects as tools that serve the well-being of individuals and society. The bioeconomy is understood not merely as a generator of profits but also as an ethical machine for solving the problems of health, regeneration, bioresponsibility, and biosecurity.

Doctors, engineers, and scientists have always played leading roles in Asian governments. Political diagnosis invariably uses sciences as both metaphor and technique for solving the myriad problems of welfare, growth, and political legitimacy.[56] The role of scientific knowledge in the success of postcolonial nations begets a powerful emotional resonance especially among the educated elite. From India to South Korea, generations of upwardly mobile parents wanted and continue to want their children to become doctors and engineers to help save and strengthen the motherland. Science and patriotism are tightly intertwined. Biotech modernity is thus the latest in a genealogy of scientific methods that have been central for enhancing and ethicalizing state-led modernization.

In polities shaped by the Confucian ethos, citizens expect the paternalistic state to set ethical norms of social well-being and moral behavior. Modern China has a tradition of mass mobilization campaigns against a variety of political foes, and more recently, for family planning and antismoking campaigns.[57] Singapore is famous as well for its civic campaigns to promote childbirth, marriage rates, and healthy living. Conduct that complies with such stated norms gives ethical visibility to these social goals. Making modern science compelling in its beneficial effects on the population and making healthy living a form of civic virtue are ways of giving visibility to ethical practices that interweave communities of shared fate.[58] Older circles of cultural, ethnic, and civic solidarity offer reinforcements for biotech innovations that raise new ethical questions about relationships between individuals, collectivities, and the nation. These emerging ethical constellations are varied and unevenly integrated across the Asian landscape. There are broad South Asian and East Asian contrasts: in Indian cases, ethical decisions about biomedical procedures tend to operate at the kinship level, whereas in other Asian contexts, individual voluntary decisions tend to take into account broader scales of ethical reasoning in thinking through benefits, risks, and the common good. In this sense, a multitude of micro conducts regarding biotechnologies help to configure new ethical imaginings of shared fate.

Asia's Sputnik Moment

"Asian biotech" refers to an assemblage of science, politics, and collective concerns that configures a realm of transcendent imaginary in which sciences in tandem with ethics shape political identities. From plant genomics to molecular science, a strong sovereign impulse runs through biotech projects in Asia, shaping political meanings of biological problems made visible and solvable by the new sciences.

In the United States, the Soviet launching of the Sputnik capsule spurred American molecular biology to disciplinary dominance in the 1950s. As Lily E. Kay has written, the Rockefeller Foundation and the California Institute of Technology (Caltech) advanced the resulting "new biology" that came to shape an American vision of science and society. The disciplinary matrix of this new biology is governed by a faith in technology over physiochemical processes and submicroscopic processes that can facilitate control of biological destiny.[59]

Conditions in the early twenty-first century are Asia's Sputnik challenge to make a definitive break from heavy industrialization to the frontiers of bioscience. The new biotechnologies originating in the West are viewed as tools not only for creating new commercial enterprises but also for re-envisioning the relationship between politics, science, and ethical regimes. Despite different biotech programs across multiple settings, the scientifically driven imagination of Asian modernity is predicated on a new articulation of sovereignty, biotechnology, and biosecurity that crystallizes a growing sense of shared fate among peoples in different nations. Specifically, the new biology in combination with politics, collective fears, and sentiments crystallizes conditions for redefining what it means to be both "Asian" and "modern."

But let us take a moment to note divergences of biotech policy, programs, and scale, specifically how individual countries relate to ideas of the region. The main contrast between India and China is the role of the state in leading biotech development. Both nations emphasize the links between biosecurity and biotechnologies, but their projects, state-market mix, and transnational linkages are very different. The Indian state focus is on nuclear weaponry (supported by the United States), since it is seen as the real assertion of Indian sovereignty in the face of First World global dominance. The fledgling Indian biotech industry has had to confront suspicion and controversy about greedy companies by the authorities, venture capitalists, religious leaders, NGO activists, and the media. As the state struggles to increase genetically modified (GM) food and cash crop production, private companies have focused on clinical trials, medical tourism, and the manufacture of generic drugs. Biotech enterprises are mostly clustered in Hyderabad and Bangalore, but they are also cropping up in Maharashtra and Goa. The private biotech sector tends to specialize in outsourced research from the United States, or is concerned about linking up with global drug companies and global medical consumer markets.

Whereas India positions itself as a biotech node networked with the West, China's biotech innovations seek to lessen the nation's dependence on the West and to strengthen its sovereign power.[60] China has raced ahead of Japan to become the second largest investor in research and development, after the United States.[61] Indeed, the Chinese state is a technocracy that dominates all aspects of biotech development, from lunar exploration to nuclear science and life sciences. Key branches of the government (including the Ministries of Science and Technology, of Agriculture, and of Education) control most research and development programs, although regional governments and the National Science Foundation of China also play significant roles.[62] The bioindustry development program is written into China's five-year plan, and there are currently fifteen major bioindustry bases including Shanghai, Shenzhen, and Beijing. Hundreds of new biotech companies—service provider, innovator, and biogenerics—emerged in 2007 alone.[63] Despite a very uneven regulatory picture when it comes to R & D, many regional or city governments forge joint venture companies by funneling funds to universities or science parks, thus influencing specific projects and directions of research.[64] Chinese political authorities also tend to shepherd projects toward collaborations with overseas Chinese sites. There are tissue sharing and research links with Singaporean institutions. Increasingly, China and Singapore are linking up over biomedical issues that are viewed as affecting ethnic Chinese on the mainland and in the diaspora.

Biotech nationalism is also pronounced in other East Asian nations. In South Korea, as Hwang's botched research illustrates, the struggle for mastery in cutting-edge science is closely associated with the nation's prestige on the global stage. In Japan, despite decades of impressive high-tech innovations, biotech research has not actively interacted with global interests.[65] The field is dominated by a scientific elite and coddled by the government.[66] This state protectionism has not exposed Japanese pharmaceutical companies to the rigors of global competition the way the Japanese automobile industry has been. In general, East Asian countries (South Korea, Japan, China, Taiwan) tend to be more state-driven in their biotech development and more oriented to regional networks of trade and research than is India, for example.

Despite these differences in types of biotech projects, degrees of state involvement and interconnections, there is a transcendental "Asian biotech" that animates a broader vision of scientific emergence. We find not an overarching biotech logic or a regional integration through science, but a constellation of shared features conditional on political, economic, and practical contingencies. Unevenly but significantly present across Asia, these shared elements are issues of excess, risk, and opportunity; development of biotech hubs; moral reasoning that involves multiple ethical scales; and the use of biosciences to promote biosovereignty.

The elements of a transcendental Asian biotech became more apparent with the formation in 2004 of the Pan-Asia SNPs (PASNP) Consortium. This genomic project was the first to be conceived, funded, and executed by Asians in Asia, as noted by Edison Liu, executive director of the Genome Institute in Singapore and one of the consortium's founders.[67] The human genetic mapping of Asia is a direct response to the grossly simplified representation of Asian genomics depicted by the Human Genome Organization (HUGO). The PASNP consortium extends the study of human genetic diversity to seventy-three Southeast and

East Asian populations. Over ninety scientists, forty institutions, and eleven countries are involved in a collective effort to plot genetic diversity in Asian populations by identifying SNPs—or "snips"—that is, single nucleotide polymorphisms, or variations in our DNA code. The study maps the range of genetic diversity in Asia and traces the genetic origins of Asian populations. A basic goal is to identify gene involvement in a disease or in responses to drugs, and thus in ethnic variations in predispositions to certain diseases or susceptibility to certain drugs.

The PASNP study is also a preemptive strike at mapping diverse Asian biodata before Western corporations gain direct access to their vast market potential. The benefits of the SNPs project will be state control of the treasure trove of biomedical knowledge and maintaining state involvement in pharmacogenetic research and ensuing profits.[68] But Edison Liu told me that "state ownership of DNA is beyond the question of individual paternity [i.e., individual ownership]. There is the ethics element, not reducible to a cash cow for foreign companies."[69] In other words, the genetic project is a regional collective that operates at multiple ethical registers as well. As the first inter-Asian scientific community, the organization promotes each participatory state's creation of a national biodata bank, to control potential drug markets, but also fundamentally to promote the development of customized medicines that will benefit Asian citizens and peoples. While still in its early stages, the consortium creates a regional ethical space that seeks to protect, at multiple political levels, the health and biological resources of Asian populations from the manipulation and predation of global pharmaceutical firms. The critical importance of scientific research and talent in emerging countries was acknowledged in 2008 when Liu was selected as president of HUGO, the Human Genome Organization, which has since moved its office from London to Singapore.

Beyond the mapping of Asian genetic diversity, other converging features crystallize conditions of possibility for the broader configuration of common interests and imagination that we call "Asian biotech."

In this section, I move from the exposition of the analytics of biotechnology and bioethics to their particular articulation in different parts of the book. Particular chapters will be discussed within the themes of excess and opportunity, the rise of biotech ventures, the ethics of communities of fate, and notions of biosovereignty.

EXCESS AND OPPORTUNITY

The "bios" in biopolitics in Asia is fraught with historical experiences of material abundance and backwardness, of susceptibilities to conquest, failures, and diseases. The elements of surplus and risk continue to haunt the ascendant megastates of China and India as they seek to grapple with double-digit growth and massive impoverished populations. In his book, *Biocapital*, Sunder Rajan stresses "surplus and symptom" to specify the place of surplus populations as experimental subjects in "*the imaginaries of the American free market*," so that the desire for excess bodies is "*symptomatic*" of global power relations.[70] Capitalist development invests Asian bodies with an "uncanny surplus," that is, as embodied commodities that promise, in Marx's formulation, the generation of never-ending surplus value and limitless desires.[71]

Biotech modernization is not, however, characterized by unambiguous outcomes of certain profits; rather, it is shaped by strategies based on probabilities and probable outcomes. Not too long ago, the demographic surplus of giant Asian nations was considered a curse, a drain on material values. The Western view of China and India as burdened by a surfeit of population defined the image of developing economies—from Indonesia to India—as caught in a Malthusian trap. In the 1960s, the Club of Rome warned that both Asian giants would founder under the weight of their population and sink deeper into backwardness if they did not rigorously curb fertility rates. Such dire judgments from outside authorities put pressure on Chinese policy makers eager for science to help their catch-up race with the West. China's uncritical embrace of high-tech science shaped a family planning policy that inflicted devastating results for the welfare of Chinese families and society at large.[72] Nevertheless, as market reforms took off on the basis of its vast pool of cheap labor, Chinese authorities continued to worry over the insufficiently high "quality" (*suzhi*) of its human resources,[73] and to promote extensive skills training from the agricultural to the highest scientific fields. Such regimes of biopolitical management cannot easily convert perceived demographic risks into human capital, but are in continual confrontation with uncertainty.

Over the past decade, Asian countries have developed new interest in the ideas of biosurplus and biosusceptibility as new realities, and a reflexive approach based on calculations of probable outcomes. The political appeal of biotechnologies and the biosciences lay in their promised though ambiguous outcomes for big nations. Gigantic populations are now viewed as a source of undervalued surplus as well as of new opportunities. Bioscience and biotechnologies have unlocked the hidden wealth of surplus humanity. Big populations articulate high-tech capitalism not only as a cheap labor pool or exploding consumer market,[74] but also as a biological source of wealth and sustainable growth.

From the vantage point of the state, biotechnologies also provide solutions to problems of human survival, living, and well-being that are delicately balanced between enormous opportunity and risk. Excess bodies are never only about presenting new opportunities for profit making, but are also openings for new political interventions that shape an economy of ideas and effects. The uncanniness of corporeal abundance is refracted through the specter of hunger and susceptibilities to crop failures and infectious diseases. But the very threats to populations create new opportunities for security interventions that continuously integrate new elements that may produce intended outcomes as well as new risks.

Bioinsecurity as a new political reality was created by political responses to recent epidemics—the AIDS/HIV virus, SARS, and avian flu—that threatened to derail booming Asian economies. These diseases originate and/or flourish in Asian ecosystems. Because migrating pathogens threaten the health and welfare of Asian populations and nations, a risk imaginary has fastened tightly on the necessity of the state in taking a big role in funding and promoting research in the life sciences. For decades, health professionals in Asia have noted limited Western interest and investments in "tropical diseases" such as malaria, dengue fever, and so on. In addition, the incompetence of authorities in handling the SARS epidemic, especially in China, exposed regional governments to their scientific unpreparedness when it came to collective health measures and biomedical sciences.

An implicit social contract of biosecurity has come to dominate public discourses as the burgeoning middle classes demand that healthy and safe bodies, not just growing paychecks, are achievable norms in Asia. The SARS epidemic, followed by the spread of avian flu and dengue fever in the past decade, has intensified the production of security-conscious subjects, and generated new discourses of ethics of modern health protection in cities such as Shanghai and Singapore.[75] As scales of ethical reasoning have moved up from the material well-being of the individual to the well-being of the state, other events have stirred a sense of collective hyperinsecurity. Especially in Southeast Asia, the series of recent financial crises, tsunamis, and epidemics have increased demands for greater state action in solving the problems of population, profits, and national survival.[76]

Indeed, the feeling of biological insecurity is exacerbated by the Western view of the Asian region as a zone of infectious diseases menacing the rest of the world. Western countries view SARS and avian flu as Asian diseases spread throughout the world by Asian travelers. Journalists refer to Asian arrivals in Australia as walking incubators of a disease epidemic,[77] and Canadian health workers traced the spread of SARS in Canada to Asian tourists. The visceral links between SARS and Asian bodies thus ignited global perceptions about the risks that threaten Asian nations and their future. The external and internal association of bioinsecurity with Asian bodies and nations seems to index their qualitative difference, a material difference that attests both to their experience and to their innovative potential as biological subjects.

Especially in places with an ethnic Chinese majority, a seeming biogenomic connection between ethnicity and SARS has given the Chinese sense of exceptionalism a new materiality. Newspaper and other media reports mediate scientific research findings, disseminating a form of social knowledge about the biological susceptibility of ethnic Chinese populations across Asia. In 2003, a research team at the MacKay Memorial Hospital in Taipei claimed that Taiwanese and other Asians, "including people from China's southern coast, Hong Kong, Singapore and part of Vietnam," have a genetic variant in the immune system that make them more susceptible than Aboriginal groups or Caucasians and Africans to SARS infection. The scientists suggest that their findings "explain why south China was the epicenter of the SARS epidemic."[78] The news was widely disseminated in Asia, producing a kind of panicked belief that "Asians" are more susceptible to an array of "Asian" tropical diseases, many of which have failed to garner sufficient research interest in the West. Asian states were pressured from within and without to control the flows of pathogens and patients that seem especially lethal to peoples in the region.

SARS was thus identified as an "Asian disease" in search of an Asian answer. The specter of Asian genetic risks stirred public perception of the need for therapies and drug markets that cater specifically to the health needs of local populations. Doctors in Singapore note that Westerners have been the dominant beneficiaries of global pharmaceuticals, and that it is time for Asian scientists to undertake research on diseases that seem to disproportionately affect populations in tropical Asia. There is also the demand for drug dosages and treatments specifically tailored to Asian patients. The Asian "ownership" of certain diseases demands Asian state solutions. For instance, Singapore's up-to-date blood storage was justified in part by the need among leukemia patients for Asian donors. Whatever the scientific bases of many of these claims, there is a growing perception of Asian health exceptionalism, of compelling reasons for the state to invest in biomedical research that address genetically inherited "Asian" diseases such as liver cancer, cancer of the lymph nodes, and nose and throat cancer. Indeed, hospitals in Hong Kong and Biopolis in Singapore are leaders in research on these diseases, as well as in developing vaccines for combating SARS and the avian flu.

By conjoining fears of mass hunger, epidemics, and economic derailments, Asian governments are redefining the contours of security. The series of health crises and perception of Asian vulnerabilities create fresh conditions that legitimize government interventions and investments in the life sciences. Hyperbiosecurity becomes the new normal, instituting necessary expertise and practices that can secure and map Asian futures. Indeed, one can say that sovereignty gains a new legitimacy in its paternalistic role, which makes a vital new connection between neoliberal logic and biotechnological expertise that can, it is hoped, protect their peoples and move Asian nations to the frontlines of global sciences.

Two chapters in this volume focus on Asian megastates, exploring how the coupling of biotechnologies and surplus populations at this historical moment shape both opportunity and risk for capital accumulation and national security. In India, the interplay of surplus and symptoms is increasingly orchestrated by state-driven interventions to technologize living labor. Sunder Rajan observes that an abundance of poor Indians has made the state desirous to "biocapitalize" its own citizens by making them available as experimental subjects of clinical trials. This is an effort to "brand" India as an ideal site for global drug testing in the context of a broader historical transition from manufacturing to speculative capitalism. The chapter investigates what (and who) becomes bioavailable to, or gets consumed by, the experimental machinery of global biocapital.

In Nancy Chen's chapter, the dynamic of population abundance and vulnerabilities is examined in the area of genetically modified food production. She notes that China's "drive toward developing new products and planting genetically modified (GM) crops" to feed a gigantic population is backlit by the recent history of crop failures and famines. Her chapter traces "the different trajectories of genetically modified rice and soy in China," and their promotion as key crops for the maintenance of national food security. The pragmatic and rapid propagation of GM foods is considered the moral obligation of the nation, an exercise of its sovereign economic and scientific capacities, finally, to ensure the survival of the masses. Thus despite pollution and displacement of older seed lines, there is barely any criticism, in sharp contrast to the debates one hears in Europe and America about the dangers of "Frankenfoods."

BIOVENTURES

Like the modernization of science in America, biotechnical innovation in Asia is a strategic political project; Asian innovations, however, have been initiated not in response to the space race but in an age of neoliberal risk calculations that anticipates infinite numbers of threats to governance and national emergence. More fundamental, unlike in North America, Asian state valorization of the sciences—from genomics to nuclear weaponry to space exploration—recreates, rather than undermines, authoritarian state power. Furthermore, the East Asia state tends to be a powerful arbiter of scientific meanings that mold how people think about themselves as ethical beings and citizens. It is the state, rather than private enterprises, that creates the moral instruction and material field for making policies for building bioeconomies.

Biotechnologies are innovations in Asian capitalism, the latest in a series of state-directed programs to create high-tech zones. Since the 1970s, China, Thailand, South Korea, India, Taiwan, and Singapore have sought to upgrade beyond the category of low-wage export economies to the rank of "knowledge economies" that will allow them to leapfrog ahead, as a World Bank report recommends.[79] Through the 1980s and 1990s, a high-tech corridor modeled on Silicon Valley emerged across Asia, from Seoul to Malaysia's Multimedia Super Corridor and India's cybercenters. These high-tech nodes are interlinked sites that assemble disparate knowledge actors and institutions to form "ecologies of expertise."[80]

At the turn of the century, neoliberal visions of Asian scientific futures spurred a biotech building spree. While many Europeans remain skeptical about focusing on the "knowledge-based bioeconomy" as a "driver of growth and competitiveness,"[81] in East Asia, there seems to be little doubt about the primacy of science in global competition. Biotech hubs have sprung up, sometimes alongside cyber and manufacturing centers, as the latest kind of special enclave for producing global values. I have argued that a neoliberal logic for administering space and population relies on zoning technologies to spatialize a graduated form of rule.[82] Science parks are well furnished with institutes, laboratories, and clinics, but they also provide special environments where social conditions foster appropriate self-enterprising conduct among the highly educated in order to link up with global markets. The state not only injects funds for cutting-edge research but also pays attention to working and living arrangements for scientists and their families. The hope is that such scientific havens may help stimulate creative work and speed up the conversion of ideas into new products.

The politics of zoning and unequal investments in national spaces reinforce existing inequalities as populations outside zones of exception, by that spatial fact alone, have limited access to state resources. In industrializing but still agrarian countries such as China and India, a string of high-tech nodes connected to global activities are practically disconnected from vast populations whose most fundamental needs have not yet been properly met. At the other extreme, there are Japan and Singapore, mainly middle-class societies where people have access to health, education, and scientific benefits, if to differing degrees.

The growth of knowledge hubs builds upon the rapid expansion of Asia's educated elite. In East Asia, there is little or no questioning of the political necessity for improving "human resources" through investments in science education and institutions. One index of a relentless development of human capital is the performance of students from different Asian countries in international test scores in the fields of science and mathematics. There is a regional competition in upgrading universities to "world-class status," with Singapore mobilizing global knowledge through strategic partnerships with American universities and scientific research institutions to form a "global schoolhouse."[83] Joint programs between Western universities and institutions from China to Singapore and Indonesia have forged many connections in engineering, medicine, and public health. Currently, hundreds of thousands of engineers and scientists join the labor markets in China and India each year, and many of them spill overseas in search of further education or jobs. Even in smaller countries such as Thailand, medical institutions produce a significant number of doctors each year to sustain a rise in sophisticated medical skills. Foreign and local scientists gathered in Asian high-tech citadels foster values associated with a fearless scientific attitude toward modernity.

The return of foreign-trained Asian experts is crucial for the rapid growth of bioeconomies. With a decade-long rate of double-digit growth, Asian countries are luring back many students educated in the United States, Europe, and Australia. The turn of the century witnessed one of the largest repatriations of global skills in recent times. Since the 1980s, over 200,000 Chinese students trained abroad, mainly in the sciences, have returned to China.[84] The significant return of the Asian scientific diaspora—especially Indians, Chinese, and South Koreans—has led to the projection that by 2010, 90 percent of all Ph.D.-holding scientists and engineers will be living in Asia. This embarrassment of scientific riches contributes to "Asia's great science experiment."[85]

Asian bioeconomies tend to move in two directions. One system is focused on establishing Asian sites as world-class research hubs; this ambition is best represented by South Korea and Singapore. The other type of project is focused on providing biotech and biomedical services to global companies and international patients. These two biotech trajectories can and do overlap in some sites, but there is a ranking of priorities that is discernable across nations, mainly in relation to the degree of state involvement. Two chapters in this book show this contrast in types of bioeconomic function.

Charis Thompson draws on ethnographic research in Singapore and South Korea as part of a broader investigation into global patterns of stem cell research. She argues that there is a tendency to think of science as being everywhere and nowhere all at once, and always of the present; yet anthropologists, sociologists, and science studies scholars have shown that there are profound regional and local differences in how "the same science" is enabled, practiced, and understood. In this spirit, her chapter compares and contrasts characteristic stem cell research and regenerative medicine facilities in these two Asian sites. The axes of comparison include a focus on differences between characteristic facilities; scientific strategies, specializations, and hoped for payoffs; the use of humans and animals; economic investment and rationales; and nationalist imaginaries. In sum, Thompson explores the question of what each nation's investment in this part of the biotech revolution tells us about the nation and region in question, as well as what these nation's engagements with regenerative medicine adds to our understanding of biotechnology and its significance.

In places where the state has not yet emerged as an initiator of biotech enterprises, private investments tend to focus on generating "low-cost, good-quality care" by health workers. Ara Wilson describes the rise of the Thai biomedical industry as a private-based assemblage that builds on earlier public projects of national development and security. Thailand's emergence as a center for corrective surgery has roots in the growth of personal services for U.S. troops and medical training by the U.S. military during the Indochina wars. Private medical companies led the way in making Bangkok an international site for cosmetic surgery, fertility treatment, and other forms of health care. For thousands of foreign patients, the high quality of Thai medical services includes the "affective labor" of Thai nurses and attendants, who excel at plying patients with care and comfort. Recent biopolitical and economic challenges have prompted the Thai state to collaborate with medical corporations in order to position Bangkok as the mecca of medical tourism.

In India, where biotech endeavors tend to be exclusively private enterprises, doctors working directly or indirectly for overseas corporations can be recruited as on-the-ground agents for overseas pharmaceutical interests. Many drug corporations, Stefan Ecks observes in his essay in this volume, are making claims to "global corporate citizenship" that aims to promote universal rights within corporate boundaries and beyond. For pharmaceutical companies, global corporate citizenship entails a promise to ease access to medications for all patients and to spread "health literacy" around the world—including Asia. Drawing on fieldwork in Kolkata (Calcutta), Ecks considers how corporate norms are translated to Indian doctors. Official and unofficial messages conveyed in a "depression awareness workshop" that he attended indicate that global norms are adapted to doctors' notions of Indian citizenship. Referring to Foucault's formulation of neoliberalism, Ecks proposes that global corporate citizenship is a form of "near-liberalism" that is not practiced uniformly across the globe, but permits switching into modes of conduct that create the opposite of consumer consciousness in the Indian context.

COMMUNITIES OF FATE

As I mentioned earlier, the ethics-as-moral-criticism approach presupposes a clear-cut division between bad guys (biotech entities and scientists) and good guys ("victims," as they tend to be characterized by impassioned anthropologists). While speaking truth to power is laudable, more sensitive analyses of ethical practices will show that in each ethnographic case, the question of "who gains, who loses" cannot be answered in advance. An anthropology that "stays close to practices"[86] stays close to the politics and pathos of how people meet challenges and resolve problems within given conditions of possibility. The nexus between biotech techniques and moral reasoning is highly variable and dynamic, and complex ethical negotiations take place in an assemblage of conflicting logics.

Some anthropologists and feminists have long argued for attention beyond abstract formulations of ethics to the moral conduct in everyday social interaction and exchange. Arthur Kleinman insists upon "relational ethics" as the grounding of responsibility and trust in the clinic encounter.[87] "Feminist ethics" also identify social relationships as the space for the generation of moral reasoning, choices, and self-image.[88] But implicit in these approaches is an assumption that a set of given principles or norms must be operative in the ethical practice of ethnographic interactions.

An anthropology of "situated ethics" therefore reaches not for ultimately universal philosophical treatments of practices, but situates ethical processes in specific milieus of politics, culture, and decision making. "Situated ethics" rejects the common assumption that moral reasoning can be simply determined by class location, or reduced to the scale of the isolated individual. In matters of biotechnology, biomedicine, and biosecurity, it is more fruitful to locate moral reasoning at the intersection of overlapping scales of risk and ethics.

For instance, biovalue and biomedical inventions are not necessarily or everywhere viewed as contrary to ethics. Ethical claims interact with degrees of risks in any context. It is the space between individual, family, professional, community, and national scales where new ethical possibilities and decisions emerge. For instance, the ethics of health self-management may articulate claims on the state to provide for the collective well-being. This situated and dynamic understanding of ethical reasoning means that outcomes cannot be noted in advance, and that tensions among divergent ethical demands engender complex solutions.

Bioethics debates in the West pivot on innovative biomedical techniques that put into question moral concerns about abortion, organs transplant, and stem cell research and genetic therapy.[89] Whereas a major focus of the bioethics debate in North America and Europe has been on individual rights and informed consent, one cannot deny that voluntary action by patients and donors tend also to be colored by the emotionally charged issues of regenerative benefits for the family, and even the community and nation.

In Asian milieus, such issues tend to be subsumed under an overriding ethical interest in the biosciences as a technology that promises to bring bioprotection and biosecurity to patients, citizens, and nations. So while biomedical enterprises are legally required to enforce bioethics, clinical and research guidelines are only the beginning of larger ethical implications of biotech innovations. Politicians, top scientists, and the media invariably link such scientific procedures to ethical concerns about collective well-being and national advancement. Indeed, the embrace of bioscience and biomedical policies has produced a new idiom of ethics that is bringing to life communities of shared corporeal needs and vulnerabilities. Biotech and biomedical procedures thus trigger emotional maps of belonging and collective fate, enhancing an awareness of the scientific and raising the security stakes of being modern Asian subjects.[90]

The spread of biomedical knowledges and practices among professionals and consumers is accompanied by the inculcation of values of bioresponsibility. The ethicalization of biomedical practices intersects with neoliberal ideas about individual capacity for self-improvement through material and scientific means, that is, by enhancing "biological capital," including at the genetic level.[91] Whether through "educated" choices as drug consumers, or readiness to donate blood or organs, people are induced to shape new ethical selves as biomedically informed subjects. But individual biomedical decision making and choices are ethically framed in relation to what is good for collective living.

Especially in South Korea, Singapore, and Japan, the state intervenes in a variety of ways to establish the apparatus of biosecurity, especially in the areas of tissue banking, regenerative medicines, and genetics research that respond to citizens' needs. This state emphasis on biosecurity measures has a cascading effect in the popularization of biomedical knowledge. Preexisting norms of ethnic consciousness and civic virtue intersect with the emerging ethics and necessity of biomedical knowledge. Pharmacogenomics popularizes a new biomedical consciousness about ethnic and racial difference, further reinforcing the necessity of biotech innovations for securing the future of communities. For instance, the use of social categories of racial/ethnic groups to frame studies of certain diseases, or the variation among groups in the metabolism of drugs, seems to make operative folk beliefs in genetic transmission, predisposition, and "risks" for certain diseases. Even well-educated politicians, medical practitioners, and scientists believe in some degree of genetic determination in relation to birth defects and mental capacities. Ethnic profiling in regenerative medicine has influenced biomedical citizen-subjects to embrace the normality of tissue donation for the good of the ethnic group, the nation, and even Asian peoples in general. This pharmacogenetic consciousness enhances the ethical embrace of "smart medicine" by the elite to protect the self, the family, and beyond. Such ethical reasoning about the value of scientific techniques becomes somewhat aligned with state interests in optimizing a vitalist order for society at large. Biomedical decisions thus take place at the intersection of many ethical scales, as contemporary science directly and indirectly poses the question, What is the value of Asian lives today?

Regenerative medicine is an area where situated ethics can overshadow universal principles of bioethics. For instance, the scandal surrounding Hwang Woo-Suk's false claim to have cloned a human embryo reveals complex ethical reasoning by egg donors. To Western critics, the research fraud was preceded by other questionable practices. In 2004, Dr. Hwang used close to 250 embryos in his cloning attempts, and it was later revealed that through an intermediary, women—among them his junior scientists—were compensated for donating eggs for the project.[92] Western observers claim that "a culture of secrecy and deference" gave Hwang influence to thwart ethical oversight in his lab.[93] Hwang was indeed celebrated as a science hero in South Korea, but while there was admission of ethical "flexibility" that allowed Hwang's project to outrace government regulations, the bioethical situation is more complex than poor lab governance. What needs to be emphasized is that the female donors acted in a voluntary capacity, less for money than in support of the Korean stem cell project. Indeed, it was later reported that Hwang had discouraged voluntary offers of eggs by his researchers, but one of them represented her voluntary act as one of historical duty: "It was an act of sacrifice. In the annals of scientific advancements, you can find again and again cases of scientists sacrificing their own bodies, using their own bodies for their experiments. When you face a new challenge, you sometimes have to leap over the ethical boundaries. Only history will judge the deed."[94] Following the international humiliation of Hwang, feminists and civic groups criticized Hwang's actions for hurting "national interests," but more women came forward to donate their eggs. One cited the Korean stem cell projects as their "only hope" for treating diseases such as spinal cord injuries. Thus, voluntary decisions to donate organs for research jump many ethical scales, linking the ethics of medical sacrifice to the ethics of national scientific achievement.

The nexus of multiple ethical decisions in the Hwang case challenges a simple argument for "the cultural constitution of bioethics."[95] Margaret Lock observes, for instance, that in Japan a diagnosis of brain death is made regularly in ICUs but the state of brain death is not equated with the end of human life, thus making the harvesting of transplant organs ethically problematic in that country.[96] Growing public pressure for the availability of high-quality organs, however, may lead to the acceptance of brain death as the cessation of life. As

I have noted above, cultural values are in a dynamic relationship to politics and in Asian contexts are frequently articulated with evolving national interests. For instance, in contrast to Westerners' skepticism over customized medicine, elite Asian populations welcome tailored medicines and the scientific imprimatur they give to popular beliefs that there is a genetic basis to social identities. Furthermore, there is an overwhelming sense that diseases prevalent in the region have not been given their due by medical research based in the West. Asian countries are now ready to reject Western one-size-fits-all models, and to conduct scientific study of genetic variants among Asian populations.

In Singapore, genomic institutes have created a stir because they promise the discovery of treatments tailored to diseases of different Asian groups, for example, early-onset breast cancer, nasopharyngeal carcinoma, and hepatitis B–linked liver cancers among ethnic Chinese; heart disease and cancer of the oral cavity among Indians; and diabetes among urban Malays. Bioethics is thus invariably linked to the protection not only of the individual patient, but of the entire ethnic community, a cultural collectivity now deeply embedded in the same genetic game of chance and fate. Scientific "facts" shape voluntary decisions in self-care and care of the family, folk notions are inveigled into clinical categories, and molecular techniques intended to undermine phenotypic differences cast in ethnic, racial, and national terms now resuscitate them. Consequently, bioethics goes beyond legal rights to stir powerful emotional bonds of distinctive biological essence and fate.

Three essays in this book explore situated ethics-making practices that legitimize or foster biotech procedures in relation to overlapping communities of fate. In China, links between private and state storage of blood are haunted by issues of sovereignty and notions of blood as a collective resource. Drawing on ethnographic research in Shanghai, Vincanne Adams, Kathleen Erwin, and Phuoc V. Le argue that the problem of "blood donation" in urban China illuminates the ways in which governance occurs in and through the management of bodies, tissues, and fluids. Unlike blood donation in other regions of the world, blood donation in China is tied to a variety of perceptions concerning blood as a vital bodily essence; obligations to family, work unit, and the larger society; and, finally, society's obligation to the donor. They claim the emergence of a regime of not "biopolitics" but rather "politicobiology," which politically constitutes fundamental ethical ideas about the body, and enables exchanges between individuals and institutions.

Transformations in the value of blood, I argue in the essay "Lifelines: The Ethics of Blood Banking for Family and Beyond," are produced by a novel configuration of biotech, ethical, and aesthetic elements in Singapore. Drawing links among official tissue networks, private banking of cord blood, the promissory marketing of blood banks, and Zhang Xiaogang's "Bloodlines" paintings, I track the revaluation of blood substances at multiple scales. Official storage of human tissues is legitimized in terms of securing citizens' future needs, part of a broader regime of biomedical citizenship. Meanwhile, commercial claims about the value of stem cells also prompt couples to bank the cord blood of their infants, a procedure that has become a performance of ethical parenting. The unwitting biomedical resuscitation of folk beliefs in fixed ethnic essences, also figured in contemporary Chinese art, led to projections of diasporic yearnings for reconnecting with ancestral, mainland China.

In Japan, the public discussion on human stem cell research is sensitive and treated with great political care. In her essay in this volume, Margaret Sleeboom-Faulkner argues that it is not stakeholders who carry the discussion on human stem cell research, but the academic, scientific, and political interest groups that support, (mis-)quote, and hijack the voices of dissenting minorities. She shows how these interest groups capitalize on their envisaged future of such research. Her argument entails an account of how past experiences are linked to stated promises, perceived risks, and doubts about recent changes in views on human stem cell research, as they link to current trends in stem cell research. In Japan, it seems, stem cell research must continue unimpeded for the good of Japanese science and the population at large.

The Rise of Biosovereignty?

The age of genomics has had the paradoxical effects of circulating economies of knowledge, on the one hand, and reinforcing nationalist goals, on the other. While the neoliberal logic of Asian states has been to make their economies more fluid, it has also enabled sovereign powers to stand up to global institutions. When anthropologists have touched on the connection between biotechnologies and sovereign power, their focus has been on the powers of drug companies and commercial rivalry. Cori Hayden, in a study of Mexico, has argued that increased activities of bioprospecting are creating new modes of inclusion and exclusion; communities are constituted either as sites for the harvesting of bioresources, or because of their potential for pharmaceutical profit making.[97] Paul Rabinow, in his study of a transatlantic project on the genetic basis of diabetes, ends with an account of how the French state broke with American partners for fear of theft and profit from the use of "French DNA."[98] Gisli Paulson and Rabinow, writing about European biotech milieus, note the "different forms of collaborations between the state, the academy and the private sector" that exist there.[99]

The biotech contexts in Asia also involve a range of public-private collaborations, but the nation-capital-genomics triangulation is differently weighted in terms of national development or biosovereignty. Some states forge a complicated relationship with global capital and Big Pharma, inviting partnerships but also promoting the development of the national economy. Furthermore, countries such as Indonesia and China recognize their wealth in biodiversity and attempt to corral and define their nation's biological resources as state property.

Tensions between property rights and sovereign rights are handled differently across Asia. In tiny Singapore, the state depends on alliances with corporations and research institutions. A strict adherence to the private property rights regime established by TRIPs (Trade-Related Aspects of Intellectual Property Rights) and the World Intellectual Property Organization attracts global corporations eager to protect patents and profits.[100] However, where government-funded agencies are involved in partnerships with foreign firms, there are contracts that split proprietary rights and profits. Countries with more natural resources seek greater control of their links with Big Pharma, especially in order to protect home-grown biomedical industries. The issue of "compulsory licensing" has become very prominent in Thailand and India lately. This process allows for opening borders for trade and securing multinational copyrights, on the one hand, and reaffirmations of national rights to allow generic production of life-saving drugs "in case of emergency," on the other. India has produced a lucrative market of generic drugs for the global South. For the Indian government, TRIPs and similar issues are usually framed in terms of rich/poor, developing/developed countries, and less in terms of national security as such.[101] Thailand, of course, is seeking to control its highly competitive medical tourism industry.

Other states are even more assertive vis-à-vis the pharmaceutical industry, and are formulating policies that lock in the potential values that can be generated from nature through scientific research. I identify "biosovereignty" as an emerging set of thinking and practices through which the state protects and leverages bioresources by placing constraints on the free market forces. Asian sovereign powers increasingly govern the distribution, uses, and compensations of bioresources that "belong" to Asian countries.[102] Biosovereign practices include a new political assertiveness in dealing with global biotech research and global Pharma, which are otherwise dominated by Western interests.

Indonesia, a latecomer to the world of modern biotechnology, expresses a form of biosovereignty that challenges the global commodification of health. In 2006, the avian flu (H5N1) crisis led Indonesia to assert political exception to the global intellectual property regime. As the country with the largest number of avian flu victims, Indonesia's health minister Siti Fadilah Supari was quoted as saying "We cannot share [virus] samples for free. There should be rules of the game for it."[103] In the face of international criticism, the Indonesian state invoked a national health law that requires an agreement prior to transferring virus samples and their limited use for diagnostic purposes. This act of biosovereign leveraging challenges the intellectual property rights of drug companies to access virus materials stored by the World Health Organization (WHO). After a period of standoff, in February 2007, Indonesia and other Southeast Asian countries pressured WHO to adopt a new mechanism on sharing viral samples and require drug companies to compensate donor countries. A Thai health official observes that nations "at the epicenter of the pandemic" should tie their transfer of H5N1 samples to "assured access to potential pandemic flu vaccines."[104] Indonesia's flexing of biosovereignty muscle resulted in a deal with Baxter International that in exchange for virus samples the corporation would help the country to produce and market bird flu vaccine. The avian flu incident crystallized conditions for the assertion of biosovereignty and the rise of a regional alliance to regulate the commercial use of health samples.

Another exercise of biosovereignty targets the flows and uses of genetic materials perceived to be distinctive to a given ethnicity, race, or nation. Cultural origins and migration stories are becoming the prior grounds for genetic mapping of peoples and nations. Genomic sciences allow for the framing of patrimony for political and economic interests, thus bolstering the stakes for nationalist pride and security interest. In China, there is increasing bioparanoia over the unauthorized use or suspected piracy of Chinese health data by foreign, non-Chinese researchers. In one heated case, Chinese scientists labeled American access to Chinese DNA materials as "the gene war of the century," that is, the theft of genetic patrimony disguised as scientific research.[105] In 1999, a Chinese law banned the export of DNA materials, and India soon followed with a similar ban.

China's image as a source of plentiful human eggs and embryos, on the one hand, and of experimental bodies, on the other, has prompted the state to more rigorously limit or channel international scientific collaborations. Beijing has a special body that authorizes international sharing of health data and tissues. Unlike India, Beijing is very slow in approving applications by global drug companies and their services to conduct clinical trials in China. Increasingly, its search for international scientific expertise is oriented toward collaborations with other Asian nations. An implicit norm of ethnic trust seems to underpin approvals for joint research projects, many of which are with overseas Chinese experts. At Singapore's universities and hospitals, more scientists are partnering with mainland Chinese clinicians in projects that range from analyzing PRC biomedical data to joint research on new therapies affecting Asian populations. In short, different forms of biotechnology are being used as tools for the management of collective national interests, reviving historical beliefs about national essences and opening up a new vital area for manifesting biosovereignty. For instance, the new genomics is being wielded for expressing nationalism and its territoriality in startling new ways.

Jennifer Liu, in her essay in this volume, investigates a biomedical laboratory project where discourses of ethnic purity and hybridity interact with notions about stem cells with uniquely "Taiwanese genetic characteristics." She maintains that these scientists seek and claim a singular truth about Taiwanese identity even though there is the recognition of population diversity and hybridity. For the researchers, stem cell research promises the hope of "pure" self-renewal in the form of autologous stem cell therapies. In discursive and laboratory spaces, ideas about purity become increasingly polyvalent, and are mobilized in new ways in making both identities and stem cells.

In the final chapter, Wen-ching Sung examines how the rise of genomics has helped substantiate the notion of "Chinese DNA," a new public imagination about nation-building in China. The notion of Chinese DNA assumes that Chinese peoples share similar biological features, which can be pinned down at a molecular level. It is a bio-cultural-geographical cluster that is entangled with China's century-long discourse and practice on race, ethnicity, and nationality. For Sung, the search for a Chinese DNA epitomizes the emergence of a certain "bio-nation" concept influential in contemporary statecraft. On the one hand, "bionation" connotes the politics of similarity, which claims that China is a unified nation because its many ethnic groups have common blood, ancestry, and genetic makeup. This narrative of "unity of diversity" shapes the Chinese notion of sovereignty and the nation's attitude toward Taiwan and Tibet. On the other hand, "bionation" identifies a mode of biopower in late capitalism that views ethnic communities as a storehouse of genetic materials to be defended and turned into products for the good of all citizens. This interplay of notions of Chinese DNA and bionation is a significant dynamic that recombines disparate cultural, political, and economic elements around emerging biotechnologies.

There are thus different orders of incipient Asian biosovereignty, and while sovereign logic actively engages biocapitalist flows, it is beginning to constrain the full exercise of global corporate powers and multilateral agencies. State biostrategies have become more pronounced in the Asian contexts of health epidemics, drug market competition, and the political ethics of collective fate. The dueling projects being undertaken in China and Taiwan on Chinese DNA show that scientific technologies cannot be pried loose from the political matrix of framing, socio-cultural obsessions, and ethics within which they are embedded and deployed. There is by no means a uniform embrace of biosovereignty, and its mapping is highly uneven and responsive to events and fluidity in the valuation and politics of bioresources.

Asian Biotech is the first study to provide on-the-ground studies of emerging biotech milieus across Asia, from India to Japan. This collection explores the political and ethical implications of biotechnologies outside contexts of Western advanced liberalism. Asia is a region of political and ethical contradictions, of population surplus and bioinsecurity, of economic backwardness and full-throttle capitalism, of memories of colonial humiliations and the cumulative force of resurgent nationalism. The life sciences, and biotechnology in particular, are becoming tools of biopolitical security and ethical claims for integrating heterogeneous peoples in ambitious nation-states. Despite sharp differences between China and India in their biotech projects, this is a transcendental moment in Asian scientific experimentation. Significant conceptual implications of Asian biotech have theoretical applications well beyond the region.

First, this collection challenges the view that the rationalities of market and science are incompatible with the "irrationalities" of feeling and identity. Rather, the proliferation of biotechnologies opens up a new question of what objects should be acted upon in the name of Asian security. Recent experiences of epidemics and the promise of biotechnologies have given a new materiality and ethical configuration to contemporary Asian exceptionalism. The chapters that follow track different vectors of biotech sciences and how they have been crucial to the regeneration of bodies, communities, and nations, giving "life" new ethical meanings at shifting scales from single nucleotide polymorphisms to ecosystems. Situated and multiscale convergences of biotechnology, politics, and ethics are involved in constructing possible communities of fate.

Second, the following chapters trace a dynamic interplay between scientific and cultural categories for shaping modern life and living that run contrary to binary nature-culture frameworks. As biotechnologies travel, specific techniques are recombined with situated cultural notions, ethical concerns, and political goals. Instead of scientific knowledge erasing social beliefs, folk categories can be applied to biomedical procedures, thus reinforcing social understanding of ethnic and racial differences. Genomic and social codes can overlap in political attempts to configure biosovereignty and deflect the incursions of global corporations.

Third, ethnographic investigations reveal that moral reasoning takes place in the midst of interacting risk calculations and ethical regimes. Scholarship on bioethics should for that reason move beyond a singular focus on individual rights, or at most, on the rights of only indigenous populations. By contrast, a situated ethics approach pays attention to actual decision-making practices at the intersection of ethical scales that can include kinship, culture, ethnicity, and the nation. Moreover, in some Asian contexts, political and individual decisions about the life sciences and biomedical innovations tend to cast biotech enterprises as a form of ethical capitalism, that is, regulated commercialized science that benefits the nation.

Fourth, the relationships among state, biotechnology, and Big Pharma vary, and non-Western contexts are not always defenseless against global science and predatory drug companies. Different biotech centers are shaping new ethical grounds for asserting state proprietorship over nature and defending against biocapitalism. At the transnational level, the SNPs consortium strengthens individual government's capacity to build their own genomic databanks and thus fend off global corporations that would otherwise freely corral living materials for commercial use.

Finally, the Asian biotech assemblages discussed in the book are contingent arrangements, vulnerable to political upsets, market meltdowns, or environmental crises. While these clusters are permutations of biotechnologies and sovereign politics, it remains uncertain whether all peoples can be drawn into the biopolitics of security. Reenvisionings of biocommunities of fate implicitly follow ethnic, majority-minority, and national lines. We can expect that unequal and uneven access to biomedical innovations will increase, and be further exacerbated by investments in biomappings of ethnic differences. Such biocollectivist claims become vulnerable to challenges from marginalized and excluded peoples as well as from individualistic claims of the burgeoning middle classes. As the life sciences open up a new world of possibilities, growing public debates about their intended and unintended outcomes will probably follow.

It is not clear if the ethicalization of biotechnologies at multiple scales implies a historical rupture in Asia's treatment of nature and biovalue, forecasting a more ethical approach to collective living systems, or whether the ethos of neoliberal self-care will undermine or unravel ethical integration. Furthermore, besides intrastate tensions between divergent ethical demands, there are also international tensions as Asian nations race to take scientific command of their nation and global influence. The biotech constellations presented in this book are based on probability calculations of economic and political outcomes that cannot be guaranteed in advance. Nevertheless, world forums should sit up and take note that the generation and crafting of genetic data are no longer a monopoly of pharmaceutical companies, nor is ethics interacting with biotechnologies only framed by Western cultural norms. Asian nations are emerging players in biogenomics and key architects of an alternative realm of biotech culture.

Notes

Thanks to Nancy N. Chen, Andy Hao, Kaushik Sunder Rajan, Anthony Stavrianakis, Janelle Lamoreaux, and Michael Fischer for comments on an earlier version of the introduction.

1. World Economic Forum, annual meeting, Davos, Switzerland, January 23–26, 2008, http://www.weforum.org/en/events/ArchivedEvents/AnnualMeeting2008/index.htm.
2. Richard Black, "Singapore High-tech Heaven Opens," BBC News, October 29, 2003, http://news.bbc.co.uk/2/hi/world/asia-pacific/3223393.stm. See also Edison Liu, "Asia's Biotech Tiger," *New Scientist* 175, no. 2360 (September 14, 2002): 54–57; and "Singapore: The Biopolis of Asia," *Science*, April–May 2003, D1.
3. David Cyranoski, "Chinese Bioscience: The Sequence Factory." *Naturenews* online edition, March 3, 2010, http://www.nature.com/news/2010/100303/full/464022a.html.
4. Andrew Pollack, "Scientific and Ethical Questions Cloud Plans to Clone for Therapy," *New York Times*, February 13, 2004, A1, A13.
5. Christopher Thomas Scott, *Stem Cell Now: A Brief Introduction to the Coming Medical Revolution* (London: Plume Printing, 2006), 187–88.
6. See Martin Fackler, "Scientist at Work: Shinya Tamanaka. Risk Taking Is in His Genes," *New York Times*, December 11, 2007, Science section, 1, 4.
7. For the concept of "global assemblages," see Stephen J. Collier and Aihwa Ong, "Global Assemblages, Anthropological Problems," in *Global Assemblages: Technology, Politics, and Ethics as Anthropological Problems*, ed. Aihwa Ong and Stephen J. Collier (Malden, Mass.: Blackwell, 2005).
8. *The American Heritage Science Dictionary* (New York: Houghton Mifflin, 2002).
9. Michael M. J. Fischer, "Four Genealogies for a Recombinant Anthropology of Science and Technology," *Cultural Anthropology* 22, no. 4 (November 2007): 573.
10. We use the term "the West" as a "native" category deployed in many Asian contexts to refer to the political and economic cluster of nations led by the United States and the European Union bloc, including Australia, New

Zealand, and occasionally, contingently, Japan, that are an imaginary geography of political domination and exemplary standard bearer of global science. Of course the emergence of "BIC"—Brazil, India, and China (sometimes Russia is included in "BRIC")—as a constellation of global power sites is another imaginary space for launching efforts to "catch up."

11. A popular example of the view is captured in Francis Fukuyama, *Our Posthuman Future: Consequences of the Biotechnology Revolution* (New York: Farrar, Straus, and Giroux, 2002).
12. Donna Haraway, "A Cyborg Manifesto," in *Simians, Cyborgs, and Women: The Reinvention of Nature* (New York: Routledge, 1991), 8–10, 152.
13. Michio Morishima, *Why Has Japan "Succeeded": Western Technology and the Japanese Ethos* (Cambridge: Cambridge University Press, 1984).
14. China's rise has realigned Asian states around its market, investments, and cultural influence. A formalization of the regional trade arrangement is ASEAN+3, or the Association of Southeast Asian Nations and China, South Korea, and Japan as an emerging economic bloc.
15. Starting in the eighteenth century, Chinese intellectuals such as Fen Guifen debated how to combine cultural essence and modern techniques (or *ti-yong*) so that wealth and power could be achieved through Western technology without eroding the foundation of Chinese civilization. See J. Mason Gentzler, *Changing China* (New York, Praeger Publishers, 1977), 70–71.
16. See Aihwa Ong, "Assembling around SARS: Technology, Body Heat, and Political Fever in Risk Society," in *Ulrich Beck: Kosmopolitisches Projekt*, ed. Angelika Pferl and Natan Szaider (Badan-Baden: Nomos Verlagsgesellschaft, 2004).
17. Harriet A. Washington, *Medical Apartheid: The Dark History of Medical Experimentation on Black Americans from Colonial Times to the Present* (New York: Random House, 2008).
18. See Pilar Ossorio and Troy Duster, "Race and Genetics: Controversies in Biomedical, Behavioral and Forensic Medicine," *American Psychologist* 60, no. 1 (2005): 116–27.
19. Nancy Scheper Hughes, "The Last Commodity: Post-human Ethics and the Global Traffic in 'Fresh' organs," in Ong and Collier, *Global Assemblages*.
20. Adriana Petryna, "Ethical Variability: Drug Development and Global Clinical Trials," *American Ethnologist* 32, no. 2 (May 2005): 183–97. See also Adriana Petryna, Andrew Lakoff, and Arthur Kleinman, eds., *Global Pharmaceuticals: Ethics, Markets, Practices* (Durham: Duke University Press, 2006).
21. Catherine Waldby and Robert Mitchell, *Tissue Economies: Blood, Organs, and Cell Lines in Late Capitalism* (Durham: Duke University Press, 2006),158–59.
22. Ibid., 31–32.
23. Kaushik Sunder Rajan, *Biocapital: The Constitution of Postgenomic Life* (Durham: Duke University Press, 2006), 7.
24. Waldby and Mitchell, *Tissue Economies*, 31–32, 185.
25. Rajan, *Biocapital*, 78–79.

26. Charis Thompson, *Making Parents: The Ontological Choreography of Reproductive Technologies* (Cambridge, Mass.: MIT Press, 2005), 155–58.
27. Sarah Franklin, "Rethinking Nature-Culture: Anthropology and the New Genetics," *Anthropological Theory* 3, no. 1 (2003): 65–85.
28. Lawrence Cohen, "Operability, Bioavailability, and Exception," in Ong and Collier, *Global Assemblages*, 82.
29. Rhonda L. Rundle, "A Daisy Chain of Kidney Donations," *Wall Street Journal*, September 23, 2008, D1, D2.
30. Paul Rabinow and Nikolas Rose, "Thoughts on the Concept of Biopower Today," *BioSocieties* 1 (2006): 195–217.
31. Nikolas Rose and Carlos Novas, "Biological Citizenship," in Ong and Collier, *Global Assemblages*, 445.
32. Nikolas Rose, *The Politics of Life Itself* (Princeton, N.J.: Princeton University Press, 2007), 3–4.
33. Michel Foucault, *Security, Territory, Population: Lectures at the Collège de France, 1977–1978*, ed. Michel Senellart, English series ed. Arnold I. Davidson, trans. Graham Burchell (New York: Palgrave Macmillan, 2007), 109.
34. Adriana Petryna, *Life Exposed: Biological Citizens after Chernobyl* (Princeton, N.J.: Princeton University Press, 2002).
35. Mitchell Dean, *Governing Societies* (Maidenhead, U.K.: Open University Press, 2007), 11.
36. In the anthropology of social medicine, see Arthur Kleinman, *The Illness Narratives: Suffering, Healing, and the Human Condition* (New York: Basic Books, 1988); Margaret Lock, *Twice Dead: Organ Transplants and the Reinvention of Death* (Berkeley: University of California Press, 2002); Emily Martin, *The Woman in the Body: A Cultural Analysis of Reproduction* (Boston, Mass.: Beacon Press, 1987); and Rayna Rapp, *Testing the Women, Testing the Fetus: Amniocentesis in America* (New York: Routledge, 1999). In the anthropology of science, see Fischer, "Four Genealogies," for a context-specific approach to ethical reasoning in scientific networks in the Middle East.
37. Stephen J. Collier and Andrew Lakoff, "On Regimes of Living," in Ong and Collier, *Global Assemblages*, 23–24.
38. Ulrich Beck, "The Reinvention of Politics: Towards a Theory of Reflexive Modernization," in *Reflexive Modernization*, ed. U. Beck, A. Giddens, and S. Lash (Stanford, Calif.: Stanford University Press, 1994), 10.
39. Michel Foucault, *"Society Must Be Defended": Lectures at the Collège de France, 1975–1976*, ed. Mauro Bertani and Alessandro Fontana, trans. David Macey (New York: Picador, 1997), 244–46.
40. Ibid., 246.
41. Foucault, *Security, Territory, Population*, 2, 11.
42. Ibid., 109.
43. Ibid., 352.
44. Foucault, *"Society Must Be Defended,"* 250.
45. Stephen J. Collier and Andrew Lakoff, "Distributed Preparedness: The Spa-

tial Logic of Domestic Security in the United States," *Environment and Planning D: Society and Space* 26, no. 1 (2008): 7–28.

46. Peter J. Spiro, "The New Sovereigntists: American Exceptionalism and Its False Prophets," *Foreign Affairs*, November–December 2001.
47. Benedict Anderson, *Imagined Communities: Reflections on the Origin and Spread of Nationalism*, 2nd ed. (1983; London: Verso, 1991; rev. ed. 2006).
48. On the concept of "civilization-state," see Martin Jacques, *China Rules the World: The End of the Western World and the Birth of a New Global Order* (New York: The Penguin Press, 2009), 196–211.
49. For a debate on the thesis of "the strong state" in Asia, see Ruth McVey, ed., *Southeast Asian Capitalists* (Ithaca, N.Y.: Cornell University Press, 1992).
50. See Tu Wei-ming, Milan Hejtmanek, and Alan Wachman, eds. *The Confucian World Observed: A Contemporary Discussion of Confucian Humanism in East Asia*. (Honolulu: Eas-West Center, 1992).
51. For a semiotic argument about the rise of "sovereign thinking" in Asia, see Lydia Liu, *The Clash of Empires: The Invention of China in Modern World Making* (Cambridge, Mass.: Harvard University Press, 2004).
52. See, for example, Yan Xuetong, "The Rise of China in Chinese Eyes," *Journal of Contemporary China* 10, no. 26 (2001): 33–39.
53. E-mail communication from Kaushik Sunder Rajan, February 18, 2008 (editors' file).
54. Michael Dillon and Luis Lobo-Guerrero, "Biopolitics of Security in the 21st Century," *Review of International Studies* 34, no. 2 (2008): 287.
55. David Held, Anthony McGrew, David Goldblatt, and Jonathan Perraton, *Global Transformation: Politics, Economics, Culture* (London: Routledge, 1999), 445–46.
56. See, e.g., Vincanne Adams, *Doctors for Democracy: Health Professionals in the Nepali Revolution* (Cambridge: Cambridge University Press, 1998).
57. Susan Greenhalgh, *Just One Child: Science and Policy in Deng's China* (Berkeley: University of California Press, 2008); and Matthew Kohrman, "Should I Quit? Tobacco, Fraught Identity, and the Risks of Governmentality," in *Privatizing China: Socialism from Afar*, ed. Li Zhang and Aihwa Ong (Ithaca, N.Y.: Cornell University Press, 2008).
58. For a similar notion of ethicalization, see Andrew Barry, "Ethical Capitalism," in *Global Governmentality*, ed. Wendy Larner and William Walters (London: Routledge, 2004), 207.
59. Lily E. Kay, *The Molecular Vision of Life: Caltech, the Rockefeller Foundation, and the Rise of New Biology* (Oxford: Oxford University Press, 1996), 17.
60. Charles Leadbeater and James Wilsdon, "South-East Asia Economies Herald a New Dawn of Technological Innovation," *Times* (London), January 17, 2007, 51.
61. James Wilsdon and James Keeley, *China: The Next Science Superpower? The Atlas of Ideas: Mapping the New Geography of Science* (London: Demos, 2007), 6.

62. Brian Salter, Melinda Cooper, and Amanda Dickens, "China and the Global Stem Cell Bioeconomy: An Emerging Political Strategy?" *Regenerative Medicine* 1, no. 5 (2006): 671–83.
63. Bioworld and General Biologic, *China Biotech 2008* (Atlanta, Ga.: Bioworld and General Biologic, 2008).
64. Nancy N. Chen, "China's Biotech Bloom," *Genewatch* 17, no. 1 (January–February 2004): 10–12.
65. Arthur Kornberg, "Whither Biotechnology in Japan: Why Biotechnology Hasn't Taken Off," *Harvard Asia Pacific Review* 106, no. 2 (fall 2002), 6–9.
66. See, e.g., Sharon Traweek, *Beamtimes and Lifetimes: The World of High Energy Physicists* (Cambridge, Mass.: Harvard University Press, 1988).
67. Dennis Normile, "SNP Study Supports Southern Migration Route to Asia," *Science Magazine*, December 11, 2009, vol. 326, 1470.
68. For a non-Asian example of the commercial use of a national health database, see Gisli Palsson and Paul Rabinow, "The Icelandic Controversy: Reflections on the Transnational Market of Civic Virtue," in Ong and Collier, *Global Assemblages*, 92.
69. Interview with Edison Liu, Genome Institute, Singapore, June, 6, 2006.
70. Rajan, *Biocapital*, 286. Italics in the original.
71. Karl Marx, *Capital: A Critique of Political Economy*, vol. 1, ed. Frederick Engels, trans. Samuel Moore and Edward Aveling (New York: International Publishers, 1967), 333–41.
72. Greenhalgh, *Just One Child.*
73. Ann Anagnost, "The Corporeal Politics of Quality (Suzhi)," Public Culture 16, no. 2 (Spring 2004): 189–208; Rachel Murphy, "Turning Peasants into Modern Chinese Citizens: 'Population Quality' Discourse, Demographic Transition and Primary Education," China Quarterly 177 (2004): 1–20.
74. Nancy N. Chen, "Consuming Medicine and Biotechnology in China," in Zhang and Ong, *Privatizing China*, 123–32.
75. See Mei Zhan, "Wild Consumptions: Relocating Responsibilities in the Time of SARS," in Zhang and Ong, *Privatizing China*.
76. For a survey of these concerns in Southeast Asia, see Warwick Anderson, ed. "Emergent Studies of Science, Technology, and Medicine in Southeast Asia." Special double issue of *East Asian Science Technology, and Society: An International Journal* (2009), 3.
77. High Flyers Think Tank, "Emerging Diseases—Ready and Waiting?," paper presented at the Shine Dome, Australian Academy of Science, Canberra, 19 October 2004.
78. Chiu Yu-tzu, "Taiwanese Scientists Find Genetic Links to SARS," *Nature Medicine* 9, no. 11 (November 2003): 1335.
79. *World Bank Development Report 1998–1999: Knowledge for Development* (Washington D.C.: World Bank, 1999), http://www.worldbank.org/wdr/wdr98.

80. See Aihwa Ong, "Ecologies of Expertise: Assembling Flows, Managing Citizenship," in Ong and Collier, *Global Assemblage*.
81. Kean Birch, "The Neoliberal Underpinnings of the Bioeconomy: The Ideological Discourses and Practices of Economic Competitiveness," *Genomics, Society, and Policy* 2, no. 3 (2006): 6–7.
82. Aihwa Ong, "Zoning Technologies in East Asia," in *Neoliberalism as Exception: Mutations in Citizenship and Sovereignty* (Durham: Duke University Press, 2006); see also Aihwa Ong and Li Zhang, "Privatizing China: Powers of the Self, Socialism from Afar," in Zhang and Ong, *Privatizing China*.
83. Kris Olds and Nigel Thrift, "Cultures on the Brink: Reengineering the Soul of Capitalism—On a Global Scale," in Ong and Collier, *Global Assemblages*.
84. Hannah Beech, "Asia's Great Science Experiment," *Time* magazine, October 23, 2006.
85. Beech, "Asia's Great Science Experiment."
86. Collier and Ong, "Global Assemblages, Anthropological Problems," 17.
87. See Arthur Kleinman, *The Illness Narratives: Suffering, Healing, and the Human Condition*, (New York: Basic Books, 1988).
88. Pat Usher, "Feminist Approaches to a Situated Ethics," in *Situated Ethics in Educational Research*, ed. Helen Simons and Robin Usher (London: Routledge, 2000).
89. Ruth Macklin, *Mortal Choices: Bioethics in Today's World* (New York: Pantheon, 1987).
90. Frank Dikotter, *Imperfect Conceptions: Medical Knowledge, Birth Defects, and Eugenics in China* (New York: Columbia University Press, 1998). Frank Dikotter argues that in contemporary China, popular views of eugenics have survived and given support to a state program that draws sharp distinctions between normal and abnormal births. Dikotter calls current health notions "eugenics," but these are individual practices of self-care and family enhancement stemming from a combination of folk medicine and the availability of modern medical techniques. This new social eugenics, if you will, is influenced by the ethos of biomedical enhancement and designer babies that originated among affluent consumers in advanced liberal societies.
91. Thomas Lemke, "'The Birth of Biopolitics'—Michel Foucault's Lecture at the Collège de France on Neo-Liberal Governmentality," *Economy and Society* 30, no. 2 (2001): 9.
92. There was also an illegal trade in ova to supply ova to mainly Japanese infertile couples. A new bioethics banning the sale of human egg cells was passed after the Hwang scandal in January 2005.
93. Herbert Gottweis and Robert Triendl, "South Korean Policy Failure and the Hwang Debacle," *Nature Biotechnology* 24, no. 2 (February 2006): 141–43.
94. Choe Sang-Hun, "Korean Lab Roiled by Egg Donor Disclosures," *International Herald Tribune*, November 23, 2005.
95. Jessica H. Muller, "Anthropology, Bioethics, and Medicine: A Provocative Trilogy," in "Conceptual Development in Medical Anthropology: A Tribute

to M. Margaret Clark," special issue of *Medical Anthropology Quarterly*, new ser., 8, no. 4 (December 1994): 448–67.

96. Lock, *Twice Dead*.
97. Cori Hayden, *When Nature Goes Public: The Making and Unmaking of Bioprospecting in Mexico* (Princeton: Princeton University Press, 2003).
98. Paul Rabinow, *French DNA: Trouble in Purgatory* (Chicago: Chicago University Press, 1999).
99. Palsson and Rabinow, "The Icelandic Controversy," 92.
100. TRIPS is an international law requiring states to provide strong protection for intellectual property rights. WIPO is a specialized agency of the United Nations to promote protection of intellectual property throughout the world.
101. E-mail communication from Stefan Ecks, March 16, 2008. Editors' file.
102. Aihwa Ong, "Scales of Exception: Experiments with Knowledge and Sheer Life in Tropical Southeast Asia," *Singapore Journal of Tropical Geography* 29, no. 2 (July 2008): 1–13.
103. "Indonesia Stops Sharing Key Bird Flu Samples," *Financial Times*, February 6, 2007.
104. Ibid.
105. Sun-Wei Guo, Chang-Jiang Zheng, and C. C. Li, "The Gene War of the Century," *Science* 278, no. 5344 (December 5, 1997): 1693–97.

I

EXCESS AND OPPORTUNITY

KAUSHIK SUNDER RAJAN

The Experimental Machinery of Global Clinical Trials | CASE STUDIES FROM INDIA

In earlier work, I have written about emergent systems of technoscientific production, value generation, and commodity circulation that concern the life sciences under the rubric of what might be called "biocapital," focusing on the sequencing of the human genome and the science of genomics that was emerging around this venture.[1] The study of clinical trials is a necessary follow-up to the study of genomics in a project on biocapital.

This is because, first, within the biomedical process itself, clinical trials are often consequent to technologies such as genomics. Genomics is important to the drug discovery process—it potentially allows for the rational screening and identification of promising lead molecules that could conceivably have a therapeutic effect. This is the "upstream" or early-stage component of therapeutic development, but it is only distantly related, epistemologically and temporally, to the production of a therapeutic molecule. Clinical trials, on the other hand, constitute the "downstream" or drug development component of the process of therapeutic development. There is no way that any new drug molecule can come to market without a series of trials for safety and efficacy in animals and humans. Clinical trials therefore constitute the *experimental machinery* of biocapital: they are necessary to conduct before a drug comes to market, are particularly elaborate in the context of the U.S. regulatory framework, and are in themselves cost-intensive and high-risk with no guarantee of success.

Clinical trials constitute the set of practices required to certify a new drug molecule as safe and efficacious for the market.[2] This set of practices serves in its rationale as a regulatory watchdog to prevent the market from being flooded with unsafe or spurious medication. In the United States, the clinical trials procedure is an elaborate one, occurring in four stages and contributing to the immense time, risk, and expense of the drug development process.

The stages of clinical trials are as follows: First, there is preclinical toxicological testing of a potential new drug molecule. This is usually performed on animals, in order to determine whether the molecule being tested is safe enough to put into a living system. This is followed by dosage studies, in order to come up with a metric that relates the dose of the drug being administered to safety and efficacy. Predictably, the efficacy of a drug increases with its dose, but so too does its toxicity, so the attempt is to find an optimum range of doses within which efficacy is maximized without compromising safety too much. If the drug is found too toxic to animals, the trial will not proceed any further, but if acceptable dose ranges can be determined within animals, then it proceeds to a three-phase trial in humans. Phase I trials are conducted on a small number of healthy volunteers to test the basic safety of the drug (since drugs that seem safe in animals may yet show adverse effects in humans). Phase II involves scaled-up, larger, efficacy and safety trials on one hundred to three hundred patients. Phase III trials are large-scale, randomized trials that may be conducted on a few thousand people, usually patients suffering from the ailment for which the therapy has been developed. These trials are usually coordinated across multiple centers, often (increasingly) globally.

Most trial sponsors are biotechnology or pharmaceutical companies because drug development in the United States (and in most parts of the world) is largely undertaken by the private sector. Universities and publicly funded laboratories in the States do play an enormous role in early-stage drug discovery—the identification of potential lead molecules and the conduct of early preclinical tests, but the institutional structure of drug development is such that they invariably license promising molecules to corporations in order to take them through clinical trials. This means that the biomedical and experimental rationales for clinical trials are completely entwined with the market value that these companies see from the drugs that eventually get developed, and with the market risk that attends the drug development process. Parenthetically, there is no epistemic reason why the drug development process should be so completely in the private sector, though this has become a naturalized facet of the biomedical economy, and is one of the factors that has allowed the seamless appropriation of health as an index whose value can be purely evaluated in terms set by the market. According to the Healthcare Financial Management Association's newsletter, "Twenty years ago, 80 percent of clinical research trials were conducted through academic medical centers. In 1998, estimates indicated the number of academic medical centers as investigator sites had dropped to less than half."[3] Health research and production is thus progressively captured by capital, and now needs to be seen as a semiautonomous sector of capital. This is an example of what Balibar and Wallerstein have described as the continual expansion of the value form and infinite process of accumulation.[4] The organizational complexity of clinical trials has however meant that it has been difficult for pharmaceutical companies to manage them, leading to the emergence of an entirely new industry segment devoted to the management and administration of clinical trials. These companies, called clinical research organizations (CROs), are now an integral part of the overall biomedical economy.

Clinical trials provide comparative insights into the study of biocapital across multiple sites globally. My own work focuses on India and the United States, two countries that are interconnected through flows of capital, infrastructure, and expertise, especially through the investment of nonresident Indian entrepreneurs repatriating a "culture of innovation" back to India. In this context, a host of CROs are emerging in India to conduct these trials, thereby providing a contracted service for (largely Western) biotech and pharmaceutical companies. If clinical trials are the experimental machinery of biocapital, then India, in this story, envisages itself as a major experimental site. Clinical trials, therefore, provide a lens through which to study the globalizing dynamics of biocapital in terms of the cost and biomedical rationales for outsourcing trials to developing country sites like India.

The Indian Clinical Trials Landscape

In this essay, I outline some of the dynamics of clinical trials in India, especially in terms of the huge amounts of capacity building taking place in anticipation of the movement of global trials there. I am interested in briefly mapping the various institutional actors and political economic dynamics at play in this arena. But I am particularly interested in showing how *ethics* is fundamental to the experimental machinery of global clinical trials as it touches down in India. It provides an engine to create ethical subjects involved in conducting clinical trials (CRO managers, employees, and researchers), but also allows the seamless creation of, and expropriation of, Third World experimental subjects, who are, I argue, "merely risked." Capacity building is certainly technological and institutional; but I want to focus on the various human capacities that are generated and/or taken advantage of as part of this experimental machinery. Ethics in the globalizing world of biotechnology is, as Aihwa Ong points out in the introduction to this volume, situated; and my interest lies in understanding the ways in which these situated ethics both structure and respond to pharmaceutical logics of value generation.

The movement of clinical trials to international (non-U.S.) locations started in earnest in the mid-1990s. Adriana Petryna cites figures that point to a dramatic growth in the number of international human subjects recruited into these trials, from 4,000 in 1995 to 400,000 in 1999.[5] A recent study by the consulting firm A. T. Kearney shows that roughly half of the 1,200 clinical trials conducted in 2005 in the United States had an international trial site.[6] In the 1990s, most of this international growth occurred, as Petryna notes, in countries that had agreed to harmonize standards in commercial drug testing with those set by the International Conference on Harmonization (ICH) guidelines. These included primarily Latin American and Eastern European countries, but interestingly not India. Over the past four years, however, India has been one of the most aggressive sites of clinical research infrastructure establishment and growth.

Indian actors currently see the country as providing an extremely attractive destination for outsourced clinical trials from the West. Contract research in the Indian pharmaceutical industry is already robust, and was estimated by the Chemical Pharmaceutical Generic Association to be worth between $100 and 120 million in 2005, while growing at 20–25 percent per year.[7] Indian actors are eagerly anticipating the further influx of global clinical trials into the country. Who are these actors, and what are their anticipations based upon?

The most central, perhaps, are members of the burgeoning CRO industry. These are the most immediate beneficiaries in terms of revenues and profits of trials coming to India, and are therefore keen to create conditions whereby the influx of these trials can grow in a sustained and streamlined fashion. CROs are the major drivers of the ramp-up in clinical research infrastructure, and are particularly influential in building a regulatory framework for the conduct of trials. It is estimated that there are approximately one hundred CROs of reasonable size operating in the country at the moment. Some of these are fairly well established, with a couple being fifteen to twenty years old. A number of the better known CROs were seeded in the late 1990s, but many of these CROs have emerged since 2005.

The Indian pharmaceutical industry is another interested party. It is in the process of retooling its business model in the wake of India becoming a signatory to patent regimes imposed by the World Trade Organization (WTO). Indian patent laws prior to WTO allowed only process and not product patents on therapeutic molecules. This meant that one could not patent a drug itself, only the specific manufacturing process that produced it. This allowed Indian pharmaceutical companies to reverse-engineer generic versions of drugs that had product patent protection in the West. Such reverse engineering is now not possible under a WTO regime for the duration of a drug's patent (twenty years). This has forced a number of leading Indian drug companies into a business model driven by research and development, whereby they, like their Western counterparts, engage in the much riskier process of novel drug discovery and development. Clinical trials become constitutive of this business model, because one cannot develop novel drugs without subjecting them to this elaborate regime of safety and efficacy testing. In other words, the Indian pharmaceutical industry has itself served as a spur to the CRO industry. Becoming signatory to the WTO has also potentially made India a more attractive clinical research destination from the perspective of Western trial sponsors seeking to outsource global trials, since their intellectual property is better protected under such a regime.

What is surprising, however, is the immediacy with which clinical trial activity has sprung into life in India post-WTO. In many ways, the real spurt in business, regulatory, and training activity around clinical trials in India started around the same time that India started implementing a WTO-based patent regime (January 1, 2005). This suggests that the elements of a robust CRO industry were already in place in anticipation of WTO compliance, and that the initial spur to this industry was perhaps not just an anticipation of Western trials post-WTO, but was more complicated and homegrown.

That initial spur did in fact come from the Indian pharmaceutical industry as it started retooling its business models in anticipation of a WTO regime. While most Indian pharmaceutical companies retain robust generic divisions even after WTO (enabling them to compete with off-patent generics in Indian and increasingly also in Western markets), a few entrepreneurial ones such as Ranbaxy and Dr. Reddy's Laboratories have moved aggressively towards an R & D–based infrastructure. Even within generics divisions, bioequivalence studies are an important subset of clinical trials, and one that Indian companies, because of their traditional expertise in generic markets, are well positioned to conduct.[8]

Ranbaxy has been responsible for the growth of the Indian clinical research industry in more ways than one. Its business model is currently twofold—first, to aggressively increase its presence in global generics markets (including the United States), and second, to try and discover its own therapeutic molecules that it might license to multinational pharmaceutical companies in exchange for the payment of various milestone-related royalties.[9] In both cases, developing clinical testing facilities became very important for the company, and Ranbaxy was one of the first Indian pharmaceutical companies to develop an in-house CRO. It also started outsourcing trials, thereby spurring the development of a CRO industry. In addition, Ranbaxy also ended up being a source of much clinical research expertise. Three of Ranbaxy's main clinical researchers left the company in 2000 to create Wellquest in Bombay (itself a CRO seeded by another major Indian pharmaceutical company, Nicholas Piramal), while two other scientists from Ranbaxy were the cofounders of another major CRO, Lambda, in 1999. In this way, certain sections of the Indian pharmaceutical industry have generated clinical research work themselves, and have provided the capital and expertise required for the industry to take off. These events again make it too simple to suggest that clinical research capacity is purely being built as a consequence of the desire of "the West" to outsource trials to cheap Indian locations, though Indian actors are certainly betting on such a desire materializing in more research contracts.[10]

A third actor consists of the regulatory agents and agents of the state. The immediate regulatory agency in India is the Drug Controller General of India (DCGI), a nominal equivalent of the U.S. Food and Drug Administration (FDA). The DCGI was, until a few years ago, indeed a fairly peripheral presence on the Indian regulatory landscape, but is now in the process of recreating itself as a serious regulatory agenda-setting organization.

Yet another actor consists of educational and training institutes for clinical research. Building the human resource capability to conduct and monitor trials in India is a key challenge, and a number of entrepreneurial ventures are engaged purely in training the labor force required to undertake this work. Finally, there are the physicians who actually conduct the trials, who in the Indian context have a relatively marginal presence compared to the CRO industry in setting the infrastructural and regulatory agenda for the conduct of such research.

There is a striking and universal interest among these actors (though not to the same extent as among physicians) not just in building clinical research infrastructure in India but also in promoting India as a clinical trial destination globally. The experimental potential of Indian populations as trial subjects melds seamlessly into the market potential that CROs perceive from an influx of these trials into India, and this convergence is facilitated by a larger historical moment that sees the Indian state branding and marketing itself to investors at global forums. Investments in the nation-state articulate with investments in biomedicine to result in capacity building for clinical trials.

Some of the enthusiasm around clinical trials within India is mirrored in the West by agents who might outsource clinical trials to the country. However, for the most part, the surge in clinical trials contracts to India is still in the realm of anticipation and potential. The infrastructure building occurring in India is very real; but it is a bet on future outcomes that, like any other speculation, may or may not pay off. Understanding the clinical trial situation in India involves understanding both the enthusiasms and the reservations that exist on the part of Western agents who may wish to contract trials out to India.

The anticipation of global clinical trials coming to India is based on the expectation that it would in various ways serve the interests of Western trial sponsors (especially U.S. biotech and pharmaceutical companies) to outsource these trials to India. This expectation is, at one level, a general market expectation—a recent McKinsey report, for instance, estimated that clinical research in India will be a one-billion-dollar industry by 2010.[11] These types of estimations are consequential in setting certain expectations as well as certain actions on the part of both Indian and Western actors in motion.

These expectations are based on the various perceived advantages involved in taking clinical trials to India. They include, among other factors, a cost advantage—estimates suggest that taking trials to India could save overall clinical trial costs by 30–50 percent for a multinational company, based on lower labor and infrastructure costs. There is also a perceived recruitment advantage—it is assumed that patients would be easier to recruit into trials, especially treatment-naïve patients. A major problem for drug companies conducting trials in the United States is that Americans are so therapeutically saturated—they tend to be on so many drugs that it is very difficult to determine the efficacy of the experimental drug being tested without having to confront a whole range of drug-drug interactions that muddy the data considerably.

There are other factors to consider while thinking about the attractiveness of a country as a clinical trials location. A recent report by A. T. Kearney, which provided an "attractiveness index" for countries as clinical trials destinations, considered three factors, in addition to cost efficiency and patient pool: "regulatory conditions," "relevant expertise," and "infrastructure and environment." These are indeed three key areas that Indian actors are focusing on as part of their capacity-building efforts; nonetheless, Kearney already ranks India as the second most attractive destination for clinical trials outside the United States after China. India scored much higher than the United States in terms of patient pool and cost efficiency, but lower on the other three counts.[12]

However, the scenario is more complicated than one in which Western multinational companies are trying to tear the door down to exploit cheap Indian populations. If anything, it is an open question as to how badly Western companies would want to outsource especially early-stage clinical trials to India. There are obvious advantages to doing so in terms of cost and the ease of volunteer recruitment; there are also downsides in terms of the relative difficulty of monitoring trials (which is very important to do properly if the data generated is to pass muster with the FDA), and in terms of the potential public relations disaster that could attend an early-stage clinical trial gone horribly wrong in a Third World context. Indeed, the Kearney report points out that in August 2005, the top twelve pharmaceutical companies reported conducting 175 ongoing trials in Germany (attractiveness index of 4.69) and 161 in the United Kingdom (attractiveness index of 5.0), compared to 26 in India (attractiveness index of 5.58). In 2004, Pfizer invested roughly $13 million into clinical trials in India, which, while sounding like a lot of capital investment, can be put in perspective by the fact that its total global R & D expenditure was $8 billion. Perhaps more than pharmaceutical companies themselves, it is Western CROs who see real value in outsourcing some of their (already outsourced) activity to other countries. Therefore, while there are convincing market rationales for taking trials to India, and an already strong movement of these trials there through the multinational CRO industry, much of the capacity building in clinical research in India is still a bet on potential future value that Indian CROs see from outsourced trials rather than a reaction to a movement of trials that has already occurred.

Capacity building here means something far more extensive than building experimental infrastructure for conducting clinical trials, which is perhaps the easiest component of capacity building for clinical trials in a country like India, where material and financial resources do not constitute anymore the rate limiting step. This most basic aspect of capacity building also generates the least amount of concern among Indian actors trying to attract trials into the country. Other aspects of capacity building include the development of the data management, human resource, and, especially, regulatory infrastructures. I elaborate briefly upon the first two, before talking about regulatory infrastructure building in some detail.

DATA MANAGEMENT INFRASTRUCTURE

One important part of the clinical trials procedure concerns experimentation—the actual process of putting experimental drug molecules into animals and humans in order to test efficacy and toxicity. The "meaning" that comes out of these trials, however, is in the data generated in these experiments; processing and managing this data is an incredibly complicated task. This mass of data is eventually the basis for the crucial end point of the regulatory process, the *package insert*.

The package insert is the label that gets put on the package of any approved drug, indicating the uses for which the FDA has legally approved a drug. Much of this data is generated by the trial sponsors themselves, and as biotech and pharmaceutical companies increasingly outsource trials to CROs, by the CROs. Annotating and presenting this data in an intelligible form to the FDA is a crucial part of the clinical trials procedure.

Independent of establishing India as an experimental site is concomitant capacity building to make India a destination of choice for managing data relating to clinical trials. This is enabled by India's strong software capabilities, which already have helped it emerge as a major site for outsourced back-end information technology (IT) service work. According to Michael Arlotto, senior vice president for corporate development at Quintiles, the North Carolina–based multinational CRO, his company sends almost three-quarters of its *global* trial data to be processed in Bangalore (the remainder of the data processing apparently occurs in Bloemfontein, South Africa, which has a renowned statistical institute).[13] The intricacies of global clinical research are suggested by the fact that, completely independent of the complexities of conducting standardized experiments on trial volunteers and patients in multiple centers across many countries is another articulated global circuit, this time of data, which (in the case of one major company at least) ends up getting concentrated in South India and South Africa in order to be made "meaningful" in the eyes of the FDA, the premier U.S. regulatory agency for drug approvals.

Not surprisingly, Indian companies have started up that focus their business model purely on the data management aspect of clinical trials. An early example of such a small homegrown start-up is the Hyderabad-based Sristek, which initiated operations in clinical trial data management in 2002, before the intense capacity building of the post-WTO era. Sristek is an example of a company that enters clinical research through the route of data management, a site at which the conduct of clinical trials comes to be quite crucially about processing and managing information. Indeed, Sristek's cofounders themselves had no background in the life sciences or health care—one was a mechanical engineer, while the other had an MBA degree. What they leveraged was their expertise in software applications, and the existence of a human resource infrastructure for those applications.[14]

Sristek's trajectory points to the constitutive importance of data management as part of the clinical research endeavor. But Sristek too is not immune to the overwhelming potential of experimental clinical research, and is indeed in the process of reinventing itself as a CRO that can also conduct trials in addition to manage trial data. Sristek's story simultaneously points to the independent importance of data management practices in clinical research, and to the ways in which the lure of experimental clinical trials overdetermines the clinical research landscape in India today.

HUMAN RESOURCE INFRASTRUCTURE

In the midst of all the infrastructure building around experimentation and data management, labor issues do not go away, and questions of vocational training, pedagogy, and human resource development are central to the concerns of Indian regulators and CROs. And so, as seen earlier in India with software, bioinformatics, and call centers, diploma courses for clinical research are opening up all over the country, sometimes in new universities set up expressly for this purpose. I wish here to briefly flag some key issues regarding human resource infrastructure.

First, there are issues of infrastructure and expertise that are called into account in the face of the challenge to train a young workforce. Second is the question of who enters such training programs in order to become clinical research managers, and who is likely to run and monitor the global trials that will likely come into India. Currently, most Phase III trials in India are run by physicians. While trials in the United States are also officially "run" by physicians, they are often not just executed but also managed by nurses, and indeed clinical research is an integral part of the pedagogy of nursing schools in the United States. So there are interesting questions as to who will get trained to manage clinical research in India, and how that will play out in terms of hierarchy (and gender) roles with doctors there.

Third is the fact that, as with work outside of the biomedical industry, work within the biomedical industry is also labor, with many of the labor conditions prevalent in other service industries replicated here. Clinical monitoring in particular is drudge work, which involves visiting multiple centers where a trial is being conducted, and ensuring that the trial protocol is being properly followed, that data entry is being correctly done, and that the inclusion and exclusion criteria set for the trial by the sponsor are being met. This involves constant traveling and has very high attrition rates in the United States. Just as call center work in India is hugely exploitative at the same time as it is creating a new socially mobile class of young professionals, so too is clinical research work likely to resolve in terms of a host of labor issues concerning quality of work, standard of living, wages, compensation, and workers' rights.

REGULATORY INFRASTRUCTURE

Perhaps the most elaborate challenge in terms of building infrastructure for clinical trials is building an adequate regulatory infrastructure. Certainly, if India is to get global trials, it is essential for its regulatory infrastructure to be much stronger than it is currently. This is especially the case with trials outsourced from a United States–based sponsor, which need to pass muster with the U.S. Food and Drug Administration's stringent regulatory criteria. In her work on clinical trials, Adriana Petryna has argued for a state of "ethical variability," suggesting that ethical practices of clinical trials resolve differentially in First World locales and Third.[15] While in practice it is quite possible that the implementation of ethical guidelines ends up being more stringent in the First World than in the Third, it is important to be attentive to the very serious attention that is being given to ethics by both the Indian regulatory agencies and the CRO industry there. Equally, it is important to be attentive to what constitutes such an ethics, and what gets left out.

An ethical trial protocol primarily concerns itself with the collection of informed consent. This includes the entire apparatus that surrounds the production of the consent process, especially an institutional review board (IRB) infrastructure. These ethical practices were enshrined in guidelines that the Indian government laid out for good clinical practice (what is known as GCP) in 2001. In 2005, these guidelines were converted into law, termed Schedule Y of the Indian Drugs and Cosmetics Act, which insists upon GCP. Interestingly, the Indian laws are the only ones in the world where the violation of GCP is deemed a criminal rather than a civil offense. At the same time, global trials that are valid in the eyes of the FDA need to be harmonized to what are known as ICH protocols (ICH being the acronym for "International

Conference on Harmonization of Technical Requirements for Registration of Pharmaceuticals for Human Use"). Therefore, Indian regulators are currently involved in a massive standardization process, driven by the Indian CRO industry, which seeks to harmonize Indians laws with ICH protocols. In the letter of the law, then, Indian ethical guidelines, legally enshrined, are likely to be at least as stringent as ethical guidelines for the conduct of clinical research in the United States, and in some ways, more so.

Members of India's CRO industry bristle at the suggestion that clinical trials move to India because it is possible to cut ethical corners there. Such suggestions have been part of the debate on the movement of clinical trials to India, and acquired salience and legitimacy because of an article published by two prominent Indian physicians, Samiran Nundy and Chandra Gulhati, in the prestigious *New England Journal of Medicine* that equated clinical trials in India to a "new colonialism."[16] CRO leaders are acutely aware of the need to build a positive media image for their industry, and are very invested in pointing out the ways in which Schedule Y goes beyond the good clinical practice demanded in ICH guidelines. Specifically, Schedule Y is concerned with ensuring extra care in gathering informed consent from illiterate subjects and in considering what might constitute "ethical" compensation for poor subjects recruited into trials (the logic here being that lucrative remuneration for participation in clinical trials can actually act as a coercive incentive for poor people to participate in early-stage trials). One Mumbai-based CRO executive, Arun Bhatt, was typically emphatic about the importance of Schedule Y and good clinical practice: "We are new. We don't want to play with the evolution of ethics."[17]

Outside the enforcement potential of Schedule Y, however, a larger regulatory body with the scope of the FDA is still absent. As mentioned earlier, the Drug Controller General of India (DGCI) is the nominal equivalent of the FDA, but one whose purview is still relatively limited to approving drugs for market or for import into the country. Part of the regulatory efforts under way in India at the moment consist in building a more substantial regulatory body with oversight powers that parallel those of the FDA, and whose conduct can further be harmonized with that of the FDA. This is, indeed, a central recommendation of the Mashelkar Committee Report of October 2005 on the regulation of biotechnology and clinical research in India, which proposes a

National Biotechnology Regulatory Authority/Commission, similar to the FDA system, which would regulate not just pharmaceuticals but also agricultural products and transgenic crops, transgenic food and feed, and transgenic animals and aquaculture.[18]

Ethics, legally enshrined and contractually enforced, is integral to the capacity-building efforts around clinical research in India. Members of the CRO industry are the biggest drivers of building an ethical regulatory infrastructure. Nonetheless, the form that ethics takes (which is, quite literally, the informed consent form) does not mitigate the fundamental structural violence of clinical trials performed in Third World contexts. I will elaborate upon this in the next section. The clinical research landscape in India is more complicated than just neocolonial exploitation of Indian populations as "guinea pigs" by rapacious multinational interests, where cutting corners is the norm and ethics is easily sacrificed. Indeed, the problematic is far more interesting, and involves analyzing the desire on the part of Indian state and corporate actors for India to become a global experimental site, as well as considering how a complete and formal attentiveness to ethics can nonetheless lead to structurally violent and exploitative structures of global biocapital.

A Critique of the Global Biomedical Economy: Expropriation, Exploitation, and the Structural Violence of Biocapital

I suggested in the previous section that Indian actors, especially the CRO industry, are seriously concerned with ethics, which gets legally enshrined in what is referred to as good clinical practice. GCP, however, is primarily concerned with proper protocols for collecting informed consent at the time of trial enrollment, and with the adequate monitoring of clinical trials in the various centers at which they are conducted. In this section, I want to lead my overview of the clinical research landscape in India toward a critique of biocapital.

Consider, for instance, the Hyderabad-based CRO Vimta Laboratories. Vimta is in many ways considered the gold-standard Indian CRO. Founded in 1991, it is one of India's oldest CROs. It is the only CRO that is publicly traded on the Bombay Stock Exchange, and the only CRO in the country that has been audited twice by the FDA (passing both times with flying colors). The clinical research manager of a U.S.-based company that I talked to suggested that Vimta was exactly the sort of company she would consider collaborating with if she were to look for an Indian partner with which to conduct trials.

Vimta's concern with and process for collecting informed consent is exemplary of the insistence of GCP in the Indian context. I visited Vimta as a part of my fieldwork. The first room I was shown was the waiting and screening room, which looks like the waiting room of a railway station, where trial subjects come in and are given their consent forms and a basic questionnaire to fill out in order to determine whether they are qualified to participate in the trial. The walls of the waiting room are empty, except for a single bulletin board that outlines all the risks that could accrue to participants in a clinical trial; it is written only in English. I was told that in order to participate in a trial, the subjects have to be literate (though not necessarily in English), and they are invariably male (Vimta only enrolls females if the trial sponsor specifies a need for female subjects).

Beyond the waiting room is a long corridor, with many rooms where different types of medical examinations are conducted on trial volunteers. First, their height and weight are recorded. If the subject weighs less than fifty-five kilograms, he is not admitted into the trial because the risk of trial-related complications becomes too high. There is then a general physical exam, after which the tests become progressively more invasive—an ECG is conducted in a third room, blood drawn in a fourth (which is sent to the pathology labs for analysis), and an X-ray taken in a fifth. I learned while being walked through this corridor that the consent forms the subjects sign in the waiting room are specifically for the medical screening procedures—if the subjects are selected to participate in the trial, they sign a separate form, which is particular to the trial they are enrolled in. A number of the trials conducted at Vimta are Phase I trials on healthy volunteers. Recruiting subjects into Phase I trials has, as I mentioned earlier, become increasingly difficult in the United States. I was told that volunteer retention is much better in India than in the States because "people trust doctors here." Interestingly, although recruiting healthy people to have risky molecules administered to them is such a challenge, the entire setup seems to emphasize "selection"—it is almost as if getting enrolled into a trial is a test that only those who are fit enough can pass. Moreover, the subjects are only ever referred to as "volunteers," suggesting no doubt their autonomous rational agency, the same agency that gets contractually codified through the consent form.

Such deep and, I believe, serious concern with informed consent and GCP, reflected both in national laws and in the practices of companies such as Vimta, does not however even touch upon the question of *access to drugs*. By this I mean the following: in the United States, clinical trials at least implicitly suggest a social contract between a few people who are put on potentially risky medication in order to garner a larger social good, the development of new therapy. People recruited into Phase I trials tend to be less well-off in the United States as well, so that the social contract is never a pure liberal contract between rational individuals in what John Rawls would call an "original position" of assumed equality.[19] Nonetheless, there is an animating liberal sentiment that absolutely presumes that therapy, if developed, will eventually be accessible (on the market, for a price—so it does raise issues of affordability and distributive justice; but those are issues that in principle can be addressed through liberal welfare state mechanisms). In the Indian context, by contrast, there is no guarantee that an experimental drug tested on an Indian population would even have to be marketed there after approval (let alone made available at an affordable cost). There have been no moves on the part of the Indian state to insist upon this through, for example, mechanisms like compulsory licensing regulations. The likely outcome therefore is a situation where Indian populations are used purely as experimental subjects, without the implicit social contract of therapeutic access at the end of the day.[20]

This issue of access to drugs is a live question in the Indian physician community, leading to critiques such as Nundy and Gulhati's referenced earlier. A leading Delhi-based psychiatrist in a prominent private hospital (who preferred anonymity) told me, for instance, that "while we understand the need for conducting trials, there is need for more uniform regulatory control."[21] This is not someone who is outside the circuits of clinical research, but rather someone who conducts a number of psychiatric trials in two centers where he has affiliations. Most of the trials such prominent physicians conduct, however, are Phase III trials on patients they are treating, which puts their practice into a different ethical calculus (having to do with pastoral care) than that of CROs who are looking to increase Phase I trials on healthy volunteers (which is a concern purely with experimental subjectivity). The relationship of trials to access to drugs is, for this physician, an acute question, especially for the Phase III trial subjects who may need to continue taking the experimental medication that is tested upon them if it is shown to have positive effects. In India the only mechanisms that exist to ensure such access, however, come from the policies of the companies sponsoring the trials, or from the concerns of the center conducting the trial. This physician told me: "In the last two trials [we conducted], the companies have said they'll try and make drugs available [after the completion of the trial]. We are yet to see if that will happen. If it doesn't happen, then we will only participate with companies who give an absolute commitment [to making drugs available]."[22]

While this physician and the hospitals where he is based might be willing to take such an uncompromising position on linking clinical experimentation to therapeutic access and pastoral care, such a linkage is less likely to figure in the calculus of CROs, especially those focused on early-stage trials, since their source of value lies directly in increasing the number of trials they can conduct rather than in seeing tangible therapeutic benefits in patient populations. As suggested earlier, it is the CRO industry rather than physicians who are currently driving the establishment of regulatory infrastructure in India. This physician told me that while there is intense debate within the psychiatric community in India over the relationship of clinical trials to drug access, there is hardly any conversation between physician investigators and regulators or the CRO industry.

This subjection to experimental regimes without an insistence on concomitant therapeutic access does not seem to occur primarily through the reluctance of Western pharmaceutical companies to market drugs in India (though admittedly, there is no great incentive for them, at this point, to consider India as a serious drug market, with 85 percent of all global drug sales accounted for by U.S., European, and Japanese markets). Indeed, the only real avenue of any sort of therapeutic access to experimental drugs is, as just suggested, through compassionate-use programs that a number of pharmaceutical companies have, whereby they make the drugs they have in Phase III trials available to the sick trial volunteers for a fixed duration of time after the completion of the trial. No one in the Indian CRO industry whom I have talked to, and no one who is actively involved in coming up with

GCP guidelines, felt that it was necessary to insist that drugs tested in India be marketed in India, in spite of the fact that the question of the relationship between clinical trials and access to drugs is a live topic of discussion amongst the Indian physician community. "Ethics," therefore, is provisional and partial, and at this point refers mostly to concerns with informed consent.[23]

Uncoupling experimental subjectivity from therapeutic access, which (through acts of omission) occurs at a legal and regulatory level, configures Indian experimental subjects in law and in practice for the cause of health, but locates them outside a regime of pastoral care. In other words, these experimental subjects contribute in some nebulous sense to health by making themselves available as experimental subjects, but this is in no way necessarily linked to their own healthiness, or to the healthiness of other Indians who might get access to new medication as a consequence of the risks to which they are subjected. The nature of these risks was brought home to me during my tour of Vimta, when I was shown a room, at the time darkened and secluded, with only four beds in it. This, I was told, is the intensive care unit where trial subjects are admitted and administered to in case of adverse events. The room looked like a medical emergency room that might exist in a factory to attend to accidents on the factory floor. It emphasized not just the high-risk nature of experimental subjectivity, but that being a trial subject is, specifically, high-risk *labor*.

Such experimental subjects, outside the circuits of pastoral care (and therapeutic consumption), come to be *merely risked*. But the very circuits of pastoral care and therapeutic consumption that these subjects fall out of *can only be constituted in the first place* through the existence of such "merely risked" subjects. These experimental subjects provide the conditions of possibility for the global (primarily Western) neoliberal consumers of therapy.

While the experimental subject, I argue, is a condition of possibility for biosociality and the neoliberal therapeutic consumer, there is an additional point that I wish to make, which is the *structural impossibility* of such a figure being a *political* subject. This does not mean that experimental subjects cannot politically mobilize; there are many conditions under which they conceivably could. But those conditions would be purely contingent, and one of the contingencies that would most likely lead to a political subjectivity for these subjects (either organized or otherwise) would be through pain and/or death, for instance through a likely scandal that would result from a serious adverse event in a clinical trial. The way in which the experimental subject *does* get figured is *ethically*. And the ethical figuration occurs through informed consent.

This merely risked experimental subject is subject to *logics of expropriation* that are constitutive of the structural logics of biocapital that I am trying to trace. These are bodies that are made bioavailable to global circuits of experimentation, circuits that are driven by value logics of pharmaceutical capital. Indeed, the very global scale of these circuits of experimentation gets constituted because of the value-considerations of capital. Without the cost rationales for outsourcing trials to Third World destinations, the globalization of clinical trials would not have become such a dynamic imperative—clinical trials have, after all, been an important part of the American drug development landscape for something in the vicinity of half a century before the rapid move to take these trials abroad started in the mid-1990s. And without the property mechanisms, harmonized and enforced globally through the WTO, that provide patent protection to multinational pharmaceutical interests, this imperative of globalizing capital would not have had the security to realize its aspirations. Similarly, capital considerations drive the Indian CRO industry to aggressively build infrastructure in India to attract these trials, to increase trial recruitment, and to uncouple these considerations from any serious concern with therapeutic access.

In this situation, the partial ethics that gets enshrined through GCP, far from mitigating the structural violence of capital, serves instead to make it possible. It does so through the instrument of the liberal contract that is embodied in the informed consent form. Just as wages becomes the materialized contractual form through which individuals are "freed" from serfdom and converted into workers in industrial capital, so too does the informed consent form "free" experimental subjects from being coerced guinea pigs by providing them with the autonomous agency that such a contract signifies. A concern with ethical variability suggests that somehow the problem with globalizing clinical trials is that ethical enforcement is likely to be less stringent and vigilant in the Third World than in the First. My attempt here has been to show that, in contrast, it is precisely the harmonization of ethical standards globally that provides the conditions of possibility for the experimental subjection of the "merely risked" Third World subject; and further, this harmonization of ethics goes hand in hand with the harmonization of property regimes globally. These two parallel movements—the contractual codification of ethics combined with the exclusionary instruments of property—together provide global capital with the security to turn even healthy Indian populations into experimental subjects, who are both merely risked and free to choose to be so.

The structural violence of clinical experimentation starts with the fact that it is a procedure that requires, in part, the risking of healthy subjects in order to be set in motion. In other words, the very epistemology of clinical trials is risk-laden—both for the subjects who get experimented upon, and for the companies who invest huge amounts of money in a therapeutic molecule that may or may not eventually come to market and realize that investment. It is a structural violence that gets exacerbated by preexisting global structural inequalities, which result in more bioavailable bodies for less cost in Third World locales than in First World ones. In other words, the structural violence of human experimentation is exacerbated by the structural violence of globalization—the former violence is epistemic, the latter historical. The third layer of structural violence is imposed in the form of the liberal contract, which, just as a wage does in industrial capital for the worker, frees the experimental subject to make his body available for experimentation.

The question to be asked of this third layer is one that is central to Marx in his analysis of capital and regards the conditions of possibility that enable the availability of workers for capital (or in this case, experimental subjects for clinical trials) in the first place. In "The So-Called Primitive Accumulation," Marx shows that this becomes possible only through pre-existing acts of violence that force people into proletarianization.[24] These acts of violence are absolutely historically specific, but they do show a consistency of form. So, for instance, subject recruitment into Phase I clinical trials in India occurs, on the face of it, through newspaper advertisements. The public face of trial recruitment cannot, however, suggest the conditions that make it attractive for individuals to consider the in fact quite lucrative inducement of risking oneself as an experimental subject.

For example, I have written elsewhere about Wellquest, which is located in the mill districts in Mumbai.[25] I learned from scientists at

Wellquest that most of the trial subjects recruited by the CRO happened to be unemployed mill workers who had lost their jobs due to the progressive evisceration of the textile industry in Mumbai over the last thirty years. The details are too elaborate to go into here; suffice to say that the mill districts are currently populated by more than 200,000 unemployed mill workers, many of whom are waiting for the payment of back wages. They are already, therefore, subjected to the violence of deproletarianization that has occurred consequent to the death of a sector of manufacturing capital. This violence is exacerbated by the fact that the textile mills are situated on prime land for real estate development, with most of the mill owners themselves turning to real estate speculation as a far more lucrative source of capital investment. This means that the workers' tenements, mainly located along with the mills in the districts (and known as *chawls*) are under threat of being torn down, so that in addition to losing wage and livelihoods, these workers are now in danger of losing their shelter as well. Tearing down the chawls was temporarily halted by a Bombay High Court verdict that stayed real estate development in the mill districts, but that verdict was overturned by the Indian Supreme Court in March 2006, thereby making it legal to tear down the mills and chawls and build middle-class housing instead. This violence occurs due to the dominance of speculative real estate, which replaces textile manufacturing as the source of value generation for capital. A number of unemployed mill workers have turned into street hawkers in order to earn a living, but there is an organized state and middle-class campaign against the hawkers, who are deemed noisy and polluting, and perhaps most important, accused of taking up valuable parking space.[26] There is no way to understand the dynamics of clinical experimentation in the mill districts of Mumbai without understanding all these prior moments of violence that act as an inducement to sign an informed consent form. First, the mill workers are removed from their factories. Then they are removed from their dwellings. Then they are removed from the streets. Only thus do they acquire the freedom to become autonomous trial "volunteers."

One way in which the situation of expropriation that I have described can be understood is as neocolonialism. This is indeed, as I have suggested, the trope employed by Nundy and Gulhati in their critique of clinical trials in India. It is also consonant with positions taken in various fictional portrayals of "biocolonialism," such as Manjula Padmanabhan's dystopic play *Harvest*, or Patricia Grace's *Baby No-Eyes*.[27] All of these accounts portray a deep historical and continuing inequity, whereby rich/First World/white subjects enrich their health (and often wealth) through the dispossession of subaltern/Third World/racially marked subjects' bodily matter. While sympathetic to the inequalities that such accounts describe, I wish to make the point that the accumulation by dispossession (to use David Harvey's term)[28] that I am trying to trace is not agential but structural, where the one thing that accumulates as a consequence of merely risking experimental subjects is *not health* but *value*.

Much of my argument rests on the fact that clinical experimentation in the Indian context is not linked to therapeutic access. It is, however, certainly possible to imagine such a situation; and if this linkage is not brought about either by the activist intervention of advocacy groups fighting for access to drugs or by the intervention of the state insisting on a biopolitical rationale of the public good/public health, then it is most likely to be brought about by market mechanisms at the point at which India is perceived as a potential market for therapeutic consumption. In such a scenario, one can quite easily imagine the coexistence of experimental subject expropriation (i.e., those who fall out of the market because they do not have the purchasing power to buy drugs) in the context of high amounts of therapeutic marketing within India itself. This latter phenomenon is traced by Stefan Ecks in this volume, in his account of psychiatric drug marketing by companies like Pfizer in India. Ecks has observed that such companies employ strategies that are not dissimilar to those employed in the United States (except that direct-to-consumer advertising, an important strategy in the States, is not allowed in India; instead, such marketing occurs exclusively to physicians).

If we are to understand biocapital from the perspective of pharmaceutical companies' logic, then what is at stake is not therapeutic access in the cause of health, but increasing therapeutic consumption in the cause of value. In parallel, from the perspective of CROs, clinical trials in the cause of therapeutic access are not at stake, but rather clinical trials in the cause of value. The global articulation of pharmaceutical and CRO logics of value generation structures and overdetermines an enterprise that purports to be about pastoral care in terms of expropriation and exploitation. (There are of course other competing logics of capital that are at play in this situation, most notably a logic of insurance that becomes particularly salient in the American context of managed care, but also in a European public health context, where paying for increased therapeutic consumption is a burden, and value logics in fact dictate an emphasis on disease prevention that is not mediated by therapeutic saturation.) It is important therefore to privilege an analysis of value, rather than assume from the outset that biopolitics, or pastoral care, is what is at stake.

At the same time, I wish to highlight my ethnographic overview of clinical trials in India to resist a too-quick denunciation of clinical trials on ethical or moral grounds. There are many incongruities that are vital to stay attentive to, not least the hyperattentiveness to ethics and regulation of clinical practice by the Indian state. The structural violence of global clinical trials, at least in its manifestations in India, is not due to a lack of ethics, but rather because value, captured by logics of capital and mediated through the pharmaceutical and CRO industries, overdetermines the practices that emerge.

Notes

A version of this essay appeared as "Experimental Values: Indian Clinical Trials and Surplus Health," *New Left Review* 45 (2007): 67–88. That version focused more on logics of global capital, while this focuses more on capacity-building efforts to attract clinical research by Indian actors. I thank the editors of *New Left Review* for permission to reproduce the article. I also thank Aihwa Ong and Nancy Chen for invaluable comments on early drafts of the essay since its presentation at the "Asian Biotechnologies" workshop in May 2006, as well as anonymous readers for comments on the earlier version submitted to the volume.

1. Kaushik Sunder Rajan, *Biocapital: The Constitution of Postgenomic Life* (Durham: Duke University Press, 2006).
2. Clinical trials have become a keen site of interest in the anthropology of science. See especially Melinda Cooper, Brian Salter, and Amanda Dickins, "China and the Global Stem Cell Bioeconomy: An Emerging Political Strategy?" *Regenerative Medicine* 1, no. 5 (2006): 671–83; Joseph Dumit, *Drugs for Life* (Durham: Duke University Press, forthcoming); Jill Fisher, "Human Subjects in Medical Experiments," in *Science, Technology, and Society*, ed. Sal Restivo (Oxford: Oxford University Press, 2005); Wen-Hua Kuo, "Japan and Taiwan in the Wake of Bio-Globalization: Drugs, Race, and Standards," Ph.D. dissertation, Massachusetts Institute of Technology, 2005; Adriana Petryna, "Drug Development and the Ethics of the Globalized Clinical Trial," working paper (Princeton, N.J.: Princeton Institute of Advanced Studies, 2005);

and "Ethical Variability: Drug Development and Globalizing Clinical Trials," *American Ethnologist* 32, no. 2 (May 2005): 183–97.

3. Indeed, the law and policy scholars Tracy Lewis, Jerome Reichman, and Anthony So have argued for public funding of clinical trials as an essential mechanism to make essential therapeutics more accessible—and therefore to move health away from being an abstract market value towards being about healthiness. See Tracy Lewis, Jerome Reichman, and Anthony So, "The Case for Public Funding and Public Oversight of Clinical Trials," *Economists' Voice* 4, no. 1, art. 3 (2007). For the Healthcare Financial Management Association's figures, see http://www.hfma.org/publications/margin_newsletter/CompetitiveFinancialAdvantages.htm (no longer available).
4. Etienne Balibar and Immanuel Wallerstein, *Race, Nation, Class: Ambiguous Identities* (New York: Verso, 1992), 180.
5. Petryna, "Drug Development and the Ethics of the Globalized Clinical Trial," Institute of Advanced Studies, Occasional Paper Series, 6.
6. A. T. Kearney, "Make Your Move: Taking Clinical Trials to the Best Location," *A. T. Kearney Report*, http://www.atkearney.com/ (accessed January 3, 2007; no longer available).
7. As cited by the Indian Brand Equity Federation on its Web site, http://www.ibef.org/industry/pharmaceuticals.aspx (accessed January 3, 2007). These figures include contract work that is generated domestically as well by foreign sponsors, and includes not just clinical trial activity but also the contract manufacturing of active pharmaceutical ingredients.
8. Bioequivalence studies test the efficacy of a generic version of the drug against other versions of the drug already on the market, which is a crucial part of the regulatory process for getting approval to market generics in the United States through the FDA.
9. In June 2008, Ranbaxy was partly acquired by the Japanese company Daitchi-Sankyo. Indications at present suggest that its business model will not change, but this is hard to predict with certainty. This is an example of some of the emergent global dynamics in the pharmaceutical industry, which is seeing the beginnings of acquisitions of Asian companies by other Asian companies. There has been speculation that some other Indian pharmaceutical companies might also be acquisition targets especially for Japanese companies.
10. Many thanks to Rakhi Jain, an independent consultant who played a big role in setting up clinical research at Ranbaxy before moving to establish Wellquest, for conversations that have helped me understand Ranbaxy's role in spurring clinical research in India.
11. *NASSCOM—McKinsey Report* (NASSCOM, 2002), http://www.nasscom.in/.
12. A. T. Kearney, "Make Your Move."
13. Michael Arlotto, personal conversations, January 25, 2006.
14. I am grateful to Ramesh Meesala, one of Sristek's cofounders, for extensive conversations about his company's trajectory.

15. Petryna, "Drug Development and the Ethics of the Globalized Clinical Trial" and "Ethical Variability."
16. Samiran Nundy and Chandra Gulhati, "A New Colonialism?—Conducting Clinical Trials in India," *New England Journal of Medicine* 352, no. 16 (2005): 1633–36.
17. Arun Bhatt, interview with the author, February 24, 2006.
18. Ramesh Mashelkar, the head of the committee that wrote this report, has for the past decade been the director general of India's Council for Scientific and Industrial Research (CSIR), which has under its purview over forty national laboratories that perform research in all areas of science and technology. Mashelkar has been one of India's most influential science policy makers since independence, and has been responsible in large measure for the aggressive embrace of global market values by India's public scientific establishment. For a longer account of Mashelkar and CSIR, see my book *Biocapital*, especially chap. 5. The Mashelkar Committee *Report on Recombinent Pharma* (2005) can be viewed at http://www.biospectrumindia.com/content/policy/10510112.asp. Mashelkar retired as director general at the end of 2006.
19. John Rawls, *A Theory of Justice* (1971; Cambridge, Mass.: Belknap, 2005).
20. In contrast, Kristin Peterson has seen in her research in Nigeria that in the West African context, the issue that is most directly on the table is access to drugs. Meanwhile, the ethical/regulatory infrastructure is far from robust. Many thanks to Peterson for conversations on clinical trials in Nigeria.
21. Delhi-based psychiatrist, interview with the author, February 27, 2006.
22. Ibid.
23. It is possible that this situation might be changing. DCGI called a meeting of key clinical research stakeholders on July 17, 2008, to consider possibilities of further amendments to Schedule Y. I was not present at that meeting, but have heard from people who were that one of the issues discussed was the question of access to experimental drugs. I cannot speculate as to the motives for this, or how this will translate into regulatory or legislative measures (and neither could my informants). Suffice to say, this discussion is occurring more than three years after the earlier regulation was drafted around GCP. Even if some attention to drug access is given now, it will happen significantly after the codification of regulation pertaining to informed consent.
24. In Karl Marx, *Capital: A Critique of Political Economy*, vol. 1, ed. Frederick Engels, trans. Samuel Moore and Edward Aveling (1867; London: Penguin, 1976), pt. 8.
25. Sunder Rajan, "Subjects of Speculation: Emergent Life Sciences and Market Logics in the US and India," *American Anthropologist* 107, no. 1 (2005): 19–30. Also see *Biocapital*, chap. 2.
26. For an account of the violence against hawkers in Mumbai, see Arvind Rajagopal, "The Menace of Hawkers," in *Property in Question: Value Transforma-*

tion in the Global Economy, ed. Katherine Verdery and Caroline Humphrey (New York: Berg, 2004).

27. Manjula Padmanabhan, *Harvest* (London: Aurora Metro Press, 2003); Patricia Grace, *Baby No-Eyes* (Honolulu: University of Hawaii Press, 1998).
28. David Harvey, *A Brief History of Neoliberalism* (Oxford: Oxford University Press, 2005). The term "accumulation by dispossession" is first used on p. 45.

NANCY N. CHEN

Feeding the Nation | CHINESE BIOTECHNOLOGY AND GENETICALLY MODIFIED FOODS

Extensive applications in agricultural biotechnology distinguish Chinese biotech projects from other countries in the Asia Pacific region. Behind China's drive toward developing new products and planting genetically modified (GM) crops lie an extensive agricultural history and concerns for feeding an ever-growing population. In this essay I will trace the different trajectories of two of those genetically modified crops, rice and soy. Although genomic sequencing of rice varieties reflects advances in Chinese biotechnology, genetically modified soy products are imported from abroad, mostly from the United States. Despite this difference, both GM foods are promoted as key for the maintenance of food security rather than considered dangerous, as in some Euro-American views.

It is hard to escape survivalist accounts where science and technology rescues China from the Malthusian fate of having too many people and not enough food. Within the next three decades, the estimated population will increase to 1.5–1.6 billion and food production must increase by at least 60 percent to match this growth.[1] Widespread starvation in the aftermath of the Great Leap Forward and other famines remains deeply etched in personal and institutional memories. Against this kind of background, biotechnology is viewed as a savior rather than a problem. Biotechnology has been touted as the best solution for meeting the needs of the world's largest population, ranging from food provisions to health care. The aggressive promotion of this new science is deemed crucial, not only for material resources but also for the well-being of the nation.

Longstanding concerns for food security have evolved in this decade to encompass biotechnology as part of a national platform for biosecurity. I propose to show how knowledge making in China, as well as China's development of biotech products, offers insights into key questions of property and how a nation engages biosovereignty to promote a vision of the public good in entrepreneurial fashion. The emphasis on GM crops and the quantity of such crops that are being produced in China also raise other questions, of safety and whether the goal of feeding the nation justifies the new world of commercialized genomics.

Making Chinese Biotechnology

The biotechnology industry in China follows a trajectory that is different from the one traced by its counterpart in the United States. The biotech boom in Silicon Valley was driven by the marriage of venture capital with university researchers. Biotechnology in China, meanwhile, depends upon several players: investors, scientists, and consumers. Venture capital from foreign firms may also be involved in the private sector. What distinguishes Chinese biotechnology from its American and European counterparts, and even from the rest of Asia, is the level of state investment and volume of investment in the agricultural sector.

Four types of state institutions engage in biotechnology research and production: state-funded research laboratories, university institutes, medical schools, and six specialized biotechnology production facilities. In total, approximately ten thousand high-level scientists, many of whom were educated or have worked abroad, are currently working on approximately one thousand biotechnology projects. One hundred of those projects are government-sponsored "key projects." Key projects, considered essential to China's development, receive priority funding from the central government. Prior to 2004, these stakeholders also included the Ministry of Science and Technology (MOST), the Ministry of Health, and military medical science departments, as well as universities headed by the Ministry of Education. Internal competition between ministries and provinces led to the creation of a top-level biotech leadership committee, the National Development and Reform Commission (NDRC), which was inaugurated in December 2004. All biotech research appropriations are subject to the approval of this centralized body based in Beijing. NDRC set up new financing mechanisms and a more beneficial tax treatment to encourage growth in the biotech sector. Jingyu Bai, a department director of the NDRC, has stated that the government funding of the biotech sector between 2006 and 2010 would increase from the previous funding period, 2001–5, which itself had jumped by 400 percent over the 1998–2000 funding level to reach 10 billion renminbi (U.S. $1.2 billion).[2]

While Chinese state institutions have been the main investor in agricultural biotechnology, many foreign biotech companies have also invested resources, mainly in the health sector, following pharmaceutical biocapital. The private sector includes over two hundred Chinese biotech firms, as well as major multinational firms. The push to build Chinese biotechnology has not gone unnoticed in other parts of Asia. Throughout Asia, science parks have been constructed to jump-start local economies that also wish to take advantage of the opportunities that biotechnology is setting in motion. Education in biotechnology and bioinformatics has been at the center of many new university initiatives. These other Asian economies, however, will focus on genomic R & D, because it will be impossible for them to compete with China's agricultural biotech, which operates on a much larger scale. There is simply not enough land in those countries to conduct field studies. Bioinformatics and genomic research, on the other hand, offer them more viable possibilities to develop market niches. China has also started to become an investor in other parts of Asia, notably India. In a strategic shift in the investment policy, China now encourages domestic entrepreneurs to move overseas in order to put in surplus funds for capital formation. This move is part of its new investment policy of encouraging domestic entrepreneurs to move into identified sectors like information technology, biotechnology, manufacturing, and textiles.

Genetically Modified Cotton and Soy

In 1988, China became the first country to commercialize a bioengineered crop: tobacco resistant to a plant virus. During 2000, the People's Republic filed patents on genetically modified organisms for crops including cotton, rice, wheat, soy, maize, peanuts, tobacco, and traditional medical herbs.[3] The most significant transgenic crops are cotton, tobacco, and rice. In 2002, Chinese farmers planted 2.2 million hectares of GM cotton, an area twice the size of Belgium.[4] One hundred and forty-one transgenic plants were developed in institutes, with sixty-five already approved for commercial use (compared to fifty in the United States). Also in 2002, the Beijing Genomics Institute published the rice genome sequence (*Oryza sativa* L. ssp. *indica* and *japonica*). Another way to measure the volume of transgenic crops in China would be to look at the relative amounts of such crops, which reflect the financial investment of the government in their cultivation. There are projections that the majority of rice, wheat, corn, cotton, soy, and canola will be transgenic by 2010.

What does it mean to have a GM crop? The most common GM traits bred in agricultural products include resistance to disease, insects, and herbicide. Despite higher costs, farmers in China find GM seeds appealing because they require fewer or lower applications of pesticides and lower labor costs.[5] In addition to the research into transgenic food crops, China's biotech industry is also working to breed sheep and goats with more meat on them; to develop human vaccines from the milk of goats, rabbits, and cows; to sequence the pig genome; and to clone goats and cows. At the same time, the government is also aware of external markets that do not want genetically modified organisms and has started to zone regions so that there will be some that can produce non-GM products for export markets. This measure does not address the issue of migration of genetic material between GM and non-GM crops. There is also the issue of GM piracy, in which farmers do not wait for permission to plant approved crops.

By looking closely at the production of GM cotton, soy, and rice in China we gain insights into different facets of state policy toward agricultural biotech. As a crop, cotton can be ecologically disastrous, because it is a monoculture crop with high water and pesticide needs. GM cotton was initially promoted to reduce the necessity for pesticides as it produces a toxin effective against bollworms and weevils, the most common pests. Chinese GM cotton continues to be portrayed as a success story over its counterparts in Indonesia and India, where Monsanto-patented seeds did not offer significantly better yields nor resistance to all pests (sucking aphids in particular). Significantly, in 2004 farmers in Andhar Pradesh committed suicide over the loss of their transgenic Bt (*Bacillus thuringiensis*) cotton crops while a bumper crop in non-GM cotton was documented. In China during 2001, over 4 million small-scale farmers planted Bt cotton over 1.6 million hectares (up from 100,000 hectares in 1998), and these figures are expected to grow. By 2002, Chinese labs had developed eighteen varieties of pest-resistant Bt cotton. Yet, in the same year, the Nanjing institute of Environmental Sciences released a report that Bt cotton crops were not as resistant to bollworms as expected and that farmers were increasingly using more pesticides. In 2004, China planted 3.7 million hectares of GM cotton in 2004, increased by nearly a third since 2003.[6] GM cotton tends to raise fewer safety concerns than GM food crops because cotton is associated with clothing rather than ingestion, though cotton seed oil is used in foods and cotton seed meal is an ingredient in animal feed

Soy presents a different aspect of China's promotion of biotechnology and GM crops. Rather than produce GM soy from its own seeds, China has been importing Roundup Ready soybeans under a series of interim safety certificates. The importation of soy reflects compliance with WTO agreements to open markets in China to foreign products and services. China recently issued a final safety certificate for the importation of soybeans and soybean products derived from this biotech-enhanced soybean seed stock. "China's decision to issue final safety certificates for Roundup Ready soybeans is good news for U.S. farmers, as well as for Chinese consumers who rely on imports of high quality soybeans to be processed into cooking oil and livestock feed," says the American Soybean Association president Ron Heck, of Perry, Iowa. "This action will help insure a steady market for U.S. soybeans, while helping stabilize meat, fish, egg, and cooking oil prices for Chinese consumers."[7] The Febuary 23, 2004, agreement is based on two years of field and food safety tests in China that confirmed the safety, healthfulness, and environmental friendliness of this variety of soybeans.

Young people are frequently portrayed in print and on public billboards to symbolize the new China of the twenty-first century and its future. During March 2005, an Archer Daniels Midland corporate advertisement featuring a Chinese boy circulated in mainstream American periodicals such as *Newsweek* and *Time*. Archer Daniels Midland is a multinational food-processing corporation that is publicly traded on NASDAQ, and proclaims itself the "world's largest agricultural processors of soybeans, wheat, corn, and cocoa."[8] In the advertisement, the image of the boy eating a dish of tofu is accompanied by this text:

Somewhere west of Shenyang, a teenager is stopping for dinner.
Which is why the soybean harvest west of Peoria is not stopping.
And why a soybean processor west of St. Louis is not stopping.
And why a ship's captain on the west coast is stopping but just for a while.
Somewhere west of Shenyang, a teenager is stopping for dinner.
A dinner rich in soy protein.
As one of the world's largest soy processors,
We like the idea that there will be no stopping him now.

The words "west" and "not stopping" are repeated throughout this ad and emphasize the continuous link between the Midwestern United States to China through the production of soy and its ultimate consumer—a teenager in China. Soy-based food products, especially tofu, are included in many Chinese dishes. Yet, ironically, many former "little emperors," now teenagers and young adults, might prefer McDonald's and KFC after a decade of rapidly expanding fast food chains in mainland China.[9] The ad revives early twentieth-century characterizations of China's population and the need to provide food for the still most populous nation in the world. It would appear from the ad that there is not enough soy being produced in China, hence the need to import soy from the Midwest. The story of soy, much of it genetically modified, and its journey to China reflect the broader story of how China's biosciences have expanded primarily in the area of agricultural biotechnology.

The perception that China's huge population needs genetically modified organisms (GMOs) in order to survive is evident also in the nation's concern about property, in its race to the GMO patent finish line. Socialist bureaucrats are determined not to become dependent upon foreign aid or food crops. For them, the pressing issues of food security and biosovereignty override the anti-GMO ethos voiced elsewhere in Europe and the United States. The Chinese biotech industry in 2000 consisted of more than six hundred companies, two hundred of which produce pharmaceuticals and another two hundred, amino acids for food supplements. In 2003, this figure grew threefold. In 2005, the value of biotech-derived products in China was U.S. $10 billion. Though the total funding for agricultural biotech in China is far lower than the investment made by multinational firms globally, China is producing the second highest number of patents related to GM foods after the United States, and it is expanding fast.

GM Rice—Made in China

GM rice is expected to soon follow GM cotton in commercial applications. China's genomic center in Beijing surprised the international science community in 2001 with its quick sequencing of the rice genome, specifically, the subspecies *indica* of *Oryza sativa*, as reported in *Science*, 2002.[10] Why rice? In addition to being the food source for over half the world's population, rice provides a model genomic structure for the eventual sequencing of other grains with larger structures, such as corn and wheat. Though the rice genome has more genes than the human genome, the repetition of certain sequences in different species (synteny) suggests that rice can be the model for sequencing grains with much longer chains despite their varying lengths. Moreover, rice is a grain with an extensive research record documenting hybrid forms, disease resistance, and adaptability.

The story of rice genome sequencing offers insights into the complexities of public-private intertwinings of knowledge making and ownership in biotechnology. Exploration of the rice genome began in the 1980s with Japan's founding of the Rice Genome Research Program. This body later advocated an international collaborative effort in 1997 to collectively participate in the sequencing of rice. (Participating countries initially included Japan, the United States, South Korea, and the United Kingdom. Canada and Thailand participated for a while, but subsequently withdrew, as did the United Kingdom. France, Taiwan, India, and Brazil then joined the consortium.) Twelve rice chromosomes were divided up among the participant countries and once a sequence was notated, the consortium would share its knowledge as public information. The disadvantage of this collaborative effort is that it is a slower approach to establishing the sequencing of genes than a centralized approach.

As with all biosciences, the role of private capital has had a huge effect on the way in which knowledge of the rice genome would become public or not. Monsanto's draft of the rice genome led to a Faustian offer to consortium scientists: they could have access to raw data on Monsanto sequencing in exchange for the right for Monsanto to be the first to obtain a license before any patents were pursued based on the resulting knowledge. The Monsanto proposal raised critical questions of how joint efforts in decoding a sequence could eventually be shared or packaged. The effort was later taken up by another biotech firm, the Swiss-based Syngenta, which used a different approach to sequencing ("whole genome shotgun") to decode the *japonica* rice subspecies. Eventually two groups of scientists, one led by Syngenta and the other a collaboration between Beijing Genomic Institute and the University of Washington, came to decode the two major subspecies of rice. The Chinese focus was on the superhybrid rice with higher yields than other subspecies. While knowledge of this genomic sequencing can be publicly accessed, the Syngenta version is held in escrow with *Science* magazine in a private databank. Scientists who wish to have access to the sequencing information must first sign usage agreements. This decision has been highly controversial, but the Syngenta agreement follows the same agreement that *Science* made with Celera for the Human Genome Project. Bioprospecting in the twenty-first century, whether of plants or animal/human genetic material, reflects ongoing compromises between the ideal of open-source information and private capital that funds highly collaborative work on a global scale. Genetic resources are open-access until certain sequences to be patented can be privatized.

In China, much research is currently being carried out in the commercial applications of GM rice. Farmers in Hubei have grown GM rice seeds with the crops sold mostly to scientists for research rather than on the open market. Initial studies indicate that 80 percent less pesticide is used for the GM rice cultivation. Though China has ratified the International Biodiversity Protocol to limit commercialization of GMOs, research on GM rice continues. The Ministry of Agriculture has allowed field studies, which must take place over two years before a tested crop can be ratified for commercial use. Greenpeace scientists have meanwhile raised concerns about gene flow, in which genetically modified varieties mix with domestic varieties, such that traditional varieties may become extinct.

Whether imported from abroad or developed as a domestic strain, GM crops constitute a considerable part of China's biotechnology applications and production. From a state perspective, engaging in genomic sequencing and developing applications enhances a China first position in biotech product lines and, ideally, its freedom from multinational agribusiness firms. This emphasis on the development of genetically enhanced agricultural products by state institutions reflects, as noted earlier, an ongoing socialist and nationalist concern for feeding the nation. But market principles of profit are also not absent from this endeavor. Farmers are enticed by the possibilities of lower pesticide applications and more labor freed up for other entrepreneurial activities. Like their counterparts in many parts of the world, Chinese farmers cultivating crops are dependent upon fluctuating circumstances like the weather and markets.

This path to biosovereignty and profitability is, however, not without health and environmental concerns. Food safety is an issue—for example, the allergens that may be present in GMOs; another issue is the ecological impact of GM crops on other species. These concerns are proving to be serious challenges to the notion that more is better, most notably in the West. But worries over food quality and purity on the part of consumers may still shift public views on GM foods even in China.

Biosovereignty and Purity

The meanings of "food safety" reflect critical categories of culture, nature, and power. Anthropologists have long considered questions of purity and danger and how these inform categories of belonging or exception. In the past decade, consumers in China have expressed much concern for the safety of their food, drugs, and drinks. Purity takes on specific material concerns in such cases. Medicine bottles and herbal supplements are carefully scrutinized to check sources of production in case they may be fake. Despite careful vetting on the part of consumers, it is not possible to entirely screen out counterfeit drugs, contaminated foods, or fake infant formula. The concerns of citizens in China are shared worldwide as product recalls have identified goods that pose hazardous consumption. Calls for more careful oversight of production lines have led to an overhaul of the Chinese food and drug administration and its safety program. Stiff penalties for individuals or institutions engaged in producing shoddy goods have been introduced including the execution of high-ranking officials at the provincial and state level.[11]

A person's degree of vulnerability continues to reflect his or her position in the economic order. Rural communities face a vicious cycle of environmental degradation, regional inequality, and poverty. Epidemics of infectious diseases such as HIV/AIDS, SARS, and avian flu also shape this landscape. In this context of limited goods and great hopes, the emerging discourse of bioethics includes a call for bans on cloning by Chinese scientists and officials.[12] There has been a sea change, where state researchers have deliberately slowed down and even adopted guidelines. In 2002, the Chinese representatives to UNESCO outlined guidelines on stem cell research restricting reproductive cloning. These guidelines were initially formulated by the Department of Ethical, Legal, and Social Issues, of the Chinese Human Genome Center in Shanghai.[13] In addition, U.K. guidelines on manipulation of material from embryos up to fourteen days old have also been addressed. The majority of bioethical guidelines emerging in China focus on human reproductive and cloning experimentation. Plant bioengineering and GM applications seem to pose less concern, and consequently have fewer bioethical guidelines.

While GM foods are actively promoted as a means to reduce pesticide use, organic foods are still produced not just for an overseas market but also for consumers at home, most notably in rural areas. Though farmers keep constant watch over crop production and aim for high crop volumes, they and their families tend to consume produce that has not been sprayed with high amounts of pesticides.[14] Notions of purity that hold organic foods as wholesome, and home-produced foods for one's own consumption, are considered key to hygiene and health.[15] The concerns for purity, food safety, and overall quality of food seem outweighed, nonetheless, by broader concerns for maintaining quantity or food security.

In the spring of 2008, amid worldwide rises in food and fuel prices, riots over high food prices occurred in Haiti, Bangladesh, Mozambique, Egypt, and many cities worldwide. The combination of poor harvests and increased fuel costs led to dwindling supplies as well as soaring prices. Several rice-producing nations, including Thailand, the Philippines, India, and Brazil, limited rice exports to ensure supplies at home. In conversations with Chinese friends and colleagues in Beijing and Shanghai just months prior to the Beijing Olympics, I was surprised by initial responses on the topic of food costs, especially rice. Most reflected that while basic costs for everyday have increased in recent years, food shortages were not present in China; there was plenty of rice available because China was a major producer of grains. While media in the United States and elsewhere were reporting problems arising from shortages, in China there were no stories of rice hoarding or panic buying, so rice was plentiful in stores. When I asked my Chinese contacts whether they would consume GM rice or any other GMOs, most of their responses were quite pragmatic. If faced with starvation, any food, GM or not, was acceptable.

Feeding the nation in twenty-first-century China has evolved from ensuring the quantity of food to accomodating ongoing concerns about the quality and safety of foods. Yet, at the same time, patents on new GMO products and genomic sequences of agricultural plants and animals are seen as a critical platform for China's push to ownership of its food sources. Ensuring the collective good in terms of adequate food and material resources has facilitated formations of biotechnology that are distinctively "made in China." Rather than situate GMOs in the monolithic categories "good" or "bad," biosecurity reflects the overarching moral duty of the state to bring different readings to GM foods. The technical elements of genetic engineering are portrayed as enhancements of preexisting foods to reduce the use of pesticides or ensure volume; they are not presented as "Frankenfoods," as GM foods have been in Western media. China has faced concerns for feeding its numerous people throughout much of its history, but because it sees this vast population as creating an exceptional situation, biotechnology and market formations can be utilized as a double helix platform in the formation of the new China and its emerging biosovereignty.

Notes

My thanks to Lesley Sharp and the anonymous press reviewers for their thoughtful comments. Special thanks to David Cleveland, who offered careful suggestions about agricultural biotech and shared information from his collaborative research with Daniela Soleri on transgenic crops in Latin America.

1. A higher figure is cited in Qifa Zhang, "China: Agricultural Biotechnology Opportunities to Meet the Challenges of Food Production," in *Agricultural Biotechnology and the Poor*, ed. G. J. Persley and M. M. Lantin (Report of the International Conference on Biotechnology, convened by the Consultative Group on International Agricultural Research of the World Bank and the U.S. National Academy of Sciences, in Washington, D.C., October 21–22, 1999),

45–50. The Population Reference Bureau projects a lower population figure of 1.476 billion by 2025 (see http://www.prb.org/Countries/China.aspx, accessed March 22, 2009).

2. Jingyu Bai, "China Moves to Reform Biotech Policies," *Nature Biotechnology* 22, no. 10 (October 2004): 1197.
3. Jikun Huang, Scott Rozelle, Carl Pray, and Qinfang Wang, "Plant Biotechnology in China," *Science* 295 (2002): 674–76.
4. Nao Nakanishi, "China Seen a Crouching Dragon in Biotechnology," Reuters, December 20, 2002.
5. Long-term benefits of GM have been questioned in recent articles, including J. Qiu, "Is China Ready for GM Rice?" *Nature* 455 (2008): 850–52. For a comparative perspective in Latin America, see D. Soleri, D. A. Cleveland, G. E. Glasgow, S. H. Sweeney, F. Aragón Cuevas, H. Ríos Labrada, and M. R. Fuentes Lopez, "Testing Assumptions Underlying Economic Research on Transgenic Food Crops for Third World Farmers: Evidence from Cuba, Guatemala and Mexico," *Ecological Economics* 67, no. 4 (2008): 667–82.
6. Jia Hepeng, "GM Rice May Soon Be Commercialized," *China Business Weekly*, January 26, 2005.
7. American Soybean Association, "ASA Welcomes Final Safety Certification of Roundup Ready Event in China," *Bean Beat*, April 2004, http://www.soygrowers.com/ (accessed August 12, 2008).
8. Quotations from 2006 edition of Archer Daniels Midland company Web site, http://www.admworld.com (accessed May 21, 2006).
9. See Jun Jing, *Feeding China's Little Emperors: Food, Children, and Social Change.* (Stanford, Calif.: Stanford University Press, 2000).
10. Jun Yu et al. "A Draft Sequence of the Rice Genome (*Oryza sativa* L. ssp. *indica*)," *Science* 296, no. 5565 (April 5, 2002): 79–92.
11. Xinhua News Agency, "China to Pose Stiff Penalties on Fake Drug Makers, Dealers," November 11, 2007.
12. John Gittings, "Experts Call for Curbs on Human Cloning in China," *Guardian* (United Kingdom), April 16, 2002.
13. Wolfgang Hennig, "Bioethics in China: Although National Guidelines Are in Place, Their Implementation Remains Difficult," *European Molecular Biology Organization (EMBO) Reports* 7 (2006): 850–54.
14. Anna Lora Wainwright, "Necessary Evil? Development, Morality, and Cancer Aetiology in a Chinese Village," paper presented at the annual meeting of the Association for Asian Studies, Atlanta, Ga., March 2008.
15. Lili Lai, "Modernization Indoors, Disorder Outdoors—Everyday Hygiene in Rural Henan," paper presented at the annual meeting of the Association for Asian Studies, Atlanta, Ga., March 2008.

| BIOVENTURES |

II

CHARIS THOMPSON

Asian Regeneration? | NATIONALISM AND INTERNATIONALISM IN STEM CELL RESEARCH IN SOUTH KOREA AND SINGAPORE

Asia is the world's most populous continent, with estimates of its share of the world's population running between 55 percent to over 60 percent, depending on the source of statistics and the boundaries of Asia being assumed. Not surprisingly, it is a leader in biotechnology and, increasingly, in biomedicine, and the impact of the latter is felt not just regionally but globally. English-language media stereotypes of emerging Asian global biomedicine abound: India is for generics, clinical trials, organ donation, and surrogate motherhood; China is where you go if you want to try something that is unproven or illegal elsewhere; while Thailand is for state-sponsored, hospital-based medical tourism. Like many stereotypes, there is probably some truth to them, but they mask much more than they reveal. In particular, all the major economies of Asia, like most of those in North America and the European Union, have thriving and rapidly growing medical tourism sectors, both formal and informal. Factors in sending as well as receiving countries—from medical insurance companies in the United States paying its insured to go to Asian countries for treatment, to EU regulations that limit the scope of intellectual property claims on life forms—also contribute to Asia as a global biomedical destination. Furthermore, several Asian countries are increasingly important in biomedical research and innovation, and this kind of research follows different patterns of global movement of people and capital than does health care delivery.

In this essay, I am interested in an example of global biomedicine that includes basic scientific research, clinical and translational research, and health care: regenerative medicine, or stem cell research and innovation. My larger project focuses on reproductive, regenerative, and genomic sciences in the United States, but I consider the United States as situated in several more global networks without which, I contend, several of the most interesting developments in these fields would be hard to understand. I work with a located but transnational comparative perspective, whereby I consider developments in other countries that are also important to developments in these biomedical fields in the United States. Among the countries of greatest salience for stem cell research are several Asian countries. I focus on two Asian countries in this essay, both known for their investment in the field, Singapore and South Korea. This kind of transnational comparative approach does not allow for extended ethnographic research in each country that is important to the U.S.-implicated narratives I am following (see below for a discussion of the linguistic, financial, and work load issues that would prohibit this), but it does require some degree of firsthand knowledge. It is precisely to go beyond easy stereotypes found, for example, in the Western press of "Eastern" attitudes to stem cell research that it is necessary to undertake even brief ethnographic research. The short-term ethnographic research on which I draw in this essay is deeply flawed relative to a more sustained ethnographic engagement, but it has one advantage: it is able to focus on some comparative and some regional and global aspects of the topics under investigation.

I propose to ask what South Korea's and Singapore's stem cell research efforts have in common, and how they differ. I also ask whether there is any kind of "Asian" regional pattern to the emerging field of regenerative medicine, and if so, how it functions in relation to the local, national, and global contexts of biomedical research in these countries. In line with the argument of this book, I find that comparing stem cell research in the two countries reveals dramatic differences—convergences and divergences—that belie the regional and economic parallels that the shared label "Asian Tiger" tends at first to suggest. Singapore engages in stem cell research in a mode that I refer to as "knowledge society internationalism." South Korea's pattern, on the other hand, is more continuous with the so-called developmental state innovation for which it is famous, and includes a brief injection of a highly nationalistic sentimentality that made the Hwang Woo-Suk scandal so gripping worldwide. A comparison between two key sites in the two countries' stem cell efforts shows that differences persist right down to the mores and organization of labs in the two places. Despite these differences, however, I find that "Asia" as an area identity remains important to both countries, albeit in different ways, enabling both to articulate positions of geopolitical and scientific saliency. I also find that, despite one strategy's being explicitly nationalist and the other's being internationalist, both further nationalistic visions of the role of biomedicine in the nation-state following the Asian financial crisis of the 1990s.

Bioscience, Biocapital, Biopolitics: Why Stem Cell Research Tells Us So Much about Globalization

Like a number of other scholars, I write about the geopolitics of stem cell research not so much to weigh in on its ethical conundrums—although the involvement of ethics in the story of stem cell research is part of what makes studying stem cell research so informative—as to understand the world of biomedical innovation.[1] Why is stem cell research so promising a site to study global patterns of science and society? First, stem cell research combines research and medicine. That is, it is "bench to bedside," meaning that it encompasses a spectrum from basic laboratory research aimed at understanding the fundamental biological properties of life, through translational research that produces clinically relevant findings, to therapeutic and diagnostic medical applications of that knowledge, including all the social and ethical issues that this trajectory implicates. Second, stem cell research exhibits, contributes to, and is in some ways a product of the emerging convergence between information technology, biotechnology, and business/finance. This convergence and the bench-to-bedside character of stem cell research are arguably two keys to understanding globalization and innovation since the turn of the century.

Stem cell research is evolving as an international field of science par excellence, because of this bench-to-bedside and convergence promise. Not only does stem cell research exhibit the international exchange of students, postdoctoral scholars, and researchers characteristic of the natural sciences in the contemporary research university; it also displays patterns of R & D, from venture capital to aggressive intellectual property activity that are increasingly characteristic of competitive transnational capital in so-called knowledge societies. And, as stem cell research moves to the bedside, it is beginning to display signs of the kinds of global regulatory and economic triage whereby some people travel to receive biomedical treatment because the treatment is not permitted, is unavailable, or is unaffordable in the sending country. This perfect storm of basic science, biocapital, and biopolitics epitomizes what I call "the innovation complex," where public and private funding and institutions ally in a welding together of intellectual inquiry, economic activity, and social engineering known and highly lauded as "innovation." Each of these three interconnected logics of innovation powerfully globalizes stem cell research. Indeed, one of the words that is most common to see in English on East Asian research campuses is "innovation," its global potential and social mandate carried in the very language politics of its inscription.

On the other hand, stem cell science is highly national, and frequently nationalistic. Given the youth and breadth of the field, stem cell science combines the potential for truly significant scientific breakthroughs in diverse fields, including molecular and cell biology, embryology, bioengineering, and biochemistry, with tantalizing medical research possibilities and enormous promise clinically. The stakes for both symbolic and economic capital are thus great. Encouraging economic growth and securing prestige are core functions of the modern nation-state and the civic nation respectively, and are twin measures of "development." For nations investing heavily in innovation, stem cell science is a relatively low-hanging fruit, given that symbolic and economic capital are both likely outcomes of the research at this stage. Ethical barriers to research in the United States and several Western European countries—relating to the field's sourcing its basic materials from human bodies, often from embryos, and to its perceived potential to tamper with humanity—have further served to make the field more genuinely competitive for other countries who may have fewer or different barriers to research. Scientists become part of brain drains and patients engage in medical tourism to follow regulatory gradients, moving to where research can be carried out or treatment obtained. For recipient countries, there is a unique opportunity to be a leader in the field, increasing national prestige and promoting government investment. For the "Asian Tigers," regenerative medicine falls into the value-added category heavily promoted in the post-1997 Asian financial crisis era, relying less on exports and low wages and more on knowledge and research priority. Furthermore, stem cell research itself is turning out to be capable of being used to answer a diverse range of social questions about the body politic that vary from country to country. Like the closely related field of genomics, stem cell research can be put to very different ends and serve national ideologies. In sum, stem cell research is, profoundly, both a national and an international enterprise.

Tyger, Tyger, Burning Bright

Singapore and South Korea are two of the four so-called Asian or East Asian Tigers (sometimes also called the "Little Dragons"), the others being Hong Kong and Taiwan, whose economies underwent rapid industrialization with high growth rates in the last four decades of the twentieth century. Singapore and South Korea share an experience with Japanese colonialism, but otherwise differ substantially in geopolitical terms. One is a tiny (a population of approximately 4.5 million) primarily English-language city-state wedged between Malaysia and Indonesia (Singapore), while the other is a Korean-language-speaking ancient nation of almost 50 million people, occupying the southern portion of a large peninsula, with a rich agricultural past. One was part of the British Empire, while the other has housed U.S. forces since the Korean War. Singapore is more multiethnic; both have several large religious denominations, including Buddhism, Taoism, and Christianity in Singapore, and Confucianism, Buddhism, and Christianity in Korea.

Both Singapore and South Korea are on the International Monetary Fund's "Advanced Economy" list; in the 2007 U.N. Human Development Index,[2] Singapore and South Korea rank twenty-sixth and twenty-seventh respectively among nations in the world. The standard account of industrialization in the Asian Tigers, as opposed to the standard account of Western industrialization, attributes its spectacular speed and magnitude to a combination of economic strategies and global relational starting conditions. The Tigers achieved this economic growth through the export of goods to rich industrialized nations; the leveraging of a period of low domestic wages relative to the countries targeted for export; a high level of state investment in national education systems, including tertiary education; government-mandated land reform to break aristocratic land tenure patterns; the use of tariffs and subsidies to control domestic spending; and investment in U.S. Treasury bonds to promote stability. The exact mechanisms accounting for the Asian economic miracle, and especially the reasons for the Asian financial crisis of 1997 are highly disputed, and are beyond my expertise. Based on my ethnographic data—what people say motivates them or explains things—it is probably reasonable, however, to designate 1997–98 a watershed in South Korea, if not in Singapore. The IMF intervention, demanding neoliberal structural adjustments to control spending, raised interests rates, permitting financial institutions to fail, and an end to favoritism in securing foreign loans, contradicted some of the characteristics of the so-called developmental state. This was especially true in hard-hit South Korea, where the *chaebols* (business conglomerates) were accustomed to oligopolistic political support and favoritism in terms of foreign loans. For Singapore to have weathered the crisis as well as it did, and for South Korea eventually to have exited the crisis, meant in both cases reduced reliance on high-capital-expenditure, export-driven growth, and a building up of foreign exchange reserves. The financial crisis marks a line in the sand, after which the kind of innovation characteristic of knowledge economies became more attractive. For Singapore, more than for Korea, investing in the new kind of bench-to-bedside biomedical research has proven very much part of the answer as to how to do this. Korea, on the other hand, has a long history of putting science and technology at the center of its development by combining private-sector R & D with governance. This form of private/public cooperation, and the Korean chaebol's original greater focus on chemicals and electronics than the life sciences, has meant that university research in the biomedical sciences has stayed under the umbrella of the Ministry of Higher Education, Science, and Technology (itself a telling grouping of science and technology), and has a less automatic path to industrial R & D than the physical and engineering sciences. Similarly, Korea's deep commitment to education as development relies on sending elite students abroad, making education more of a qualification for taking a place in the private sector and government upon return than in promoting an innovation space that encompasses Korean university labs and the private sector.

It is not uncommon to list cultural factors, especially "Chinese influence," among the traits that unite the Asian Tigers. Given the different colonial and imperial relations and forms of nationalism pertaining in the four countries/territories over the last fifty years, and given the rapidly changing politics of China over this time and the relevant diasporas, and the consequent difficulties in attributing changing cultural Chinese influences to Chinese ethnicity or historical influence in the countries in question, I have not found this hypothesis helpful to my analysis. Ethnographically, I found a number of Singaporeans who attributed a role to Chinese ethnicity in producing growth and productivity. Among Koreans I heard relations with Japan and the United States mentioned, whereas China came up more as a synonym for remnants of the class system, often through its association with Confucian elites and the regional dominance of some parts of Korea over others. Jennifer Liu, in her groundbreaking work on stem cell research in Taiwan, documents an active process of de-Sinicization evident in attempts to pin down biologically a distinctly Taiwanese population (this volume). For these reasons I do not emphasize the idea of Chineseness in this brief summary of prima facie similarities between Singapore and Korea.

The economic factors listed above (export to the West, a period of low wages, state investment in education, land reform, and tariffs) produced and were in turn produced by a relatively high level of state authoritarianism or paternalism, combined with a high level of so-called economic freedom, and resulted in a trade surplus with highly industrialized countries and sustained high growth rates. In short, the pattern that for many in the West has become a stereotype of East Asia and its people—an extraordinary educational drive, high productivity, paternalistic government and social policies, along with a business-friendly culture—has a recent history and was produced in relation to the already highly industrialized world.

The similarities between the historical time scale of the Tigers' industrialization and their resultant place in the global economic order might lead one to expect a prima facie similarity between the countries' stem cell research efforts in this "post-Tiger" time. Instead, one finds stark differences. To borrow a metaphor from evolutionary theory, this is analogous rather than homologous evolution; innovation makes sense to both countries being considered here, in part because of their similar regional location and time scale of development, but if advanced economic activity is the equivalent of, say, the power of flight, Singapore and South Korea are insects and birds, solving the problem of flying in ways that show functional isomorphism to shared evolutionary pressure, but which differ fundamentally in underlying design. What it is to have been an Asian Tiger and now be participating in the age of biotechnology is a heterogeneous affair.

Stem Cell Research in South Korea and Singapore: A Comparison

I carried out fieldwork in Seoul, South Korea, and in Singapore in 2005, and again in South Korea in 2008. For all the usual reasons that limit transnational comparative work by full-time academics—language, funding, teaching and administrative schedules—these visits were brief and my research questions correspondingly focused.[3] Constraints on ethnographic data collection for transnational comparative work are somewhat offset by the perspective that comes from moving between sites. My observations of Korea and Singapore and other countries are informed and to some extent framed by my experience researching the biopolitics and bioethics of stem cell research, as a scholar and as a member of a multidisciplinary stem cell training program and of ethics committees in California, with which they stand in contrast.[4]

My original aim in 2005 was to compare the flagship laboratories of the two countries' respective stem cell research efforts, Hwang Woo-Suk's laboratory in Korea and the newly constructed Biopolis in Singapore. This was part of an abiding interest in biomedicine as governance, and in "innovation" as a propulsive force of globalization. In the short term, I wanted to lay to rest an idea that was circulating at the time that, put crudely (and it usually was), stem cell research was patterning in one way in "the West" because of Christianity's objections to the embryo destruction involved in deriving human embryonic stem cell lines, while stem cell research in "the East" was developing apace, in a relative regulatory oasis, because Eastern religions did not recognize the preimplantation embryo as a person and saw cloning as akin to reincarnation.[5] Among the weaknesses of the explanation from religion, the account ignores the importance of Christianity in Asia, conflates Eastern religions, ignores the political and regulatory aspects of religion such as efforts on the part of some East Asian stem cell ethicists to come up with Confucian ethical precepts to guide stem cell regulation, and sidelines politically enforced Confucian revivalism.[6] Other weaknesses include equating North American and European left-progressive views against tampering with nature with a post-Christianity that reveres nature as God, despite the fact that most adherents of these views use nonreligious idioms; failing to distinguish between abortion politics in Catholicism and in evangelical Prostestantism; ignoring nonreligious or differently religious reasons for supporting or opposing stem cell research; and ignoring political, legal, economic, and scientific reasons for regulatory gradients for stem cell research.

The comparison, if it found variation within Asia, would suggest that a more sophisticated analysis was required: if two Asian Tigers were different, how could the entirety of Asia (and the entirety of the West) be accounted for by referring to "Eastern versus Western" religion? Once the Korean stem cell scandal broke, however, the comparison took on an additional aspect, familiar from science journalism, in attempting to account for the scandal: how/why did this happen in South Korea (as opposed to the United States or Singapore)? When I returned to Korea in 2008, it was apparent that the reasons for which Hwang had risen and fallen were also symptoms of some key differences between South Korean and Singaporean stem cell research, and of the complexity and regionality of Asia writ large.

A South Korean Laboratory

Hwang Woo-Suk was a researcher and faculty member at Seoul National University (SNU). SNU is considered the top university in South Korea, in a country that valorizes education; it is notorious for pushing its students to excel in exams and its workforce for productivity, the two being seen as twin pillars of development. The summer of 2005 was the height of Hwang Woo Suk's fame in Korea and around the world for having reportedly succeeded in creating the world's first patient-specific human embryonic stem cell lines through the process of somatic cell nuclear transfer, or therapeutic/research cloning. It was still a few months away from his "fall" (as it was subsequently to become known), first for revelations about the allegedly "coercive" practices of procuring eggs from women, and then shortly thereafter for scientific fraud.

CHARISMATIC NATIONALISM

During those months Dr. Hwang was one of a handful of the best-known scientists in the world: mediagenic, and possessed of an extraordinary knack for narrating his work in a manner that was both modest and charismatic. Who could not be seduced by the story of hard work, Korean rural values, fame and honor from achievement rather than from being rich or a celebrity? Not to mention his comprehensible and medically relevant scientific breakthroughs. In a time when the line between CEOs and scientists was becoming increasingly blurred in countries that were most aggressively adopting the innovation model in university life science departments, this was the kind of scientific hero that the world longed for again. And in a country where educational achievement and recognition abroad is a key currency of symbolic capital, Koreans themselves both envied and fervently promoted Hwang, in a campaign that culminated in the government's naming him Korea's "Supreme Scientist."[7] Even after Hwang's disgrace over the following months, many Koreans, including Korean women who had volunteered to be egg donors for his research, continued to believe in and support Hwang.[8] Many abroad, myself included, also wanted his research to be vindicated, as a rejoinder to the threat of corruption posed by the innovation model, and as a decentering of an imperialist, West-centered, English-language-dominated economy of scientific research.

Like others visiting Hwang's lab, I felt privileged to be there and to be witnessing a great breakthrough.[9] Despite his ascendancy, Hwang was not entirely without critics in Korea at the time. In fact, several people mentioned the casualties of what one person described to me as "the cult of Hwang," including the erasure of the contribution of his high-level collaborators (among them at least one prominent woman scientist who got little notice), and widespread envy of Hwang for his rise as well as his funding success in what is widely taken to be a zero-sum Korean science funding system. Pride may come before a fall, but so too does envy. Likewise, the rumors about ethical lapses in egg procurement were already widespread, and had reached me in California through my feminist networks before I left for Korea.[10] I was interviewed with a Korean feminist scholar and prominent bioethicist by a Korean newspaper during my visit, and my interlocutor openly voiced skepticism of Hwang's rise to the reporter. The charismatic nationalism, then, was all-encompassing, more in its emotional than its rational grip, and this in part accounts for its mythic exaggeration and the potential for fraud opened up by many parties wanting the phenomena to be real.

Visitors entering Hwang's lab were required to put on a protective light-weight jumpsuit over their clothes, to wear shoe covers, and to tuck hair into a scrub hat, as well as to pass through an air lock to decontaminate them. It is not entirely clear what functional value these protective practices held, apart from creating a general environment of care: the lab was designed such that visitors entered down a central hall on one side of which was the human embryonic stem cell research and the other side of which was the training facility where the team worked on porcine ova. The porcine side was the one through which visitors toured. Visitors were encouraged to imagine an isomorphism between the side they were visiting and the human embryonic stem cell side by the symmetry of the layout and by screens on the wall on the human side showing images of the work going on inside. It is not likely that anything being done on the porcine side would lead to human therapeutic biomaterials (cells that might be transplanted into a patient, for example), which might have made it important to protect tissue from contaminants carried by visitors. Nor is it likely that the petri dishes of pig eggs, embryos, and stem cells posed a risk to us. On my visit, the rigorous contamination standards reminded those of us touring of sterile medical facilities, on the one hand, and of silicon chip manufacturing, on the other. The difficulty and mode of entering also seemed to mark the esteem in which Hwang and the lab were held.

HWANG'S CHOPSTICK PASTORALE

Once inside the facility, we were taken around two adjoining rooms that together made up each of the stages of somatic cell nuclear transfer techniques and embryonic stem cell line derivation. The first station involved sorting and grossly preparing pig eggs, and the postdocs seated at that station literally had their hands in a large plastic basin of porcine ovarian material from the abattoir. Subsequent stations involved microscope and micromanipulation work representing the different stages of fertilization, incubation, and derivation of stem cell lines. Taken together, the lab resembled an artisan's workshop, with its apprentices in training. Our guide, a lab member, described the time and dedication necessary to master each step, citing six months as the time it might take to become good at a particular micromanipulation skill. No one could move on to the next skill until the previous one was mastered. The highest standards of care were taken with the materials at each stage, conferring a profound embodied sense of the potential value of the materials and the techniques as they were transforming them.

This layout and these mores had deep resonances with the charismatic nationalist narrative of Hwang perpetuated by Hwang himself and others in the media. Hwang was already known for citing his rural, livestock veterinarian roots, and his rise from modest beginnings to supreme scientist. He credited the values of the Korean countryside with his work ethic, in a prelapsarian bucolic narrative appealing to inhabitants of advanced capitalist cities, myself included. His work ethic—a stated readiness to work 365 days a year, night and day if need be—was expressed in terms of there being not a second to lose to find life-saving and life-altering cures, in contrast to the capitalist "24/7" work ethic compelled by profit and self-interest. Above all, he had famously made the statement that he and his colleagues had succeeded in deriving embryonic stem cell lines from patient-specific cloned embryos because of national characteristics of the Koreans. Referring to the heavy metal chopsticks Koreans typically use to eat with and the slippery foods such as glass noodles they are required to pick up with these chopsticks, he was frequently quoted around the world for claiming that this conferred a superior degree of manual dexterity in the Korean population as a whole. As such, the breakthrough in question, which required hitherto unattained manual skill, was naturalized to the Korean people. Hwang's honor and glory was deflected from himself and onto the whole nation, only further fueling his rise. The ethos of care and the guild-like apprenticeship of the lab reflected and exemplified these values of sacrificial hard work and pastoral humility. At the same time, the evident hierarchy and the presence of non-Koreans from other Asian countries such as Bangladesh (itself an interesting and important phenomenon, differing considerably from the kinds of science diasporas of Singapore's stem cell research—see below) contradicted this picture. When I asked our guide about the egg procurement allegations, his answer was evasive and noncommittal, making it clear that for me to ask further would be disrespectful.

FIRST-IN-CLASS THERAPEUTIC PROOF OF CONCEPT

The scientific payoff of Hwang's lab was not primarily progress in basic cellular and molecular research, advancing understanding of pluripotency and regeneration, or the advancement of tissue engineering prowess. Rather, it was being the first to succeed in applying a difficult veterinary technique to human cells; namely, to get an enucleated human egg to begin dividing and differentiating after manually giving it the nuclear DNA from an individual afflicted with a condition in need of a cure. The promise of this technique was to be able to customize the DNA fingerprint of stem cell lines so as to treat individuals down the line with cells that bore their own DNA and so would not be rejected by the patient's immune system. While industrial scale-up seemed (and still seems) to be a daunting prospect, the therapeutic value was apparent. The technique, known colloquially as "therapeutic cloning," is the one that had been introduced to the world in Dolly the sheep almost a decade earlier. What Hwang et al.'s results appeared to demonstrate was that this procedure was possible in and viable for humans. It would have been a scientific first. Hwang's credentials for carrying out the work were emblemized by his success in cloning the world's first dog, an Afghan hound named Snuppy, for "Seoul National University puppy." Dogs, like humans and other primates, have notoriously difficult reproductive endocrinology, and so the feat was considerable. That Hwang's team should prevail in the race to clone human embryos and derive stem cells from them was plausible because of this existing expertise. But this difficult mammalian reproductive and embryological micromanipulation achievement far exceeded the veterinary cloning prowess from which it gained its credibility. (The distance of this difference is evident in the activities to which Hwang had been consigned before my 2008 visit, namely, the commercial business of pet cloning, in which he was busying himself while applying to reenter mainstream science.) Success with human cells would have meant both proof of principle—patient-specific cells could in principle be made—and would have had almost limitless therapeutic value: given that embryonic stem cells can give rise to almost all the cells of the body, each of us would have the possibility of an infinitely replenishable cellular repair kit in Hwang's hands.

Hwang et al.'s apparent achievement was personal and national, the promise therapeutic and universal, and the ethos one of humility with glory, and meritocratic rather than economic success. This was a scientific priority race won by a charismatic scientist in university lab facilities, rather than the basis for a biotech start-up and the procurement of intellectual property. Once Hwang's team attempted to extend the achievement beyond Korea to found a worldwide stem cell hub, the rest of the world resisted, and joined Korean whistle blowers in uncovering the fraud that was exposed rapidly thereafter. One U.S researcher who had gotten his name on one of the suspect publications despite perhaps having been less than a full coauthor (illustrating the symbolic stakes and the international dimensions of scientific authorship) scrambled to dissociate himself and also became the subject of an investigation at his home institution.

The ethos, lab layout, and scientific goals, even the iconic animal, were radically different in Singapore.

Biopolis, One North, Singapore

The city-state of Singapore has been an independent republic since 1965, following brief periods of occupation, stewardship, or incorporation by Japan, Britain, and Malaysia respectively. Since then it has capitalized on the international potential of its English-language educational and legal system, and dealt, through intense social planning, with extreme housing and land shortages. Biopolis is the name of Phase I of a huge custom-built biomedical research facility collectively known as "One North," signifying Singapore's latitude and its aspirations to be a research and finance hub at the center of Southeast Asia.[11] Biopolis was built at the turn of the new century and displays a degree of social planning at once continuous with preexisting waves of social planning and yet radically new. When I visited in 2005, Phase I of building had been completed and its buildings, Chromos, Helios, Centros, Genome, Matrix, Nanos, and Proteos, were still being filled.[12]

CIVIC SCIENCE REAL ESTATE

Biopolis's newness for Singapore lies in part in the way in which it posits biomedical research as a way of life: somewhat as in a Silicon Valley company such as Google (but without the Peter Pan syndrome), one can get one's laundry done and socialize without leaving one's place of work. More significant for my argument here, though, is the turn-of-the-century "mind meld" between the public and private sectors that its physical structure posits: two of Biopolis's seven buildings are occupied by biomedical companies from the private sector, while the remaining five buildings are occupied by the various biomedical research institutes of Singapore's A*STAR (the Agency of Science, Technology and Research). The seven buildings are connected by sky bridges, making concrete the lofty connections between each unit. Similarly, all seven buildings share infrastructure and a basement and parking lot, in a single foundation.

A second aspect of the newness of Biopolis that is central to my argument here is its organizational structure. A*STAR oversees Biopolis. It falls under the Ministry of Trade and Industry, yet is made up of the Biomedical Research Council, the Science and Engineering Research Council, Exploit Technologies Pte. Ltd., the A*STAR Graduate Academy, and the Corporate Planning and Administration Division, mixing public and private, educational and corporate. As A*STAR's very name suggests, it puts research together with/as science, encompassing what it calls a "full spectrum of R & D activities and graduate training."[13] That academic training, scientific research, and industrial R & D activities are seen as part of a single organizational entity stands in contrast to the Korean case.

This infrastructure for innovation has resulted in new areas of interdisciplinary biosciences research: of the five research institutes that make up the public part of Biopolis—the BioInformatics Institute, the Bioprocessing Technology Institute, the Genome Institute of Singapore, the Institute of Molecular and Cell Biology (IMCB), and the Institute of Bioengineering and Nanotechnology—four were formed at the turn of the century, the exception being IMCB, which dates back to the mid-1980s. A*STAR states as its vision: "A prosperous and vibrant Singapore built upon a knowledge based economy," responsible for "fostering world-class scientific research and talent for a vibrant knowledge-based Singapore," and made up of "today's research scientists and future generation of aspiring scientists who dare to race with the world's best towards the very limits of modern science."[14]

FILLING BIOPOLIS: MODEL SPECIES AND AN INTERNATIONAL ELITE

I was taken around Biopolis by one of its researchers, just as at Hwang's lab. Being shown around Biopolis was rather like getting a real estate tour of an expensive new development, with the emphasis on filling the space with the right kinds of people. Unlike at Hwang's lab, there were no sterility procedures; instead, entry was regulated by security, and I was required to sign in and to wear a badge while on the premises. The researcher showing me around emphasized the spaciousness, the layout that included the sky bridges and shared facilities, and the residents and research projects of the various lab spaces we visited. The most salient aspects of the tour concerned the residents, both animal and human, of the lab. High-status researchers from overseas headed up many of the populated labs. Europe, North America, and Asia were all represented as sending countries, and not all of these lab heads were in residence all year round, some managing to keep academic positions elsewhere while being involved with a lab at Biopolis. Singapore universities are famous for paying expatriate faculty higher salaries than nationals, in a bid to lure faculty with international credentials and reputations, so the pattern of having foreign-born and/or -trained heads of the labs had precedent. Most of the students, however, seemed to be from Singapore.

If Snuppy the cloned Afghan hound was the totem animal of Hwang's lab and all it stood for, the zebrafish holds this position at Biopolis. The zebrafish is one of the world's most commonly used research animals, because it is considered to be a good model of vertebrate development, including the basic biology of stem cell research. A species with a long history as a valued tropical fish in Singapore, the zebrafish became central to Singapore's research infrastructure in the early 1990s in fish farming research. Biopolis's massive zebrafish research facility was established in 2004, and had apparently taken a certain amount of trial and error to set up.[15] It was still relatively new when I visited and was clearly a prize exhibit. The room was by far the largest model animal facility I had ever seen. Far from Hwang's guild-like and heavily peopled lab, the zebrafish facility had no one in it when we visited. And far from being told how the hoped-for scientific achievements of this space would be made possible by the national characteristics of researchers, as occurred in Hwang's lab, the zebrafish facility was explicitly organized to allow researchers to choose which international style of zebrafish maintenance they preferred.

The fish tanks were organized into two sections, one kept in "the American style," and one in "the German style." I was told that there are two major schools of thought on establishing zebrafish populations for research: the American one, which enables food, light, and temperature to be individually adjusted for each tank, as part of the experimental conditions, and the German one, which standardizes food, water and ambient temperature, and light, against which to measure experimental effects. After some joking about the stereotypes involved—Americans and endless choice versus Germans and standardization—my guide told me that this layout enabled them to appeal to major overseas researchers, no matter their preferences or country of training/origin. In other words, the zebrafish also displayed the international real estate for science and technology design and organizational structure of the whole of Biopolis.

While the ethics of human egg procurement dominated the unspoken space at Hwang's lab, Biopolis suggested that foundational biological questions could be answered through research on model species. Neither individual charisma nor contested ethics was in evidence, even though many of the major figures behind Biopolis were important and well-known figures in Singapore society, and even though Singapore was actively in the process of writing and revising regulations to deal with the ethics of stem cell research, like so many countries around the world at the time.

A FULL SPECTRUM OF STEM CELLS

Biopolis's stem cell research, a central part of its biomedical research activities, reflects its organizational structure. Our guide, an A*STAR researcher, told me that a full spectrum of stem cell research, not just human embryonic stem cell research, is encouraged, and that they are trying to benefit from having basic science research and translational and clinically relevant stem cell research all in the same site. In using the term "spectrum" to characterize Biopolis's fundamental approach to stem cell research, he echoed A*STAR's description of its research mandate as covering the "full spectrum of R & D activities and graduate training." The recurrence of this metaphor during my visit was striking. Framing different kinds of research and different sectors by placing them on an imagined spectrum suggests that these activities and sectors naturally go together. This tends to obscure just how original (and how unlike the situation in South Korea) it is to place these elements together in this way and demonstrates that Biopolis's existence is original precisely for uniting these very elements.

The use of the spectrum metaphor also suggests that the spectrum itself is the real payoff, rather than lab results coming from a single point on the spectrum. At Biopolis, the various spectrums used to describe the place plot the parameters of the innovation hub being imagined. Not surprisingly, then, when I tried to find out what researchers and administrators were hoping would be the scientific payoffs of the stem cell activities at Biopolis (were there some goals equivalent to the Hwang team's attempts to make patient specific stem cell lines, for example?), the answers were more about "generating innovation," or at least producing a research environment indicative of innovation, in general. A success would not be judged by sensational newsworthy feats, but more by productive teams led by the right people and working in synergy, whose output in publications and conferences would display the rapid growth patterns of the value-added location. The practice of successfully luring major figures from abroad was jovially referred to as "serial kidnapping," and I was quoted facts and figures indicating productivity, hub-like activity (such as the number of published reviews of research in a field, high concentrations of scientists in a subfield, and the hosting of major conferences), as well as percentages of the facilities in use. More than being the first to do something the clinical relevance of which the public could understand, the three researchers I talked to hoped to develop basic science research tools (such as a better understanding of the gene regulation of stem cell differentiation) that would be feedstuff for the onsite R & D chain and also positively reinforce onsite and Singapore's knowledge infrastructure.

STEM CELL RESEARCH AND KNOWLEDGE SOCIETIES

Singapore has set itself up as the central business and research and financial hub of Asia and beyond by seeking to recruit the most highly qualified international experts it can to train its youth, while Korea has moved much more slowly to open up its faculty positions to foreign researchers, and still sends a huge number of its elite students abroad to train. In the city-state of Singapore, business, education, research, and social planning are different facets of the same civic mission; at Biopolis, world-class stem cell and other biomedical researchers are training a young largely Singaporean group of researchers to be the new citizens of its knowledge society. In Hwang's lab, the emphasis was on the Koreanness of Hwang himself, not on his lab's role in a knowledge society.

In South Korea, much of university research, including most of the life sciences, falls under the Ministry of Higher Education, Science, and

Technology, and is an additional arena for displaying national educational competitiveness as a developmental strategy, rather than part of the powerful private but state-protected industrial conglomerates that do most of the nation's R & D. The formation in 2008, under President Lee Myung-bak of the new Ministry of Knowledge Economy (MKE) represents an aspiration to more effectively integrate older developmental nation-state practices with newer calls for financial deregulation, globalization, and innovation. The name of the new ministry is deceptive, however, as it replaces the older Ministry of Commerce, Industry, and Energy, and is separate from the Ministry of Higher Education, Science, and Technology.[16] Despite calls from some quarters to bring about a convergence between bio- and information sciences, and to move toward a knowledge society, university life science and translational biomedical research is much harder to integrate into the knowledge economy in South Korea than in Singapore because that's not where it started. The protectionist and nationalist basis of its previous decades of economic growth is also hard to change; only in 2008, with the establishment of the Ministry of Knowledge Economy, did South Korea change its policy to open up directorships of Korea's powerful research institutes to nonnationals.

Even where both Singapore and South Korea reacted to similar global and regional trends by doing similar things, such as responding to the Asian financial crisis by moving somewhat away from high-expenditure, foreign-export manufacturing toward value-added knowledge economies, bench-to-bedside biomedical research such as stem cell research played a different role in the two places. Biomedical research, especially stem cell research, is a cornerstone of Singapore's effort in this regard, while South Korea, later and less enthusiastic in this response in the first place, has relied more on transforming its already highly advanced information and communication technology sector to accommodate World Bank demands, while stem cell research initially flourished in its national educational system. South Korea produced and then participated in the emotional nationalist drama of the fall of its "Supreme Scientist," because its university research labs are more part of its educational meritocracy, which has in turn been central to South Korea's development strategy, rather than part of its R & D sector.

Singapore built and began to fill a facility devoted to a lifestyle of integrated research that embodied both the bench-to-bedside trajectory and the convergence of business, information, and biosciences, while taking care of all the living needs of its civic entrepreneurs. The prize of one was, or could have been, glory; as the then president of Seoul National University expressed it after the fall of Hwang Woo Suk, "Most of us, in the name of national interests, exaggerated Dr. Hwang's research to make it an aspiration of the nation."[17] The prize of the other is its potential to be Asia's, if not the "world's easiest place to do business," thanks to its stable legal, political, and economic environment.[18] While Singapore has led the way in regional intellectual property law and finance reform, South Korea has been urged by the European Union and others to strengthen its intellectual property regimes. While Singapore continues to pay foreign faculty more than its nationals and to recruit superstars from prestigious universities overseas, South Korea saw one of its own nationals become a household name around the world, and boasts the most successful education system in the world. Both represent different ways of being Asian Tigers.

The aspects of the ethnographic comparison above—lab layout and mores, scientific strategies and strengths and weaknesses—reflect and produce this situation.

Conclusions

Science is everywhere and nowhere all at once. Yet anthropologists, sociologists, historians of science, and science studies scholars have shown that there are profound regional and local differences in how "the same science" is enabled, practiced, and understood. In this spirit, my study has compared and contrasted characteristic stem cell research and regenerative medicine facilities in two Asian Tiger countries. I compared each lab's version of this small part of biotech revolution, asking what it tells us about the nation in question, as well as what these nations' engagements with regenerative medicine add to our understanding of biotechnology, knowledge societies, and their significance. While there is no unified "Asian biotech" in evidence—each country's pattern is in stark contrast to the other in many respects—both countries are operating within geographic, historical, and economic patterns that are importantly located in and as Asia.

In conclusion, then, it is not time to do away with area studies in undertaking transnational comparative analyses of networks of scientific research; to the contrary, we still suffer a serious lack of regionally informed comparative research on science. The comparison I have presented here suggests, rather, that we need to be more alert to the different roles that "the same" area or regional identity can play, and the interrelations between them, especially the specificities of historical and emerging connections among the economy, scientific epistemology, and the polity. The study of science and technology promises to be a fruitful site for transnational comparative analysis. The intrinsic global aspects of scientific knowledge and its international social organization facilitate access and comprehension, while the dominance of the English language as the lingua franca of scientific research and as a first or second language around the world somewhat reduces linguistic barriers to studying scientific field sites to growing numbers of English-speaking scholars. Put together with the increasing importance of science and technology in all aspects of modern society, this suggests in turn that transnational studies of science and technology have much to teach us.

Notes

1. For exceptional accounts of the geopolitics of stem cell research, see Sarah Franklin, "Stem Cells R Us: Emergent Life Forms and the Global Biological," in *Global Assemblages: Technology, Politics and Ethics as Anthropological Problems*, ed. Aihwa Ong and Stephen J. Collier (New York: Blackwell, 2005); Jennifer Liu, "Asia Modern: Stem Cells, Ethics, and Contemporary Taiwan," Ph.D. dissertation, University of California, Berkeley, 2008; Ruha Benjamin, "Culturing Consent: Science and Democracy in the Stem Cell State," Ph.D. dissertation, University of California, Berkeley, 2008; and Ong's essay, "The Ethics of Blood Banking for Family and Beyond," in this volume.
2. The United Nations Human Development Index is calculated using a combined measure of education, life expectancy, and GDP, whereas the IMF "advanced economy" designation uses the macroeconomic criteria of per capita income, export diversification, and integration into the global financial system.
3. Sheila Jasanoff's brilliant defense and exemplification of transnational comparative work is my guide (*Designs on Nature: Science and Democracy in Europe and the United States* [Princeton, N.J.: Princeton University Press, 2005]).
4. A transnational comparative perspective alerts the ethnographer to the strengths and weaknesses of her/his own insider/outsider perspective. Working in the United States, I am probably in general more inclined to attribute causal agency to cultural and detailed institutional patterns in the United States that I know well, and less inclined to notice macroeconomic and global trends than in East Asia. An exercise in symmetry can perhaps improve both

sides of the implicit comparison: it may be worth giving more weight to macroeconomic factors when investigating the growth of stem cell research in the United States, instead of relying as strongly as most commentators are inclined to on political and religious aspects of the rights to life of the embryo. Likewise, actively seeking archival and ethnographic evidence for political and religious voices in the East Asian stem cell research avoids taking for granted a U.S.-centric perspective on Asia that primarily sees freedom from the regulatory burden of abortion politics in the United States.

5. E.g., Lee Silver, "The God Effect: America's Religious Conservatives Aren't the Only Ones Who object to Science on Spiritual Grounds—So Do Europe's Greens. The Big Winner Is Asia," *Newsweek International*, April 2004; these simplistic Eastern-religions-versus-Western-religions accounts have not entirely faded, e.g., John Tierney, "Are Scientists Playing God? It Depends on Your Religion," *New York Times*, November 20, 2007.
6. See Liu, "Asia Modern"; and Hae-joang Cho, "Constructing and Deconstructing Koreanness," in *Making Majorities: Constituting the Nation in Japan, Korea, China, Malaysia, Fiji, Turkey, and the United States*, ed. Dru Gladney (Stanford, Calif.: Stanford University Press, 1998).
7. For a helpful account of the Hwang scandal, see Sungook Hong, "The Hwang Scandal That Shook the World of Science," *East Asian Science, Technology and Society* 2 (2008): 1–7.
8. For a sensitive reading of the relation of Korean women to Hwang's rise and fall, see So Yeon Leem and Jin Hee Park, "Rethinking Women and Their Bodies in the Age of Biotechnology: Feminist Commentaries on the Hwang Affair," *East Asian Science, Technology and Society* 2 (2008): 9–26.
9. During this research, given its time frame, I opted to work with conditions of anonymity for those who graciously showed me around labs and talked to me. For personnel at SNU's lab and Biopolis, this means I give neither names nor ranks of scientists, so as to minimize the risk of recognition.
10. As an advocate for the payment under some circumstances of women for donating eggs for research (e.g., Charis Thompson, "Why We Should, in Fact, Pay for Egg Donation," *Regenerative Medicine* 2, no. 2 [2007], 203–9), I am less concerned by the charges that some egg donors had been paid than by the construction of good and bad practice around egg donation. The payment scandal, which emerged as proxy for a lack of consultation of women and possible coercion of junior colleagues, took part in an emerging international discourse about bioethics in this area. A major aspect of the scientific breakthrough attributed to Hwang and his team was the ability to reduce the numbers of eggs used to succeed in cloning, so the misrepresentations of the numbers of eggs used was also of great interest to me (see Thompson, *Making Parents: The Ontological Choreography of Reproductive Technologies* [Cambridge, Mass.: MIT Press, 2005], 245–76, on ethical issues around waste and profligacy of valued tissue in cloning).
11. On the nature of Singapore as a "hub," see Ong, "Ecologies of Expertise:

Assembling Flows, Managing Citizenship," in Ong and Collier, *Global Assemblages*.

12. See Paul Smaglik, "Filling Biopolis," *Nature* 425 (2003): 746–47, on the luring of international science stars to this research real estate.
13. Agency of Science, Technology and Research (A*STAR), http://www.a-star.edu.sg/biopolis/9-Biopolis (accessed August 15, 2008).
14. A*STAR, http://www.a-star.edu.sg/a_star/2-About-A-STAR (accessed August 15, 2008).
15. On the establishment of zebrafish colonies in Biopolis, see the article by two researchers from Proteus: May-Su You and Vladimir Korzh, "Zebrafish in the Tropical One-North," *Zebrafish* 1, no. 4. (March 1, 2005): 327–34.
16. The English-language Web site of the Ministry of Knowledge Economy says: "In 2008, with the launch of the administration of President Lee Myung-bak, the Ministry of Knowledge Economy (MKE) was born. Formerly the Ministry of Commerce, Industry, and Energy, MKE incorporates certain functions that were previously the responsibility of other Ministries (Information and Communications, Science and Technology, Finance and Economy). MKE is making painstaking efforts to develop Korea into a knowledge-based economy, one that is driven by technological innovation." MKE, http://www.mke.go.kr/language/eng/about/history.jsp (accessed August 15, 2008).
17. Quoted in Anthony Faiola, "Koreans 'Blinded' to Truth about Claims on Stem Cells," *Washington Post Foreign Service*, January 13, 2006, A10.
18. Michelle Tay, "S'pore Is Easiest City in the World to Do Business; It Is Also Top in Region for Economic Stability and Legal/Political Framework: Survey," *Straits Times* (Singapore), June 10, 2008.

ARA WILSON

Medical Tourism in Thailand

The quotation below, a stock paragraph from a company text, comes from a press release announcing a Bangkok hospital's contract for a "wireless infrastructure project" with Motorola, Inc. The hospital—Bumrungrad International—is more accurately described as a corporation, a cluster of health-related financial, service, and managerial projects; like many major Thai corporations, Bumrungrad International is publicly traded while also remaining largely under the control of a Chinese Thai family empire.[1]

> Bumrungrad International is the largest private hospital in Southeast Asia and one of the world's most popular destinations for medical tourism. It offers state-of-the-art diagnostic, therapeutic, and intensive care facilities in a multi-specialty medical center located in Bangkok, Thailand. Opened in 1980 the hospital was Asia's first to pass the demanding review of the Joint Commission International, the highest US standard for hospital accreditation. Newsweek recently included Bumrungrad on its list of 10 leading international hospitals, calling it "one of the most modern and efficient medical facilities in the world."[2]

This public-relations prose, echoed in media commentary, establishes Thailand as a globally competitive site of medical modernity. The term "medical tourism" most often describes the recent trend in which international elites obtain modern medical care in countries that are not associated with the pinnacle of biotech: countries such as the Dominican Republic, India, and Thailand. These Third World sites nonetheless offer advanced equipment, expertise, and management in a secure, sanitized environment—the "gleaming" interiors described in media reports—all at lower costs than in industrialized nations.

Discussions of medical sites like Bumrungrad Hospital emphasize the international nature of their biotechnological facilities, reinforcing the notion that such resources are imported from, or at least certified by, Western sources. Yet medical tourism is not imported wholesale. In the case of Thailand, for example, it should be seen as a domestically situated, transnational assemblage that redeploys capacities already available in the country.[3] Understanding medical tourism in Thailand as an assemblage calls attention to the ways that already available domestic capacities help to establish the nation's "comparative advantage" in applied biotech. Such capacities include an available medical infrastructure: Bumrungrad, for example, had been popular with foreign residents in Bangkok decades before new flows of medical tourists. In addition, beyond medical technologies, other forms of labor, technology, and investments underwrite biotech in Thailand. Without symbolic and "affective labor," in particular, medical modernity could not be marketed from such an unevenly developed Asian metropolis as Bangkok. Thus, in line with recent analyses of the "local" creation of "universality,"[4] Thailand's achievement of "international" biotech is a national product.

Thailand's provision of state-of-the-art allopathic medical services to global consumers is one example of the recent relocation of biotech modernity to Asia. As with biotech projects found elsewhere in Asia, medical tourism in Thailand represents a national biopolitical strategy for addressing domestic uncertainty, geopolitical conditions, and global capital flows. Biotech is less fully under government control than it is in more centralized Asian states (e.g., the cases of Singapore or China described in this volume). Rather, state agencies collaborate with private corporations like Bumrungrad International to foster medical tourism in ways that reflect the changing nature of governance in Thailand over the past decades. This context requires attention to the political economy of governance, that is, to intersections of state projects and corporate practices.

The first part of this essay unpacks the phenomenon described as medical tourism. It details the social infrastructure for Thai biotech, that is, the diverse resources that have been marshaled to market state-of-the-art medical care to foreigners. I emphasize the ways that the nonbiotech features, including the state investments and affective labor, have been key to realizing the "international" standards that enable the relocation of medical modernity to Thailand. These enabling conditions have a biopolitical history, which I trace in the next section of the essay. Over the twentieth century, the state's involvement with medicine transformed as national governance shifted from kingdom to bureaucracy to entrepreneurial state. The investments in medicine were shaped by geopolitics—particularly in relation to the United States. Notably, U.S. engagements with Thailand during the Indochina war generated a tourist industry and medical resources, the key elements to the new assemblage of medical tourism. The essay finally turns to the emergence of medical tourism in the 2000s as a collaborative public-private strategy to secure the national economic future in the aftermath of the Asian economic crisis.[5] This overview chronicles changing national conditions—state governance, capital investments, and a plurality of labor—that have been deployed in establishing Thailand's global medical modernity.

Medical Movement

The consumption of health care by foreigners in Thailand has grown markedly over the 2000s. In 2006, more than a million foreigners received medical treatment in the country. Foreign patients account for more than half of Bumrungrad's revenue.[6] A number of these are foreign nationals, but reside in the region. This fact highlights the misleading nature of the term "medical tourism," which implies that citizenship and nationality can be equated with location or distance traveled, among other connotations.[7] Yet the number of people who travel to Thailand for medical care has increased, reflecting a deliberate strategy on the part of medical corporations and state policies to globalize select medical sites in Thailand.

In 2006, eighty thousand Americans went to a single Bangkok hospital, the majority of them women.[8] The United States and Great Britain informally—and in some cases, formally—outsource citizens' medical care to Thailand. While many representations of medical tourism highlight such Western travelers, a great share of foreign patients in Thai hospitals comes from Asia. In 2001, the largest group of medical tourists to Thailand came from Japan.[9] There are growing numbers from

China, joined by smaller flows of elites from such countries as Bangladesh or Nepal. In recent years more patients have come from the Middle East, a rise attributed to the consequences of the post-9/11 constraints on travel to the United States.[10]

The most popular surgery sought by foreign patients is cosmetic surgery, leading to the spin-off phrase, "scalpel tourism." Many are seeking to refashion raced and gendered embodiment with breast implants, penile enhancements, eye reshaping, nose jobs, liposuction, or sex reassignment surgery (SRS), which is one of Thailand's specializations.[11] Some are seeking reproductive technologies, generating a subcategory called "fertility tourists." The services that most exemplify medical tourism are considered elective: routine checkups or cosmetic surgery. But procedures include those acknowledged to be necessary as well.

There are many factors producing the willingness to travel for medical care, including internationally uneven medical conditions, national legal contexts, worldwide transformations to state entitlements and health plans, and the practices of finance capital. Those who seek medical care in Thailand often do so because the Thai medical resources are superior to those in their home country. In other cases, patients cannot afford the procedures in their country, often because they lack health insurance or the procedure is not covered by their insurance.[12] The cost of medical services in Thailand is lower than in the industrialized world. A comprehensive package of up to twenty-three different exams (including lab work) cost about U.S. $600 in 2007.[13] In vitro fertilization (IVF) costs a third of the rates in the United States or Europe.[14] Fees in Thailand are also lower than those in Singapore, the country's main regional competitor.[15] The outsourcing of citizen's health care to foreign sites is beginning to be formalized by finance capital. Some American medical tourists can have expenses covered by their U.S. health insurance, for example, BlueCross BlueShield of South Carolina.[16] In addition to cost, people also travel to bypass constraints of national medical policies. Procedures available in Thailand may be illegal or procedurally onerous in their home country, notably, sex reassignment surgery or the test that allows sex selection before IVF implantation (which is not permitted in Australia, for example).[17]

The demand for medical tourism is an anxious demand. Consider the following set of rhetorical questions posed on a Web site about medical travel: "We understand that just the idea of going overseas can be a frightening one. Are the doctors well qualified? Are the hospitals safe? Does the food taste good?"[18] When someone asks whether hospital food abroad is going to taste good, it is time to wonder what other concerns are at play. Gathering relevant information and making arrangements across continents with native speakers of a different language can be daunting. The stakes for bodily transformations anywhere, but especially in a foreign location, are high. And when it comes to medical and dental care, actual and imagined geography matters. Foreigners' perceptions of the risks of health care in Thailand reflect entrenched notions of the global distribution of modernity. The technological modernity that ensures medical security has long been conflated with the West or global North, the locus for "international" standards. Beyond simply being attracted by lower costs alone, global consumers must be persuaded that modern biotech *can* be located in a developing Asian nation like Thailand. Such persuasion depends on a range of labors and technologies beyond those of medical biotech. (For one, it requires the symbolic labor mobilizing the signs of modern technology.) In the next section, I discuss the labors that enable biomedicine to be effectively deployed and marketed, showing how medical tourism is a globally oriented national project that assembles existing capacities.

Socializing Biomedicine

Medical tourism leverages resources that are available in Bangkok to achieve a comparative advantage in global health care. It uses the relative underdevelopment of the economy to market Western technologies to the developed (and developing) world. It makes use of state resources and affective dispositions, including orientations to hospitality honed in the service sector and in cultural codifications of social hierarchy.

Thailand's comparative advantage derives from offering international standards at low cost. Lower costs are the consequence mainly of lower wages, secured by Thailand's location in the global economy: salaries make up one-sixth of an elite Thai hospital's budget, compared to half of U.S. hospital budgets.[19] The legal context, notably the place of litigation, also affects cost, since Thai doctors do not hold costly malpractice insurance policies. As I discuss below, hospitals have also received direct or indirect assistance from the state in set-asides or tax credits, which helps keep down costs. The political and economic context produces the competitive advantage in cost. The medical tourist assemblage overcomes the geographic deficit of its location in a developing nation by leveraging the advantages of a less developed economy.

While medical tourism prospers through privatized medical care, it depends heavily on public resources. Credentialed medical staff are a socialized product: most doctors, nurses, and technicians at Thai institutions were trained from the age of eighteen or so at state medical schools attached to state universities. Although a private institution, Bumrungrad has affiliated with a state university to provide teaching and training for Thai medical students, with the express goal "of easing the doctor shortage in rural Thailand,"[20] and perhaps also because an association with university-based research and training constitutes competitive medical credentials. State-funded universities are key to the private health care sold in medical tourism. In addition, state medical facilities provide medical staff for medical tourism. Many of the available doctors are on the public payroll at state medical facilities and moonlighting as consultants at private medical facilities like Bumrungrad.

Those nervous questions—Are the doctors well qualified? Are the hospitals safe? Does the food taste good?—convey the interconnected anxieties about various facets of embodied security. The ten Thai medical centers that appeal to global consumers must address these concerns. I consider how they do so mainly through the example of Bumrungrad.

The qualifications of doctors are established by references to Western training and certification, mostly in the United States or United Kingdom. Bumrungrad's materials continually refer to the international experience of medical staff, such as its "US trained medical director." Safety, too, is conveyed through a reliance on international standards. Throughout its elaborate Web site, the hospital announces its accreditation with the American-based Joint Commission International, a body that certifies "international" standards for health care institutions, and the hospital incorporates the JCI logo and name on every Web page. Most viewers are unlikely to recognize this agency's name or symbol: the reference to JCI nevertheless not only recognizes, but constitutes, the legitimacy that accreditation by this agency confers. The company's name, Bumrungrad International, is the outcome of a 2005 "rebranding" effort of the old "brand," Bumrungrad Hospital.[21] International modernity is thus realized not only through equipment and medicine but also through marketing and accreditation—the medical tourism assemblage relies heavily on such immaterial labor.

Indeed, while Thai medical sites aim to match global (Western) standards for biotech, Thai hospitals are considered *superior* to those in the global North in the qualitative dimensions of healing, hospitality, and leisure. The superior qualities of medical care in Thailand derive from a full spectrum of services associated with hospitality and travel industries. Bumrungrad's lobby is characterized as like that of a five-star hotel. The hospital takes pains to ensure the food tastes good: it meets the dietary requirements of various populations by offering certified halal food, "spa cuisine," or meals prepared by a European-based food-service company.

Tourist services and medical services are often linked. In 2000, Bumrungrad partnered with the government-owned airline, Thai Air, to offer combined travel-medical packages. Now Cathay Pacific and Royal Orchid Tours also offer travel packages that include medical checkups.[22] The Bangkok Hospital, which is connected to a hotel, offers spa visits, Thai massage, and sightseeing tours for visitors accompanying a patient. Bumrungrad Hospital also supports patients' role as elite global workers through a range of resources: secretarial support (including a private secretary and bookbinding), translation, printing, laptop rental, Internet access, courier and messenger services, faxing, and photocopying.

What achieves "high quality, affordable healthcare with no waiting"[23] is a plurality of labor,[24] including nurses, subcontracted cleaning staff, and translators. Bumrungrad employs more than 2,600 workers, which includes 1,000 workers beyond the 700 nurses and 900 physicians and dentists.[25] It pays five people to answer e-mails from around the world.[26] The security of patients is achieved not only through biomedical equipment and privacy, but also through labor in an ambiance of care. Safety is created by certified doctors, subcontracted sanitation crews and hired security personnel, by information technologists, and food managers working with sound food policies. It is also fostered by the often-noted level of attentive care that patients receive from medical providers and support workers in the hospital.

As much of the imagery surrounding medical tourism to Thailand shows (see figure 1), a significant form of labor that fosters the security of foreign visitors is affective labor. Former patients speak of the

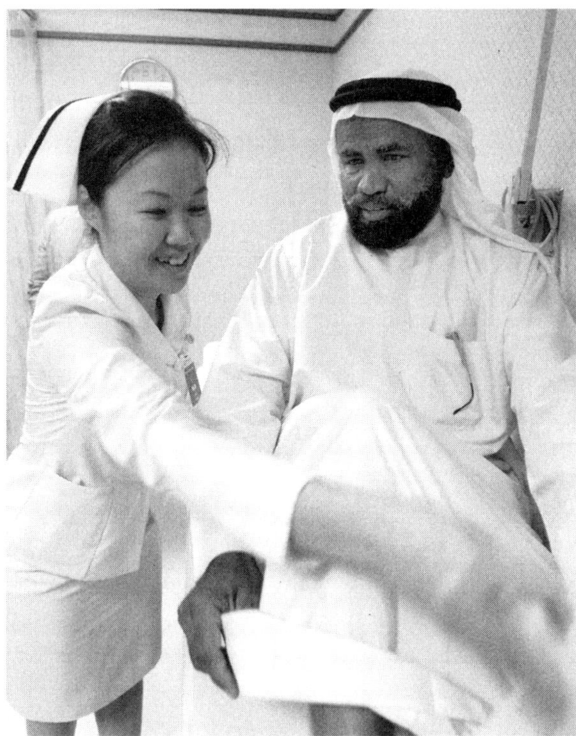

Figure 1 This stock photograph shows an attentive nurse and a foreign patient in Bumrungrad International, illustrating two key elements—national difference and affective labor—that produce the modernity of medical tourism. PHOTOGRAPH BY SAEED KHAN. COPYRIGHT GETTY IMAGES.

attentive and reassuring care they received. In *The Managed Heart*, the sociologist Arlie Hochschild described the increasing reliance on such affective labor in U.S. industries (such as airlines). Her analysis explores the implications of the commodification of the ability to manage emotions, for example, producing friendliness.[27] As I note below, in its sex trade and tourist industries, the Thai economy has also relied on affective labor to massage foreign visitors, literally and figuratively. Standards for solicitous service are quite high in Thai retail, hospitality, and travel industries. The literature on affective labor does not generally address postcolonial geography, or the place of national identity in commodifying relationality. In the case of Thailand, the modes of hospitable engagement found in medical tourism—or sex tourism—are often attributed to Thai culture. The labor involved in gracious caretaking is naturalized in this cultural attribution. Without denying the possibility that structures of feeling or the effects of social hierarchies might produce patterned modes of comportment and interaction, it remains worth considering their commodification, particularly in the transnational, interracial, and imperial contexts of medical tourism. Nor are these attributes only the fantasies of white or other foreigners. The Thai state has reinforced this association through its codification of Thai culture in terms of monastic Buddhism, customs such as the *wai* (the prayer-like greeting), and assertions of forms of hierarchy as traditional Thai values.

Medical tourism has bundled a range of services—food service, hotels accommodation, visa extensions—into the "campus" of the global hospital. Biotech is embedded in, and realized through, this assemblage. In particular, affective and immaterial labor—provided by nurses, food service staff, copywriters, or portfolio managers—are critical to realizing biomedical modernity in the global South. The low cost of biomedical care is subsidized by the state and a function of Thailand's economic underdevelopment. In these ways, the international standards that authorize biotech in Thailand are realized through, not despite, "local" conditions, understanding the local to have been constituted in relation to transnational forces. In the following sections, I discuss how some of these local capacities—including medical expertise, the tourist sector, and Thai capital and labor—developed over the twentieth century, and then will turn to the strategic redeployment of such resources into the medical tourism assemblage.

Medical Infrastructures

Medical tourism assembles national capacities in medicine, tourism, finance, and state resources. In what follows, I trace the history behind these capacities. The infrastructure enabling medical tourism developed through national projects of governance in relation to global forces—economic nationalism, urban-centered development programs, and global capitalism. The navigation of geopolitics by public and private enterprises generated an interacting complex of sex work, medicine, and tourism that was a precursor to medical tourism. Thus, twentieth-century biopolitical projects concerning national well-being produced capacities used to provide biotechnological services to foreigners.

The emergence of "modern" medicine in Thailand reflects the shift in national governance in a global context: from sovereign royalty in a context of European imperialism to a bureaucratic polity navigating the hot wars of the cold war, to the managerial and CEO state characterized by public-private navigations of globalization. As with so many of Thailand's august institutions, medical facilities are credited to the initiative of the ruling nobility. The first hospital was founded by royalty on the grounds of an old palace, and the first medical school was the Royal Medical School. Individual members of the aristocracy are credited with advancing medicine, including both parents of the current king of Thailand. The king's mother, a commoner, studied nursing in Thailand (then called Siam) and the United States. Prince Mahidol, father to the current king, is dubbed "Father of Modern Medicine and Public Health of Thailand." His career coincided with early twentieth-century engagements of European resources to advance modernity and centralized rule in Siam/Thailand. He pursued military training in Germany and took up roles in the Siamese military and state before studying for degrees in public health and medicine at Harvard University in the 1920s. The relationship to the United States was integral to Thai medicine: Prince Mahidol enlisted the Rockefeller Foundation to finance medical and nursing education,[28] a project that aimed "to bring the medical school up to international standard," described in both physical and pedagogical terms:[29] "Major construction work began and many old wooden structures were replaced by concrete buildings. The medical curriculum was updated periodically, in keeping with the progress of medical science in the West."[30]

As the Thai state shifted from sovereign king to bureaucratic governance and military rule (which incorporated or alternated with popular democracy), narratives about royal involvement in Thailand's allopathic medical infrastructure remain part of the discourse about how the royal family nurtures the nation. Indeed, any description of the leading public hospital and medical school, or the large snake farm producing venom for rabies vaccines, highlights royal investments. The stream of reverently sentimental narratives about the royal deployment of international modernity for the well-being of the nation, including medicine, have helped reconfigure monarchy, and sovereignty, in Thailand.

As Thai governance shifted from monarchy to state bureaucracy governed by military dictatorships, the state used medicine in projects oriented to domestic well-being and also geopolitical security. The Southeast Asia Treaty Organization (SEATO), a transnational anticommunist alliance in which Thailand was a key Asian participant, created a medical laboratory in Thailand in 1959, as a response to the destabilizing threats of cholera epidemics. The SEATO lab later transformed into the Armed Forces Research Institute of the Medical Sciences (AFRIMS), a U.S. military enterprise that relies on Thai collaboration (it is housed in the Royal Thai Army Medical Center); AFRIMS is the largest of a global network of U.S. Department of Defense overseas biomedical research laboratories. With thirty field sites and an animal lab, AFRIMS conducts research on "infectious diseases of military importance," including HIV/AIDS.[31] This U.S.-Thai military institute also houses the largest medical library in Southeast Asia. Thus, the development of medical technologies in Thailand was part of military security in relation to regional and domestic threats. (The Thai state has used U.S. military investments to consolidate authority over its territory.) Military activity has been integral to advancing Thai medical technologies, including the skills used in elective cosmetic surgery. Thai plastic surgeons were produced during the Vietnam War, when the United States sent Thai doctors to America for specialized training.[32]

The consequences of the U.S. military presence in Indochina in the 1960s into the 1970s had other lasting effects. The abundance of American GIs at bases or in R & R sites led to sexual services that developed specifically for the military, practices tolerated (or encouraged) by the U.S. armed forces. Militarized prostitution, once in place, makes the health of heterosexual men a political concern—as much social history has shown, sexually transmitted diseases pose threats to military bodies. (AFRIMS investigates such diseases as AIDS, chlamydia, hepatitis, and herpes.) The state's response has often involved surveillance and regulation of female sex workers, usually through the domain of public health services.[33] The variegated Thai sex trade has, in fact, been articulated with the medical system since the Vietnam War. Indeed, when prostitution became illegal, albeit widespread, in the later twentieth century, the state regulated it through public health surveillance. Clinics conducted medical examinations for communicable diseases, and sex workers were recruited for protocols testing forms of contraception. In essence, then, it was the development of militarized sex work for foreigners that enabled the expansion of two key sectors relevant for medical tourism—public health and tourism.

Following the departure of U.S. troops from Thailand, state and private-sector efforts installed a large-scale tourist industry as a strategy of economic development. This collaboration expanded air travel, improved roads, and welcomed European hotels. By the 1980s, tourism brought more foreign currency into the country than agriculture. And where would Thai tourism be without sex work? The "nightlife" of former R & R sites of the U.S. military, like Bangkok and Pattaya, became a staple attraction not only for the infamous "sex tourists" but for other travelers. Guidebooks present it as one more part of local Thai scenery. Medical migration built on these flows, but also transformed them. For example, the gendered flows of businessmen and sex tourists from Japan, Korea, and the Middle East have been altered, perhaps even inverted, with the increased number of women travelers, or family visits, connected with medical tourism.

Sino-Thai firms spread wealth derived from agricultural enterprises into manufacturing and urban services. Their investment, coupled with Bangkok-centered policies, created an expanding urban class of male and female laborers. Workers in go-go bars represented one part of a stream of young people coming from the countryside, others of whom drove taxis, cleaned houses and offices, did light assembly in factories, or provided private security. Their work was subsidized by family farms, which took them back when they were unemployed or sick. To global investors, the business environment became characterized by graceful service, nimble handiwork, and limited union organizing. Tourism, linked with sex work, produced populations of workers skilled in deferential service for foreigners.[34] The traffic of country peasants to urban worksites ultimately supported flows of foreigners coming into Thailand for business, spiritual quests, pleasure, and eventually health care.

City and country presented challenges to Bangkok's rule, particularly the management of population growth and sprawling urban slums. The scope of public health programs extended beyond regulating sex workers to address a range of social effects of modernity. By the 1980s, Thailand was pronounced an international success story for population control, which was the World Bank's recommendation for it to achieve economic take-off.[35] These programs limiting population growth or curtailing sexually transmitted diseases had the effect of linking the health of Thai populations and foreign visitors to economic development. Investments in medical resources were also investements in domestic security in a number of ways, including controlling borders and remote regions. One example is the Thai military's collaboration with the U.S. military to support "syndromic surveillance" at Thailand's national borders[36] and on a medical civil assistance program (MEDCAPS).

In 1988, I attended the first Thai conference on AIDS, an event that expressed the different orientations of the medical establishment (however uneven their grasp of transmission, risk, and social categories) and other branches of the state, which at the time was concerned with the effects that HIV/AIDS would have on the tourist sector and on investments. HIV/AIDS became a specialized arena for medical care, government policy, and nongovernment organizations. Early on, some of this work was associated with gay male communities, and even as the epidemic became associated with heterosexual transmission, the global HIV/AIDS projects articulated Thai participants with international gay discourse.

The scope and skills of the medical profession that enabled medical tourism were in part produced through state interests in sexuality: in population control, regulation of sex workers, and containment of HIV transmission. The expansion of medical resources, the increased participation of Thai medical practitioners at international conferences, and the close links between economic development, marketing, and evaluations of Thai and foreign bodies all inform the medicalization of the tourist economy in Thailand. Another way to present this is to highlight the contributions of marginalized populations to the establishment of globalized biotech in Thailand: sex workers, the objects and agents of public health; Thai women who experimented with, and were used in experiments on, contraception; or gay men and NGOs that pushed the medical industry to develop better responses to HIV/AIDS.

In addition, Thais generated a demand for sex reassignment surgery (SRS, also known as gender reassignment surgery, GRS). For example, male-to-female *kathoey* (to use the Thai term) sought reconstructive surgery from the leading university's hospital in the late 1970s. Patients were for the most part Thai until the 1990s. Over time, particularly with the advent of transgender Internet communities, Thailand developed an international reputation among male-to-female (mtf) transsexual communities for sex reassignment surgery. One specialist now concentrates on foreign patients who come mainly from the United States and Japan.[37] Preecha Aesthetic Institute has conducted public demonstrations of mtf surgery for foreign surgeons and for international media.[38] Although in few numbers, some Thai ftm transsexuals have also sought the longer and more expensive surgery to become transsexual men and the Preecha Aesthetic Institute Web site includes a page for those seeking female-to-male surgery.

Demand for sex reassignment surgery, coupled with military-generated plastic surgery skills, produced the particular niche specialization, arguably the first of Thailand's biotech services to be globally competitive. In this way, deviant sex/gender subjects—Thai sex workers, HIV-positive (or at risk) gay men, kathoey, tom, and foreign transsexuals—cultivated the expertise that generated Thailand's comparative advantage in medical tourism.[39]

This brief sketch outlined the emergence of the infrastructural conditions, the capacities in tourism and health care that underwrote medical tourism. In this final section, I consider their assemblage into a strategic investment in global biotech as a way to address national crisis and foster national security.

Curing Crisis

Most of the 1990s were years of economic boom in Thailand. Opening the Thai financial market in 1992 allowed an influx of loans and short-term investments. The business class that managed and profited from global finance was made of established Sino-Thai family corporations with a history of advantageous connections to the political power structure and transnational relations with "foreign capital and trade/finance networks established outside of Thailand."[40] These kin-based corporations responded to changing political and economic conditions connected with globalization, and during boom years, expanded into retail, real estate, information technology, and in some cases, transnational medicine.

One of those old Sino-Thai family firms was the Sophonpanich family, which exemplified the postwar transition from Sino-Thai merchant communities to a consolidated capitalist class. The Sophonpanich family is behind a major Thai bank, Bangkok Bank.[41] In the 1980s, the family and bank created Bumrungrad Hospital as an investment; in 1989, the hospital became a publicly traded company, but the family and bank remain major shareholders.[42] From the start, Bumrungrad Hospital attracted foreign residents in Thailand. During my fieldwork in the early 1990s, this was the choice for health care for a number of my international acquaintances. Other Thai family firms invested in medical care as well. Nourished by the money streams of the 1990s, private hospitals blossomed, resulting in an abundance of private medical resources. The outlook for medicine as a mode of capital accumulation looked bright, and in early 1997, Bumrungrad undertook a major expansion, constructing a large new hospital in the center of Bangkok with more than five hundred beds and twenty-one operating theaters.[43]

By July 1997, a currency crisis began with Thai banks such as Bangkok Bank, and it expanded across the region, generating what was known as the Asian economic crisis (a crisis often described through medical metaphors of contagion, in a symbolic linking of bodily, national, and economic well-being). The crisis led to unemployment, business failures, and the fire sale of Thai enterprises. Banking and real estate crises were soon compounded by other challenges from the region, including SARS, avian flu, the 2005 tsunami, and violent conflict in the south of Thailand, now recast through a post-9/11 lens in terms of Islamic terrorism. These upheavals discouraged tourists from coming to Thailand, a downturn with significant effects in a country in which the spending of foreign travelers is a substantial source for national revenue. Well-heeled international visitors are a critical source of foreign currency and medical tourists, in particular, spend more than other visitors to Thailand. For private hospitals, this diminished traffic impacted revenue. In addition, Thais, facing financial difficulties, opted for state-run hospitals for their personal health needs over private ones. With an oversupply of empty beds, many private hospitals faced bankruptcy and downsizing.[44] Bumrungrad, having just expanded and relying on foreigners and Thais of the capitalist class, faced a particularly dire situation, as its major shareholder was a bank implicated in the crisis itself. These conditions created a classic crisis of accumulation for Thai capitalists and a situation of domestic instability that presented challenges to the Thai state.

In the aftermath of the crisis, with companies declaring bankruptcy or being bought by foreign investors, Thai enterprises looked for strategies to restore their viability. Bumrungrad was jeopardized as it lost middle-class Thai patients (its mainstay). The company chose a global strategy, intensifying the focus on foreign patients. In 1997 it launched a Web site that allowed users to search for doctors by specialty as well as nationality. It sent sales representatives to Asian cities and established "authorized overseas representative offices" in a dozen countries in Asia, as well as in Ethiopia, Canada, and Oman. It also expanded internationally by selling medical managerial services and investing capital in medical sites in Asia and the Middle East.

Following 9/11, Bumrungrad executives saw an opportunity, as elites in the Middle East were now uncertain about seeking health care in the United States. The hospital took out advertisements in Arabic newspapers in the region, worked with travel agents, and made arrangements for the Saudi Arabian government to direct patients to it.[45] Staff of Bumrungrad underwent sensitivity training about Islam. In addition to offering certified halal food, the hospital also installed a prayer room and offered prayer mats in rooms.[46] In this way, the security of Arab Muslims became a paramount concern for globally oriented biomedicine in Thailand at the same time that the Thai government stepped up militarized policing of Muslims in southern Thailand.

Inviting foreign patients from outside of the country required a concern with visas and immigration policies. Bumrungrad's Web site features a photograph of a signing ceremony with the commissioner of the Immigration Bureau and hospital staff, which marked a new program institutionalizing weekly visits by immigration officials to expedite applications for extensions of visas.[47] This arrangement, just one example of the public-private collaborations in this sector, converts state procedures for regulating national borders into a hospitality service for this new category of medical tourists. It also suggests that the orientation to global medicine in Thailand was not only the vision of Thai kin-corporate capital, but also a project of the entrepreneurial state.

The governmental role can be seen particularly through the figure of the postcrisis prime minister, Thaksin Shinawatra. A billionaire turned politician, Thaksin promised to chart a new course for Thailand using the know-how of a successful globetrotting tycoon.[48] Thaksin had the support of fellow business families, notably, the Sophonpanich family, major shareholders of Bumrungrad.[49] In a political trend that can be found across regions, Thaksin combined a (selective) proglobalization orientation with the cultivation of rural populism. He couched his campaign in nationalist aspirations, as indicated by the name of his political party, "Thai love Thai" (Thai rak Thai). Such nationalism included a capitalist nationalism, which meant supporting Thai businesses' engagement with global markets as a way to restore national economic growth. His nationalist, neoliberal populism addressed Thailand's political and economic troubles through dual commitments to Thai capital and countryside.

Thaksin's bifurcated agenda was concretely realized in public policies, most notably in a "dual track" for medicine comprised of privatized fee-based care and public state-funded care. The "populism" part of Thaksin's program was an initiative for universal health care[50] through a program charging Thai users a thirty-baht payment, roughly one U.S. dollar. The thirty-baht program, however incompletely realized, is said to have increased access to health care from 76 to 96 percent of the population.[51] It also injected state funds into the medical system as a whole. The thirty-baht program was supplemented by such policies as low-cost universal access to anti-retroviral HIV medications.[52]

The global track of Thaksin's bifurcated medical policies involved promoting Thai medical resources to international markets.[53] With a five-year plan reminiscent of earlier development plans, the government launched a project to turn Thailand into a regional medical hub, an Asian center of health care excellence. Providing medical services to foreign patients is categorized as a mode of export. The Ministry of Commerce's traveling exhibits to promote Thai exports included representatives of Bumrungrad. In 2002, Bumrungrad won the Prime Minister's Export Award for its success at recruiting foreigners. In this way, Thailand's dual track in medical care was offering both import substitution (the HIV medications) as well as export-oriented services (cosmetic surgery). As with export manufacturing, globalized medical services are seen as a technique to accumulate foreign currency and to drive economic growth. Medical tourism is widely acknowledged to be Thailand's strategic national response to competitive global conditions. (One international headline said, "Want to Fix Thailand's Ailing Economy? More Sex Change Operations!")[54] Medical tourism creates a zone of exception for tourists and corporations, similar to export processing zones. The Thai state underwrote the medical hub project, investing millions of dollars in it. Hospitals have been given inexpensive loans or tax breaks in order to purchase expensive technologies.[55] The government also subsidizes medical tourism by funding infrastructure, promotion, and training. A number of state agencies are involved, including the Immigration Bureau; in addition, the Tourist Authority of Thailand, the Export Promotion Board, and Thai consulates abroad cultivate the global demand for medical services in Thailand.

The collaborative state-corporate project to globalize Thailand's biomedicine has been a successful strategy for achieving economic growth and regional significance. Bumrungrad International is one of the best-known sites for medical tourism and a well-regarded "small-cap" investment sustaining impressive growth in revenues. While it faces competition from Singapore and India, Thailand is well established as a leading site for medical tourism, particularly for its specialties in cosmetic surgery. Medical tourism has been credited with "providing a windfall for the travel and hospitality sector,"[56] bringing in high-spending medical travelers from new areas. In this way, investments in biotech have helped restore national economic outlooks. Medical tourism has also generated a steady stream of positive publicity for the country, a relief after the representations of the Asian economic crisis, the tsunami, and SARS. Thailand's biomedical services, exported at home, offer a hold on future security by enhancing national development and advancing Thailand's position in the region.

At the same time, the effort to globalize Thailand's medical care has generated new problems. The dual track of public/private health care clearly creates a tiered medical system. In much public discourse, this dual track is often signified through nationality: it is portrayed in the contrast between high-tech medical care for foreigners and socialized medicine providing basic health care for Thai citizens. Medical tourism, moreover, gets equated with elective cosmetic surgery. The nationalist differentiation between elective care for foreign elites and routine care for Thais ignores the well-off Thais who are often the majority of private hospital patients. (It also neglects the health care available to other "foreigners"—the poor Burmese, Lao, or other migrants in Thailand.) The economic nationalism used to criticize Thaksin's dual-track health care policies resembles the post-1997 anti–International Monetary Fund nationalism that allowed the billionaire Thaksin to appeal to Thai capitalists and rural peasants alike and underwrote the regime that the Thai economist Pasuk Phongpaichit calls "neoliberal populism."[57] (Thaksin's corporate and political practices made him a controversial head of state and led to support for his ouster in 2006.)[58]

The investments in private hospitals, and the orientation to foreign patients, have exacerbated differences between public and private health care in Thailand. Thaksin's populist thirty-baht program increased workloads at state-run clinics, which was said to cause the flight of staff to higher-paying positions at private institutions, constituting an internal brain drain on the scale of the mid-century traffic of doctors to the United States. State-run hospitals tend to focus "on cost reductions, generic drugs and making limited investment in upgrading medical equipment," while the fee-based hospitals are "increasing capital, investing in new medical equipment and honing skills primarily to capture cash-rich patients."[59] According to the president of Bangkok Hospital, "privately owned hospitals would rather play a critical role in fulfilling the government's goal of becoming the regional medical hub, as they are more attuned to catering to international patients."[60] In this way, neoliberal health care of medical tourism contradicts the populist demands of universal health care. The biopolitical use of biotechnology to address economic crisis and secure political support is thus generating further economic and political challenges for the nation.

Many states are mobilizing biomedicine as a domestically based export in order to enrich a national economy's future. In Asia, these include India, Singapore, and Thailand; internationally, countries include various postcolonial, postsocialist, and postcrisis sites. Specific medical-tourist assemblages carve out specialty niches—cosmetic surgery here, dentistry there—but they also share features, notably, an emphasis on manifesting international (i.e., Western) standards and a history of leveraging knowledge, infrastructure, and labor generated through public health care systems to underwrite globalized and privatized medical services. These two shared features are linked: leveraging the "local"—instrumentalized versions of culture, inexpensive material and immaterial labor, contingent expert knowledges—is what allows Thailand and other sites to produce the universal elements, the gleaming biotech, five-star lobbies, and accreditation by global/Western standards. The history behind this process is a specific biopolitical history that is local, regional, and global. In the case of Thailand's medical-tourism assemblage, this history includes military medicine and public health and laboring bodies in tourism and sex work, and points to the role of kathoeys, toms, and sex workers—sex/gender deviants marginal to authorized national history and excluded from national futures in shaping the enabling conditions for Thailand's medical tourism project. Thailand's medical tourism is one of two national/medical/economic tactics in the aftermath of the Asian economic crisis; the other is domestic universal health coverage—and its prospects conflict with those of medical tourism. Through these intricate histories, Thailand's medical tourism offers one example of the ways that Asia is producing biotechnology's global futures.

Notes

I would like to thank Aihwa Ong, Chris Roebuck, and Elizabeth Roberts for encouraging me to write up the earliest phases of a new project. This essay was much improved by the assistance of Brian Carr, Alexis Gumbs, Kinohi Nishikawa, and Netta Van Vliet at Duke University. Although primarily relying on secondary sources, my discussion draws on long-term fieldwork in Bangkok, beginning in 1988 and most recently in 2005.

1. The major shareholders of Bumrungrad International are connected with the Bangkok Bank and the Sino-Thai family behind it, the Sophonpanich family. Bumrungrad's chairperson and director are from the Sophonpanich family as well. For information on Bumrungrad, see Center for Management Research (ICMR), *Bumrungrad's Global Services Marketing Strategy* (Hyderabad, India: ICFAI Center for Management Research Case Collection, 2003).
2. "Next-Generation Healthcare Comes to Life at Bumrungrad International Hospital," Motorola Media Center News, http://www.motorola.com/media center/news.
3. Discussions of global assemblage or global projects are predicated on critiques of frameworks that emphasize a binary, one-way flow between global and local scales. See, e.g., Aihwa Ong and Stephen J. Collier, eds., *Global Assemblages: Technology, Politics, and Ethics as Anthropological Problems* (Malden, Mass.: Blackwell, 2005); Anna Tsing, "The Global Situation," *Cultural Anthropology* 15, no. 3 (2000): 327–60; Saskia Sassen, *Territory, Authority, Rights: From Medieval to Global Assemblages* (Princeton, N.J.: Princeton University Press, 2006).
4. E.g., Tsing, "The Global Situation"; and Tim Choy, "Articulated Knowledges: Environmental Forms after Universality's Demise," *American Anthropologist* 107, no. 1 (2005): 5–18.
5. My use of infrastructure draws on work in science studies, for example, Susan Leigh Star, "The Ethnography of Infrastructure," *American Behavioral Scientist* 43, no. 3 (1999): 377–91. Star refers to the high-tech infrastructure of informational technologies, but her work in "structural inversion"—"foregrounding the truly backstage elements of work practice" (380)—and the work of other ethnographic analyses of science are helpful in thinking about the backdrop to Asian biotech.

6. Charoen Kittikanya, "Foreigners Still Flock to Thai Hospitals, Attracted by Highly Skilled Doctors and Lower Bills," *Bangkok Post* "Economic Year-End Review 2007," http://www.bangkokpost.com (accessed March 14, 2008).
7. The term "medical tourism" is misleading. Many object to the "tourist" label, because it appears to trivialize the medical concerns involved. Some have suggested "medical travel" as a substitute, but the phrase "medical tourism" has endured. Moreover, the term confuses identity and location. It applies to select relatively elite noncitizens, as opposed to noncitizen migrant laborers or refugees. The "medical tourism" term hinges on the identity of foreigner: in Thailand, of the non-Thai subject. The emblematic figure is the wealthy East Asian or Western (white) tourist who combines cosmetic surgery with recovery on a beach resort. But the category includes those who come primarily for specialized medical treatment, foregoing sunbathing, and also elite non-Thais who live in the region and seek medical care. (The term "expat" is a racial/national/class marker, distinguishing European or Western residents, documented or not, from less valorized migrant workers.) Many of those patients counted as "foreign" are actually residents of Thailand seeking routine health care. Also, the well-equipped facilities seeing well-off foreigners also see elite Thais, who can remain the majority of patients and income. Medical tourism might best be seen as elite global health care situated in the developing world. "Medical tourism" thus establishes a national/ethnic divide between medical care for foreigners and for "Thais," rather than a class divide. Although venues for medical tourism also serve Thai elites (and through charity work, nonelites), the phrase "medical tourism" differentiates a sector of health care defined by, and attributed to, foreigners (rather than a transnational elite class of medical consumers). For the purposes of this essay, I use the prevailing discourse that distinguishes a sector of the medical industry in relation to privileged foreign citizenship and currencies. However problematic, the construction of a medical tourist sector does highlight the place of the nation-state and national imaginaries in Thailand's embrace of biotech.
8. Molly M. Ginty, "Women Flock to Thai Hospital for Affordable Care," Women's eNews, http://www.womensenews.org/article.cfm?aid=2705 (accessed March 14, 2008).
9. The percentages of foreign patients in Thailand in 2007 were estimated as the following: Japanese 15 percent, U.S. 10 percent, South Asian 8 percent, Middle Easterners 8 percent, other Southeast Asian nationalities (from the ASEAN bloc) 6 percent.
10. Middle Eastern patients outnumbered Japanese in Bangkok Hospital in 2005: Tourism Investigation and Monitoring Team, "Opinion Divided over Benefits of Medical Tourism," *new frontiers* 12, no. 3 (2006); Third World Network Web site, http://www.twnside.org.sg/title2/nf123.doc (accessed March 14, 2008).
11. Sex reassignment surgeries are performed at a few sites in Bangkok and in

the beach resort areas of Phuket and Samui. A well-known plastic surgeon at the premier university hospital reported that he had conducted five hundred sex reassignment surgeries between 1980 and 1997; fifteen to thirty of those were female-to-male, all for Thai women. Aren Z. Aizura has done research on the sex reassignment surgery/gender reassignment surgery (SRS/GRS) field in Bangkok. See Aizura, "The Romance of the Amazing Scalpel: 'Race,' Labour and Affect in Thai Gender Reassignment Clinics" (unpublished manuscript, copy in possession of Ara Wilson); other sources include Mick Elmore, "Thailand's Plastic Surgeons Cut a Niche for Themselves," *International News*, Deutsche Press-Agentur, February 7, 1997 (printout in possession of author); Andrea Whittaker, "Pleasure and Pain: Medical Travel in Asia," *Global Public Health* 3, no. 3 (2008): 279; and "Thai Doctor to Open Sex-Change Surgery Clinic," International News, Deutsche Presse-Agentur, November 10, 1997 (printout in possession of author).

12. The greater expenses of medical care outside of Thailand are produced by structural adjustment and privatization of state services, pharmaceutical company strategies, intellectual property, and (at least in the First World) insurance industry profits.
13. The comprehensive exams include up to twenty-three procedures: physical, eye, pelvic exams; fifteen lab tests (including kidney function panel, thyroid panel, pap smear, tumor markers); and several other exams and tests (EKG, abdominal ultrasound).
14. "Thailand Offers Less Expensive Fertility Treatment, Preimplantation Genetic Diagnosis, Attracting 'Fertility Tourists,'" Kaiser Daily Women's Health Policy, http://www.kaisernetwork.org/Daily_reports/rep_index.cfm?DR_ID=38986 (accessed April 17, 2007). Spain also offers reproductive technologies that are less expensive than in the United States. Preimplantation genetic diagnosis (PGD) is used to determine the sex of the embryo and allow sex selection. The Thai Medical Council has advised Thai providers against offering PGD, but it is not illegal.
15. Charoen Kittikanya, "Dual-Track System," *Bangkok Post* "Mid-Year Economic Review 2004," http://www.bangkokpost.com/midyear2004/health01.html (accessed March 14, 2008). As noted, Thailand's comparative advantage with First World medical treatment depends not only on the cost of doctors but on the range of labor costs and availability of personnel (e.g., nurses) that constitutes quality care.
16. "BlueCross BlueShield and BlueChoice HealthPlan Pioneer Global Healthcare Alternative," BlueCross BlueShield Association, http://www.bcbs.com/news/plans/bluecross-blueshield-and.html (accessed April 17, 2007).
17. See "Thailand Offers Less Expensive Fertility Treatment, Preimplantation Genetic Diagnosis."
18. PlanetHospital, http://www.planethospital.com/?page=home (accessed April 19, 2007). PlanetHospital is a clearinghouse for medical tourism information, with an informational Web site and "concierge staff" in each country.

19. Ginty, "Women Flock to Thai Hospital."
20. "Bumrungrad Hospital and Naresuan University Sign MOU to Train Doctors," Thai News Online, http://www.tivarati.com/ (accessed March 14, 2008; no longer available).
21. "More than Just a Hospital—Bumrungrad Hospital Relaunches as Bumrungrad International," press release, http://www.free-press-release.com/news/200504/1112773662.html (accessed March 14, 2008). The change in the hospital's "identity," according to a press release, involved a foreign creative agency that "envisioned the rebranding as more of a brand elevation." The use of "international" reflected the corporation's diversification into hospital management in Bangladesh, Myanmar (Burma), the Philippines, and United Arab Emirates.
22. "Health in Thailand: What If I Get Sick?," Royal Orchid Holidays (Thai Air), http://www.thaiair.com/ (accessed March 14, 2008; no longer available). The numbers have increased at a high rate, from 630,000 visitors in 2003 to more than a million today.
23. "Welcome," Bumrungrad International Hospital, http://www.bumrungrad.com/ (accessed April 17, 2007).
24. Saskia Sassen highlights the diverse range of laborers who produce globalization. See Sassen, *Globalization and Its Discontents: Essays on the New Mobility of People and Money* (New York: New Press, 1998).
25. "Factsheet," Bumrungrad International Hospital, http://www.bumrungrad.com/ (accessed March 14, 2008; no longer available).
26. ICFAI Center for Management Research. *Bumrungrad's Global Services Marketing Strategy*, ICFAI Case Collection (Hyderabad, India: Institute of Chartered Financial Analysts of India Center for Management Research, 2003), 10.
27. Arlie Russell Hochschild, *The Managed Heart: Commercialization of Human Feeling* (Berkeley: University of California Press, 1983).
28. Prince Mahidol Award Foundation, "A Complete Biography of His Royal Highness Prince Mahidol of Songkla," http://www.princemahidolaward.org/complete-biography.en.php (accessed April 17, 2007).
29. Kanokporn Chanasongkram, "Siriraj Hospital Continues to Lead the Way in Healthcare," *Bangkok Post*, September 21, 2007. The article outlines a new cardiology unit in the hospital that offers tiers of service based on cost.
30. Ibid.
31. AFRIMS regional projects include a Global Emerging Diseases Surveillance system; a GIS biosurveillance infrustructure in the Philippines; and technical support for the Royal Thai Army's syndromic surveillance system on the Thai border with Burma, Laos, Malaysia, and Cambodia. AFRIMS runs thirty field sites in Thailand, Nepal, Cambodia, Vietnam, and Bangladesh. It also has a research animal facility accredited by the Association for the Assessment and Accreditation of Laboratory Animal Care, International. See the AFRIMS Web site, http://www.afrims.org, and U.S. Embassy, "US Army Medical Component of the Armed Forces Research Institute of the Medical Sciences," Em-

bassy of the United States, Bangkok, Thailand, http://bangkok.usembassy.gov/embassy/usamc.htm (accessed April 20, 2008).

32. Elmore, "Thailand's Plastic Surgeons." Thailand is also considered a "world leader in penis reattachment," attributed to the "numerous cases of wives and girlfriends mutilating partners by cutting off penises." See Chris Pritchard, "Want to Fix Thailand's Ailing Economy? More Sex Change Operations!" *Medical Post* (Canada) 34, no. 5 (February 3, 1998): 59.
33. On sex work, militarization, and medicine, see, e.g., Cynthia H. Enloe, *Bananas, Beaches, and Bases: Making Feminist Sense of International Politics* (Berkeley: University of California Press, 1990).
34. Ara Wilson, *The Intimate Economies of Bangkok: Tomboys, Tycoons, and Avon Ladies in the Global City* (Berkeley: University of California Press, 2004), chap. 2.
35. Population control was locally reconfigured as family planning at the same time it was applied with heightened vigor to sex workers, not as members of a family, but as risks to the nation, as vectors for infecting Thai men (and their wives) and foreign customers, which would damage the tourist economy.
36. AFRIMS brochure 2008, Armed Forces Research Institute of Medical Sciences, http://www.afrims.org/media/af-brochure2008.pdf (accessed April 18, 2008).
37. Aren Z. Aizura, "The Romance of the Amazing Scalpel: 'Race,' Labour and Affect in Thai Gender Reassignment Clinics," unpublished manuscript in possession of the author.
38. See the Preecha Aesthetic Institute Web site, http://www.pai.co.th.
39. On the impact of marginal communities on medical science in the United States, see, e.g., Joanne J. Meyerowitz, *How Sex Changed: A History of Transsexuality in the United States* (Cambridge, Mass.: Harvard University Press, 2002); Steven Epstein, *Impure Science: AIDS, Activism, and the Politics of Knowledge* (Berkeley: University of California Press, 1996); and Jennifer Terry, *An American Obsession: Science, Medicine, and Homosexuality in Modern Society* (Chicago: University of Chicago Press, 1999).
40. Akira Suehiro, "Capitalist Development in Postwar Thailand: Commercial Bankers, Industrial Elite, and Agribusiness Groups," in *Southeast Asian Capitalists*, ed. Ruth McVey (Ithaca, N.Y.: Southeast Asian Program at Cornell University, 1992), 41.
41. Chin Sophonpanich migrated to Thailand from China. He became a successful trader moving with ease among the overseas Chinese business communities in Hong Kong, Singapore, and Vietnam. Collaborating with other Sino-Thai traders in China as colonial European banks receded during the Second World War, Chin engineered a near monopoly on migrants' remittances back to China. His transnational projects evolved into Thailand's most powerful financial institution, the Bangkok Bank. He also formed strategic, mutually enriching alliances with the shifting military regimes (Pasuk Phongpaichit, "Thailand under Thaksin: Another Malaysia?" [Perth, Australia: Asia Research Centre at Murdoch University, 2004], http://wwwarc.murdoch.edu

.au/wp/wp109.pdf [accessed March 14, 2008]; and Chris Baker, *Thailand: Economy and Politics* [Oxford: Oxford University Press, 1995], 22–23, 125). Although the Bangkok Bank's relations to the state diminished as some of its functions were taken over by the Thai government from the 1970s onward, the bank parlayed its strength into influence in all economic arenas. It remained dominant by introducing new financial instruments, cultivating "modern" (though still heavily kin-based) managerial strategies, and opening overseas branches in Asia, Europe, and the United States (Suehiro, "Capitalist Development in Postwar Thailand," 62). For portraits of other Sino-Thai family firms, see Wilson, *The Intimate Economies of Bangkok*, chaps. 1 and 4.

42. Bumrungrad's Web site (http://www.bumrungrad.com) includes pages on investment relations and stock quotes, and offers e-mail alerts for announcements relevant to investors.
43. ICFAI, *Bumrungrad's Global Services Marketing Strategy*, 4.
44. Suwit Wibulpolparsert, "International Trade and Migration of Health Workforce: Experienced from Thailand," paper presented at the Joint WTO–World Bank Symposium on the Movement of Persons (Mode 4) under GATS, World Trade Organization, Geneva, April 11–12, 2008, www.wto.org/english/tratop_e/serv_e/symp_apr_02_suwit_e.doc (accessed March 14, 2008).
45. Kittikanya, "Foreigners Still Flock to Thai Hospitals." On Thai hospitals' arrangements with Saudi Arabia, see Petchanet Pratruangkrai, "Saudi Health Scheme Inked," *The Nation* (Thailand), http://www.nationmultimedia.com/2006/05/20/business/business_30004463.php (accessed April 30, 2007).
46. ICFAI, *Bumrungrad's Global Services Marketing Strategy*, 6.
47. G. Satish, "Thai Hospitals Take Professionalism in Medical Tourism to Another Level," Travel Video Television News, http://travelvideo.tv/news/more.php?id=A9299_0_1_0_M (accessed April 20, 2007). Visas are subject to differentials of labor and profession: not all nationalities qualify for visa extensions. The United States issued a memo to U.S. consulates to make additional inquiries about applicants for U.S. visas seeking medical care to ensure that their treatment and follow-on costs were covered. See Colin L. Powell, "Nonimmigrant Visas for Medical Treatment," U.S. Department of State, http://travel.state.gov/visa/laws/telegrams/telegrams_1533.html (dated November 1, no year specified; accessed November 5, 2006).
48. On Thaksin, see Wilson, *The Intimate Economies of Bangkok*, chap. 4.
49. Kevin Hewison, *Pathways to Recovery: Bankers, Business and Nationalism in Thailand*, Working Paper Series no. 1 (Hong Kong: Southeast Asia Research Centre, City University of Hong Kong, April 2001). However, not all of the Sophonpanich family supported Thaksin throughout his tenure. As a progressive Democrat M.P., Kalaya Sophonpanich criticized Thaksin's free-trade agreements, arguing that the U.S.-Thailand free trade pact allowed foreign advantage in medical domains (e.g., on patents for native herbs). See also Preeyanat Phanayanggoor Apinya Wipatayotin, "PM 'Failed to Consult the Public,'" *Bangkok Post*, January 9, 2006.

50. The universal thirty-baht program was provided through 1051 "service units" covering 46 million people. The 2004 budget allocated 1,447 baht per capita (15–17 billion baht overall); in 2005 it increased slightly to 1,500 baht per capita (Kittikanya, "Dual-Track System").
51. Ibid.; Arthit Khwankhom, "Bt30 Health Scheme Still Lacks Funds, Says Official," *The Nation* (Thailand), http://www.nationmultimedia.com/2006/07/14/national/national_30008668.php; and "Bt30 Health Fee May Be Scrapped," *The Nation* (Thailand), http://www.nationmultimedia.com/2006/10/13/national/national_30016065.php (accessed March 14, 2008). Populist gestures like the thirty-baht universal health care program targeted the long-term marginalization and discontent of people in the countryside. At the same time, medical and government authorities criticized the universal policy. It resulted in increased workloads for health care workers and was inadequately funded, said critics. For example, 2004 allocations for HIV/AIDS, drug addiction, and accidents were inadequate and were exhausted before the year was complete. The ruling junta of 2006–7 continued the populist promise while criticizing Thaksin's scheme as a ploy to curry favor.
52. HIV/AIDS rates of infection appear to be in decline in Thailand. Despite the availability of the "cocktail" medications, there is concern that agreement to free market policies with the United States would eliminate the low-cost generics.
53. The government set aside 2.6 billion baht (Charoen Kittikanya, "Health," *Bangkok Post* Economic Year-End Review 2004, http://www.bangkokpost.com/ecoreviewye2004/health.html [accessed March 14, 2008]).
54. Pritchard, "Want to Fix Thailand's Ailing Economy?"
55. The Thai state provides "necessary funds in order for it to stay ahead of competition from rival companies, especially Singapore" (as well as tax exemptions for imported equipment). Kittikanya, "Dual-Track System," 3.
56. Tourism Investigation and Monitoring Team, "Opinion Divided over Benefits of Medical Tourism," *new frontiers* 12, no. 3 (2006), Third World Network Web site, http://www.twnside.org.sg/title2/nf1123.doc (accessed March 14, 2008).
57. Pasuk Phongpaichit, "Thailand under Thaksin: Another Malaysia?" (Perth, Australia: Asia Research Centre at Murdoch University, 2004), http://wwwarc.murdoch.edu.au/wp/wp109.pdf (accessed March 14, 2008).
58. Prime Minister Thaksin was ousted by a military coup in September 2006, replacing the CEO state with an updated version of the militarized state bureaucracy. The explicit reasons for his ouster were corruption and profiteering, especially from the sale of his company to a Singapore government investment company, Temasek (which also bought shares in Bumrungrad International around the same time).
59. Kittikanya, "Dual-Track System," 2.
60. Ibid.

STEFAN ECKS

Near-Liberalism | GLOBAL CORPORATE CITIZENSHIP AND PHARMACEUTICAL MARKETING IN INDIA

While doing research on pharmaceutical uses in Kolkata in 2005, I had the opportunity to take part in a "depression awareness workshop" organized by the Indian branch of the world's largest pharmaceutical company, Pfizer Inc. Invited to the workshop were twelve general physicians who had private chambers in an upwardly mobile area of South Kolkata. The event took place in the back rooms of a fancy restaurant and lasted for around three hours. After a brief welcome, Pfizer representatives showed a fifteen-minute teaching video. Then a buffet lunch was served, lasting for about forty-five minutes. Afterward, a Kolkata psychiatrist gave a PowerPoint presentation on the epidemiology of depression and on the best available treatments (which happened to coincide with Pfizer's brand of sertraline). This was followed by a teaching session with diagnostic case studies. Based on patients' answers to a questionnaire, the GPs were asked to identify which patients should be labeled with "MDD" (major depressive disorder) and be given antidepressants.

The stated aim of this workshop was not to advertise Pfizer's products, but to teach the GPs on how to use a particular diagnostic questionnaire, called PrimeMD Today™ (PrimeMD is the abbreviation for Primary Care Evaluation of Mental Disorders).[1] Pfizer suggests that this questionnaire be given to patients in the waiting room and be filled in by them before they speak to the doctor. Together with the patient, the doctor would then go over the answers and make a diagnosis. The video that opened the workshop showed that leading American psychiatrists developed this questionnaire in order to "enhance the ability of busy physicians to diagnose mental health problems." Because GPs were heavily pressured for time, they needed a "quick, easy to use" diagnostic tool to figure out if a patient should be given antidepressants. PrimeMD promised to give them an "advanced algorithm" with which a diagnosis would not take longer than one or two minutes. The Pfizer material stressed the pivotal role of GPs in the global fight against depression: most patients' first point of contact were GPs and other nonspecialists, but since they often did not recognize depression, it remained heavily undertreated. The video underlined that "depression *should* and *can* be treated by GPs" and called on the doctors to use it daily: "Believe it or not, it is easy to learn, and you can diagnose depression in less than one minute." The video went on to state that PrimeMD, while based on American diagnostic criteria, was now also available in eleven Indian languages (Hindi, Marathi, Bengali, etc.). Translations were tested with three hundred patients in each language to adjust them perfectly to local idioms.

One of the case studies enacted in the video is the story of Mrs. Rao. A general physician introduces Mrs. Rao as a patient who is "not well educated." She has to support the whole family because her husband is an unemployed alcoholic. Mrs. Rao complains of backaches and headaches and has previously undergone an operation. When the GP gives Mrs. Rao the PrimeMD questionnaire to fill in, he detects an "underlying depression." The video shows how the doctor and the patient interact (slightly abridged here):

> PAT: What is the cause of this?
>
> DOC: We will come to that. First let's go over some of your answers in the questionnaire. . . . You are not feeling so well . . . you are responsible for the whole family. . . . I think your symptoms are caused by depression.
>
> PAT: No, no, no! I just have a headache! I am not going mad!
>
> DOC: You are not going insane. Depression is treatable. It will take six months to cure.
>
> PAT: Six months! Oh no! A few days, and I will be all right.
>
> DOC: Depression is a medical condition. You wouldn't let a medical condition go without treatment, would you?

The fictional patient, despite being resistant to a depression diagnosis, is being educated by her physician and made to understand that her problems did not come from her family problems, but from depression.

The message conveyed by the video is that the GPs' educational mission is greatly enhanced if an awareness-raising questionnaire like PrimeMD is put at the center of the doctor-patient encounter. Moreover, Pfizer claims not to push as many pills as it can, but to be a "good citizen" and to fulfill a public service by raising awareness about medical conditions. In the teaching video, a voice-over states that "Pfizer's commitment goes beyond developing effective therapies. The company works closely with patient groups and opinion leaders to increase awareness, as well as creating disease management programs. Part of this program is the development of one diagnostic tool, PrimeMD Today."

While enjoying a plate of Bengali curries with the other doctors after the first part of the workshop, I thought I was witnessing a moment of what Clarke and colleagues call "biomedicalization": a process of turning patients into flexible, self-caring health consumers who are able and willing to buy all the latest pharmaceuticals.[2] Whereas old-style medicalization was driven by the state, continuing processes of *bio*-medicalization presented a different situation. In line with neoliberal transformations of society at large, biomedicalization was shifting the governance of health from the domain of the state into the domain of corporations and self-responsible individuals. A reformulated imperative to "know and take care of thyself" biomedically was creating new "technoscientific identities." Biomedicalization is defined, to use a term defined by Michel Foucault, as a form of governmentality: a comprehensive set of techniques aimed at regulating and optimizing the "conduct of conduct" of both populations and of individual selves.[3] Biomedical governmentality captures "particular kinds of power often guided by expert knowledge, that seek to monitor, observe, measure, and normalize individuals and populations."[4]

At first sight, PrimeMD seemed like a good example of such biomedical governmentality. Instead of targeting doctors only, Pfizer aims to involve patients on a new level of self-responsibility. Doctors are told not only to give pills but to raise awareness among patients as well. The educational mission was not driven by the state but by capitalists: disease-conscious people promise to be better customers for the pharmaceutical industry. In short, PrimeMD appeared to exemplify an emerging "neo-liberal consumer discourse that promotes being 'proactive' and 'taking charge' of one's health."[5]

But what was said at the workshop *beyond* the teaching video put all this into question. In his lecture, the invited Kolkata psychiatrist told the GPs that they *might* try giving the questionnaire directly into the hands of patients, but that this would cause more problems of patient resistance than necessary. Hence his advice was not to hand out the questionnaire, but to leave the diagnosis entirely with the doctor. The psychiatrist's recommendation did not raise any eyebrows among the Pfizer representatives present. Indeed, the psychiatrist's whole performance was put on stage by them: they had supplied him with the PowerPoint presentation upon his arrival at the venue and during the first part of his talk he did nothing other than read out bullet points. Their tacit consent to the psychiatrist's advice was further reaffirmed when I asked one of representatives if he had a Bengali version of PrimeMD with him. He said that he did not bring any versions, because giving the questionnaire into the hands of patients was not really the point of PrimeMD. Patients might use the questionnaire in irregular ways, misunderstand it, and even misdiagnose themselves. Besides, he said, PrimeMD was a "strictly scientific" tool for diagnosis, and as such only meant for doctors, not for patients. In other words, Pfizer's PrimeMD was *not* about letting patients know and take care of themselves.

But why does Pfizer go through all the trouble of devising this questionnaire, translating it into eleven Indian languages, and testing it with 3,300 patients, but then neither makes it available to patients nor encourages the doctors to do so? Is Pfizer's talk of educating patients only a façade, nothing but corporate PR? Or were only a few isolated Indian marketing representatives sabotaging the agenda set by Pfizer's American headquarters? PrimeMD could be easily criticized either as brainwash (of consumers) or as whitewash (trying to "look good" in annual reports). But as I want to argue here, it is important to take the invocation of "good citizenship" seriously and to look at its implications.

Global Near-Liberalism

Pfizer says that "patient-focused health information" increases patients' own abilities to prevent and manage disease. To educate patients —both those currently ill and those potentially ill—about diseases and available drug treatments is part of Pfizer's corporate strategy, and global corporate citizenship (GCC) is the general header under which this is now grouped. Since the values of good citizenship are seen as universal, they apply to Asia just as much as to Euro-American countries.

Global corporate citizenship is a recent avatar of corporate social responsibility (CSR). To understand a company as a "good corporate citizen" has been part of CSR programs all along, and substantial differences between GCC and CSR are hard to spot.[6] Indeed, these two terms are still used more or less synonymously.[7] But over the past years, many companies found the language of "citizenship" more appealing than that of "social responsibility." A move from CSR to GCC is also noticeable in the publications of international lobby organizations. For example, CEOs from sixteen countries signed the first agenda for GCC at the World Economic Forum 2002.[8] Academic research is trailing this trend; for example, a *Journal of Corporate Citizenship* was launched in 2001. In business studies, GCC is described as the highest level of corporate ethics, transcending the mere "egoism" of pure market competition.[9]

Pfizer's U.S. Web site states that "citizenship defines our role in local and global communities and how we strive to conduct business responsibly in a changing world." Pfizer sees GCC as a dialogic engagement, as "listening to, understanding, and responding to our stakeholders about their needs." This engagement takes several forms. The company works with NGOs to hear their concerns about Pfizer's international operations. The Pfizer Medical Humanities Initiative conducts town hall meetings across the United States to find a "balance between humane care and scientific expertise." Pfizer points out that it is the first (and only) U.S.-American pharmaceutical company to join the United Nations Global Compact, a collaboration of governmental and nongovernmental organizations that endorse human rights, fair labor relations, environmental sustainability, and corruption-free business. According to Kofi Annan, former secretary general of the United Nations and one of the organizers of the Global Compact, the goal is "to unite the power of the market with the authority of universal ideals."[10] By signing the compact, Pfizer committed itself to ten principles of good citizenship. The first two principles relate to human rights. Principle 1 is that the company will "support and respect the protection of internationally proclaimed human rights"; principle 2 is that the company must be "not complicit in human rights abuses." The other eight principles relate to good labor standards, the environment, and anticorruption measures.

Concerns about "society," "rights," and "responsibility" are present in all the company's national Web sites, but with different emphases on GCC. The Canadian Web site focuses on "corporate philanthropy." Pfizer UK uses the term "corporate responsibility." The German branch translates "corporate citizen" literally as *Unternehmensbürger* and states that the company wants to be a trusted partner for multiple stakeholders. The French site underlines that Pfizer is an *entreprise solidaire* (yet does not declare itself as a corporate *citoyen*). Despite these divergences, "good citizenship" is the cardinal rule for all the company's global employees.

Pfizer India focuses less on individualized citizenship than on the company's "constructive interaction with society." These interactions were not just about "providing access to medicines," but also to give "support to patient groups," "providing health literacy," "spreading disease awareness," and "building communities." In recognition for its work, the Federation of Indian Chambers of Commerce and Industry awarded Pfizer India a "Certificate of Commendation for its social responsibility efforts."

The "citizen company" seems to contradict current critiques of neoliberal capitalism. David Harvey holds that neoliberals try to make personal freedom dependent on markets and to reduce elected governments to an apparatus whose sole mission is to "facilitate conditions for profitable capital accumulation."[11] For Pierre Bourdieu, neoliberalism is "a programme for destroying collective structures which may impede pure market logic."[12] It tries to cut out "social realities" to give business free rein in all spheres of life. Instead of social collectives arriving at consensus decisions that benefit all, neoliberal capitalism spreads a new "moral Darwinism" that rewards winners and discards losers. But instead of being the *opposite* of neoliberal capitalism, as Harvey and Bourdieu suggest, I would argue that corporate citizenship is a novel form of reconfiguring profit maximization through notions of "citizenship" that had previously been either neutral or even inimical to free-market capitalism.

Corporations have strong reasons to portray themselves as global citizens. Being good and asking for something in return is easier in a language of "citizenship" than in one of "social responsibility." Whereas CSR implies duties without rights, "citizenship" lets a company appear as good without forgetting its own benefits. A definition of GCC as "listening" to stakeholders also means that businesses want to be listened to in return. Good citizenship can yield good economic profits. The simplest is that a convincing program of GCC inspires consumer loyalty. Interacting with potential critics and pressure groups serves as an early warning system to avoid damage to a company's reputation.

GCC aims to boost the standing of Big Pharma among both citizens and national governments to justify demands for industry-friendly regulations.[13] For example, pharmaceutical lobbies are arguing that restrictive regulations are causing a dangerous bottleneck of innovative drugs reaching the market. Companies estimate the cost of developing a new drug at U.S. $800 million (although critics put the figure at below half of this). High costs and fewer successes are used to demand an increase in public-private partnerships. A Brussels-based association called Emerging Biopharmaceutical Enterprises (EBE), which represents sixty-five global biopharmaceutical companies, asks the European Union for an "improved climate of innovation."[14] One of EBE's goals is to receive funding for pharmaceutical R & D within European Union funding schemes. It is a bold move for an already profitable private industry to lay claim to public research funds. The language of "corporate citizenship" is part of a strategy to make such requests more plausible.

There has always been a tradition in anthropology to show the diversity of values. Some recent writings try to shift the focus from cultural relativism toward exploring how the "conceptual lucidity, simplicity, and universalism" of rights become a fulcrum for social movements today.[15] This is a fruitful approach, but it overlooks the fact that the simplicity of rights is obscured once powerful players, such as corporations, also lay claim to them. This is what is happening to "citizenship": already a perplexing notion, corporate claims to global citizenship make it even fuzzier.

From a historical perspective, the corporation was always already some sort of "citizen" with global aspirations. From its inception, the capitalist corporation had ambitions for worldwide reach. Marx and Engels saw this clearly when they described how constantly expanding markets force capitalists to "nestle everywhere, settle everywhere, establish connections everywhere."[16] Further, the emergence of the modern business corporation in the nineteenth century was made possible by an extension of citizens' rights into domains previously reserved to individual persons. The corporation required a notion of "juridical personality" to let it assume a legal standing similar to a private individual, with the rights to hold property, to enter into contracts, to be taxable by the state, to sue and be sued in court. Thus the corporation was from the start a "global citizen," though only in relation to the right to earn and possess private property worldwide.

That corporations pursue profits is not new. But what is new is that corporations do not appeal only to the right of private property, but also to what T. H. Marshall[17] called the "social rights" of active and equal participation in the wider community.[18] The usual counterpart of these social rights is the nation-state. However, GCC makes no reference to nation-states. It is framed entirely on the supranational level. GCC often appeals to "local communities," but the values it propagates are cosmopolitan. The Global Compact, as signed by Pfizer, is under the auspices of the United Nations and national governments are no more than miscellaneous "partners."

At the same time, GCC is introduced as an entirely voluntary act of kindness. It remains unclear what legal mechanisms would apply if a corporation broke any of the principles it had underwritten. Within the boundaries of nation-states, corporations can be sued for breaking national laws. But the legal commitment in being a global corporate citizen is minimal, if not absent. This is very different from being a "citizen" in the usual sense of the word, whose rights and duties can be enforced by the state.

These ambiguities partly disappear once the corporation is not seen as a citizen, but as its counterpart: a state. Probusiness theorists see the rise of GCC as part of a shift in how governments run public services. In times when national administrations are reluctant to provide welfare and ensure social rights, corporations are taking on some of their responsibilities: "As one of the actors most central to globalization . . . corporations have tended to partly take over certain functions with regard to the protection, facilitation and enabling of citizen's rights."[19]

GCC aims to be both "global" and "corporate." It is a type of governance that is not defined by control over a territory, nor is it exercised by a body that represents a political constituency. One way to understand this is through the concept of "transnational governmentality" developed by James Ferguson and Akhil Gupta.[20] By applying Foucault's notion of governmentality to transnational and nongovernmental domains, they describe how NGOs and supranational organizations take over functions for which previously only national governments would have been held responsible. In a similar vein, I would describe GCC as a form of transnational governmentality through which private corporations fashion themselves as "citizens" to open new terrains of government. GCC draws on established norms and forms of citizenship and statehood, yet reinscribes them in new ways.

That GCC is a way of governing people is most obvious in its application *within* companies. In a survey of CEOs of global companies, 90 percent of respondents named "communicate values internally" as the best implementation of GCC, far ahead of other uses.[21] Klaus Leisinger, president of the Novartis Foundation and a special adviser on the U.N. Global Compact, points out that GCC is introduced by a company's top management and is then implemented throughout all levels of the company "through normal corporate-management processes, from individual target setting to performance appraisals to compliance management to auditing to reporting."[22] The conduct of conduct stipulated by GCC policies should not be understood as superficial "icing on the cake" of real-world business. GCC can only be successful if its principles are turned into individual performance targets. To make salaries and promotions dependent on citizen-like conduct shows that GCC is a form of government *internal* to business organizations.

But GCC is a form of governmentality that reaches beyond corporate boundaries. The inclusion of nonbusiness "stakeholders" is critical for its legitimacy. This is a two-way process. On the one hand, those outside of corporations who enter into GCC alliances have to agree to many of its forms of governance. On the other hand, these nonbusiness allies must not be fully subsumed by corporate interests, as this would undermine the purpose of the project. The whole point of a corporation adopting a GCC regime is to let it appear as a good citizen *among* other good citizens. This cannot be achieved without recognition from those other citizens. Even if it coopts others, it must still appear as a fellow citizen.

GCC cannot be successfully contained within corporations, since its goals are oriented toward standards defined *outside* the business domain. This is most evident in discussions about how to audit GCC compliance. To verify a company's good financial bookkeeping, the usual auditing firms might be employed. But to let business auditors inspect human rights standards lacks credibility. In turn, human rights organizations do not have the required auditing capacities. More to the point, nongovernmental organizations, such as Amnesty International, would probably be unwilling to become a Pricewaterhouse-Coopers of Human Rights Auditing.

In response to this, human rights institutes are trying to fill this gap. For example, Novartis is working with the Danish Institute for Human Rights to develop a compliance assessment that covers core areas of the GCC agenda.[23] The institute's Human Rights Compliance Assessment (HRCA) comes in the form of computer software that assesses human rights compliance along one thousand indicators.[24] It asks questions such as "Does the company have mechanisms for hearing, processing, and settling the grievances of the local community?" It then gives scores for various levels of compliance and prompts corrective actions. It is likely that these not-for-profit types of audit will develop a competitive market similar to the competition between national drug approval agencies.[25]

With its emphasis on "compliance," it seems that GCC aims at establishing a uniform code of behavior within corporations and beyond. It appeals to universal values and claims to apply them in all countries. But I would argue that GCC, as a form of neoliberal governmentality, is *not* about normalizing individuals and populations across the globe. Rather, it is a way of creating *difference*. GCC is an example of what Aihwa Ong calls "neo-liberalism as exception."[26] Ong analyzes the emergence of new alignments between business and politics that are "neither state nor market."[27] Corporations that subscribe to GCC seek to draw on the credibility of nonbusiness allies. Corporations do so most successfully if they do not aim at "normalizing" its collaborators.

Some passages from Michel Foucault's little-known work on neoliberalism are helpful to understand this. From 1978 to 1979, Foucault delivered a series of lectures on "the birth of biopolitics" at the Collège de France.[28] For the most part, these talks analyze different forms of liberal and neoliberal forms of government. In the lecture of March 12,1979, Foucault discusses whether neoliberalism is a form of normalization. Contrary to the kinds of positions that most anthropological writings take as Foucauldian, in this lecture Foucault points out that neoliberalism does *not* aim at normalizing or disciplining people.[29]

It does not target inner selves, but regulates the structure of incentives on which actors base their decisions. Neoliberalism replaces forms of *inner* subjectivation (*assujettissement interne*) with interventions that target actors' external environment (*intervention de type environnemental*). It fosters different and irregular ways of behavior because it sees this as the best way to exploit hidden opportunities. As Foucault explains, neoliberalism fosters minority views and leaves fields of action in a state of oscillation. Because of this, neoliberal society is *not* a social order where "the mechanism of generalized normalization and the exclusion of what cannot be normalized is required."[30]

Foucault's analysis brings out nuances in neoliberal governance that have received little attention yet. To put even more emphasis on the difference-making power of neoliberalism, I suggest calling it by another name: "near-liberalism." The term stresses the oscillating form of neoliberalism in several ways. Near-liberalism emphasizes that freedom, emancipation, and autonomy are always held out as future goals, even if they are not yet realized in the present. It suggests that neoliberalism is not a uniform practice, but that it tends toward nearness and local differentiation. It also accentuates that neoliberalism can switch to restrictive modes of governing at any moment. Near-liberalism is not a program to get rid of the social and political from the sphere of economics, but one that seeks to produce new alliances between markets, states, and citizens. These alliances need to remain as flexible as possible, to allow moving into new directions at once, and to allow severing ties from stakeholders that have become liabilities. Near-liberalism tends to promote biomedicalization, as described by Clarke and colleagues, but it is not shy of suspending notions of patient "awareness" and "self-responsibility" if need be. To show how near-liberalism allows corporations to form flexible alliances with dissimilar outside actors, I want to return to Pfizer's depression awareness workshop.

Pharmaceutical Near-Liberalism in India

What goal is Pfizer pursuing with its workshops on "depression awareness"? Pfizer is an established company in India. With drug sales of over U.S. $100 million in 2004, Pfizer is India's second-largest pharmaceutical multinational corporation after GlaxoSmithKline. This total, however, is still small compared to sales by Indian companies. For example, the Indian company Ranbaxy sold over eight times more medicines (U.S. $823 million) in 2004 than did Pfizer India.[31] The drug advertised to the doctors in the Kolkata workshop, sertraline HC (Indian brand name Daxid), has fierce generic competition, which makes brand building difficult. There are at least thirty brands of sertraline available in the Indian market, making it impossible for Pfizer to demand high prices (indeed, Daxid is cheaper than some of its generic competitors, e.g., Torrent's Serenata and Ranbaxy's Serlift). The relative weakness of the Daxid brand partly explains why awareness workshops aim less at pushing this particular brand as opposed to growing the market for antidepressants more broadly.[32] Inviting local doctors over for a meal and a chat is primarily meant to build good relations with them.

The conventional wisdom held by the World Health Organization is that there is a large "treatment gap" between developed and less developed countries in regard to mental health treatments.[33] The WHO assumes that doctors in developing countries do not yet know much about mental health problems and mostly misdiagnose mental problems as physical ones. Indian newspapers frequently make the same point. For example, almost daily a suicide is reported, and often "unrecognized" and "untreated" depression is presumed to be behind it. A recent article on depression in the Kolkata newspaper the *Telegraph* (March 2, 2008) quotes an associate professor from the All India Institute of Medical Sciences: "Depression is grossly underdiagnosed and undertreated in India."

This line of argument is actively promoted by drug companies. As is pointed out in Pfizer's PrimeMD information pack, general physicians "fail to diagnose and treat 50–75% of patients suffering from common mental disorders" because of their "inadequate knowledge of the diagnostic criteria." This rather aggressive statement was not repeated verbally in the workshop for the Kolkata GPs, but the underlying message was still clear: the first group that needs better education about depression are the general physicians, not (yet) the patients. All information about PrimeMD—as being developed by cutting-edge American psychiatrists and so on—suggests to the local doctors that they need to prescribe far more antidepressants in order to catch up with global standards. PrimeMD subtly promises to turn them into "world-class" diagnosticians of depression. Pfizer wants to train them without confronting them openly about their alleged lack of knowledge. At stake in Pfizer's depression awareness workshop is the "global citizenship" of Indian doctors, not yet the inclusion of patients.

If the Pfizer workshop officially aims at aligning its citizenship project with that of Kolkatan doctors, what is the reason for unofficially discouraging them from using PrimeMD? To answer this question, it is necessary to separate the views of psychiatrists from those of GPs. As the theory of "biomedicalization" would lead one to expect, it would surely be in the interest of both the pharmaceutical industries *and* the doctors that patients become cued into mental health problems and become more willing to be treated. As I want to argue in what follows, psychiatrists do indeed share Pfizer's agenda of patient education—but not GPs. The success of Pfizer's workshop lies in speaking to the interests of both groups of doctors.

Kolkatan psychiatrists are aligned with Pfizer's GCC agenda, especially its drive to raise disease awareness among patients. Let me quote, as an example, a Kolkata psychiatrist whom I interviewed in 2005. When I asked him about what should be done most urgently in Indian psychiatry over the next few years, he stressed the need for much greater public awareness of mental disease and for a transformed perception of psychiatry: "What has not yet come to India is the transformation from patienthood to personhood. I would like to see that more and more people come to psychiatry saying: 'I want to function at my best, I want to contribute my best, so tell me: in what way can I make improvements? What nutrition do I require for my brain, and what do I require so I can give the best to my family, my society, my country?' "

In this statement a specific coconstitution of pharmaceuticals, citizenship, and Indian nationalism is formulated. Taking psychotropic drugs is framed not just as a right, but as every Indian citizen's *duty*. The low demand for psychotropics in India—compared to Western countries—is turned into a call for a utopian politics of national development *and* self-development, through drugs. For this psychiatrist, psychotropics should be used like food supplements, not only to treat disease but to become "better than well." And the aim should be not to think just of individual betterment but of the improvement of the whole country.

Even if these views seem excessive, this particular doctor is one of the most influential psychiatrists in Kolkata. He is the founder of the city's first so-called NGO for mental illness awareness, a place where patients come together to talk about their problems in the fashion of Euro-American self-help groups.[34] The terms "NGO" and "self-help" should be taken with caution, as his organization is directly funded by pharmaceutical companies. For this doctor, India is poised to enter a new era of medicine and citizenship, an era in which the taking of neuropsychiatric substances should become just as much the duty of the good citizen as the sharing of food is the duty of every good member of a family. As one of the doctor's assistants asked me rhetorically: "Why be opposed to brain nutrients?"

While none of the other psychiatrists with whom I talked was quite as ambitious as this doctor, they all agreed that more mental health awareness was needed. At the most minimal level, this meant that every patient prescribed with antidepressants should be told about depression and why medication was needed. Once patients had taken the difficult decision to go to a psychiatrist, there was no stigma attached to hearing the diagnosis.

Like other doctors, psychiatrists look at patients from their specialized viewpoint, so they tend to discourage patients who believe that their problems are *not* psychiatric. For example, one of the most common forms of experiencing and expressing distress in Bengal is to complain about one's stomach and digestive problems. Here is how one of the psychiatrists phrased it: "In our culture, most problems are tummy-related problems: 'I don't get a clear bowel movement.' This is, I think, a state characteristic of Bengalis. If you ask someone in the morning, 'How are you?,' the first thing he will say is 'I didn't get a good motion this morning.' Or he is looking very satisfied: 'Yes, I got a good motion in the morning.'"

All the psychiatrists pointed out that "gas" and other digestive problems were such common symptom presentations that they tended to disregard them altogether. When I observed a psychiatrist in an outpatient clinic in Kolkata in 2005, a forty-five-year-old man came and complained about various bodily problems, above all about a twitching feeling around his navel. During the ten-minute consultation with the doctor (who gave him a depression diagnosis), the man pointed to his tummy almost throughout, saying that the pain goes here, then there, then goes up, and so on. When I later asked the psychiatrist if this patient's digestive problems were relevant for the diagnosis, he said plainly "no": "This is just obsession. It is nothing." And although he did not take this particular patient very seriously, the psychiatrist informed him about his diagnosis and treatment. It is fair to say that psychiatrists see their relations to patients as hierarchical, and do not usually look at them as "equal citizens." All the same, their specific position in the medical field makes it more likely that they will inform patients about depression than nonspecialists. Hence their idea of educated health citizenship and that of the drug companies are not too different.

That still leaves the question open why both the Pfizer representatives and the lecturing psychiatrist discouraged the GPs from using PrimeMD. As discussed earlier, the psychiatrist told them that using the PrimeMD questionnaire might cause trouble with patients. But this advice hardly taught the GPs anything that they did not know before. It rather reaffirmed what they were thinking about the questionnaire from the start of the workshop: that it is impossible to use it as envisioned by Pfizer. Far from handing out a questionnaire with depression symptoms directly to patients, the GPs do not only leave "education" out of their consultations: they prefer to tell their patients nothing at all. When I interviewed GPs, they said that they told their patients *neither* that they had been diagnosed with depression *nor* that the prescribed pills were antidepressants. It was common opinion among them that patients had too many superstitions about psychiatric disorders to make it possible for them to talk straight with them. Giving a depression diagnosis "upset" patients for no good reason and made them hesitant to take the drugs prescribed to them. The situation shown in the Pfizer video, of Mrs. Rao getting offended by being told that she was suffering from depression and that she had to be on medication for a long time, resonates with the GPs' experience, except that they tend to go into the exact opposite direction from the doctor shown. Instead of confronting patients, trying to educate them, or even handing out questionnaires to them, the doctors avoid any mention of "depression" or "antidepressant." Otherwise they risk to become known as a "mental" prescriber. Being seen as a *pagoler daktar* (Bengali for "madman's doctor") would mean losing precious clients. Private GPs are directly dependent on patients' fees, paid in cash after the consultation. A doctor who unnecessarily "upsets" patients risks losing them to competitors. Mrs. Rao's shock at the news that she is supposed to take pills for at least six months echoes patient fears of side effects, high costs, and the suspicion that biomedical drugs only suppress symptoms but do not cure the underlying causes.

Faced with such resistance, the GPs have various strategies to prescribe antidepressants without telling patients openly about them. The most common is to highlight physical symptoms of depression, such as sleeping too much or too little, having too much or too little appetite, and so on, and then telling patients that these pills make them sleep well, or increase their appetite. To quote from one of the GP's replies: "No, I don't tell my patients, they take it very badly. Let's say someone [with depression] is suffering from insomnia, then I say: take this for insomnia."

When I asked the GPs why they were not telling their patients about antidepressants, they often argued that it was impossible to treat Indians like Europeans or Americans. They said that India is a developing country and that Indian patients were different. Western-style standards of informed consent could not be applied. Another line of argument taken by the GPs is that the relation between themselves and their patients was strictly hierarchical. This hierarchy was constructed in filial terms: just as parents should treat their children *as* children, for their own good, so should the doctors treat their patients as children. Those who suffered from depression, especially, simply did not have the same amount of insight and knowledge as the doctors. A third line of defense voiced by the GPs was that going into long and adversarial discussions with their patients is a waste of time. They saw their role in prescribing drugs, not in educating patients. Trying to argue with them was seen as a disservice to all others waiting to be treated. In a context of limited time and resources, the GPs implied that it was unfair toward other patients to spend too much time with any one individual. Everyone had to pay the same fee for a medical consultation. If a doctor spent too much time with one, it ate into the time for all others. Therefore, not arguing with depressed patients was constructed as an act of fairness toward all other patients.

Most GPs mentioned that the introduction of SSRIs (selective serotonin uptake inhibitors) during the 1990s shifted prescriptions of psychiatric drugs from specialized psychiatrists to general practitioners. The GPs said that with previous forms of psychotropics, it was difficult to get the dosage right. SSRIs, by contrast, were "easy" and "safe" to prescribe.[35] But apart from therapeutic reasons, the GPs also have tangible economic benefits from telling patients as little as possible while prescribing as many pills as possible. The main one is that they can directly earn from prescribing antidepressants. A patient on antidepressants is expected to be buying medicines for several months, if not years. That is why these drugs can be very profitable for companies, and in return, pharmaceutical companies reward doctors for such prescriptions.

In India, pharmaceutical companies systematically monitor the prescription patterns of individual physicians through, for instance, quizzing staff in medicine shops. Depending on what kinds of drugs they prescribe and how many, they get classified as, for example, "A" (high) or "B" (low) prescribers. Those in the "A" category are rewarded with gifts, travel, and consumer commodities. As some doctors told me, there are many instances when a company offers to give them money for prescribing a higher number of its products. The few regulations that exist to curb such complicity between prescribers and the industry are never enforced.[36]

With more producers going into the psychopharmaceuticals market, there is now an intense competition for market share, and more money is lavished on Indian doctors than ever before. While the biggest benefits are earned by high-volume prescribing psychiatrists, GPs are also benefiting from this shift. That a company like Pfizer gives so much attention to antidepressants is just one symptom of this. And these marketing efforts have not been in vain. When I asked the GPs to how many of all their patients they were giving antidepressants, many of them said "up to 20 percent," and that they "routinely" prescribed these drugs to certain categories of patients, especially the elderly and those suffering from chronic and incurable diseases. Indian GPs have become ready prescribers of antidepressants.[37]

But the GPs' idea of citizenship does not entail engaging patients as informed equals. This is why the Pfizer representatives did not care to bring copies of the PrimeMD questionnaire to the workshop: they knew that the GPs were not interested in using them. Seen superficially, it looks as if PrimeMD, and with it Pfizer's agenda for global corporate citizenship, is failing in India. What happens instead is that Pfizer's representatives make deliberate exceptions from the global principles to accommodate Indian doctors' preference for keeping their relations with patients free from patient awareness. That the marketing reps of Pfizer India exempt the GPs from using PrimeMD shows how global corporate citizenship is a flexible regime of governmentality that works on outer incentives rather than on inner normalization. It allows adjustments and realignments whenever it seems fit. It can do so best if liability remains with self-responsible "stakeholders" rather than within corporations. Near-liberal corporate citizenship can excuse its participants from the agreed rules at any moment and endorse doctors that have no time for "patient empowerment" of any kind.

Notes

1. PrimeMD is also the template for the self-evaluation questionnaire on Pfizer's Web sites; see http://www.zoloft.com/ (accessed March 13, 2008).
2. Adele E. Clarke, Janet K. Shim, Laura Mamo, Jennifer R. Fosket, and Jennifer R. Fishman, "Biomedicalization: Technoscientific Transformations of Health, Illness, and U.S. Medicine," *American Sociological Review* 68 (2003): 161–94.
3. Michel Foucault, "Governmentality," in *Essential Works of Foucault, 1954–1984*, vol. 3: *Power*, ed. James Faubion, ser. ed. Paul Rabinow (New York: New Press, 2000).
4. Clarke et al., "Biomedicalization," 165.
5. Ibid., 181.
6. Grahame F. Thompson, "Global Corporate Citizenship: What Does It Mean?" *Competition and Change* 9 (2005): 131–52.
7. "Corporate citizenship" and "corporate responsibility" are the most commonly used terms, but there are many similar terms, e.g., "corporate social performance," "business citizenship," "business ethics," "stakeholder management," "stakeholder relationships," or "stakeholder engagement."
8. See https://members.weforum.org/pdf/ppp.pdf, p. 3 (accessed March 13, 2008).
9. Thomas Donaldson, "Decompacting the Global Compact," paper presented at the All-Academy Symposium, "The Global Compact: Building Corporate Citizenship in a World of Networks," at the 2002 Academy of Management Conference, Denver, Colo., August 12, 2002.
10. See the United Nations Global Contact Web site, http://www.unglobalcompact.org/ (accessed December 12, 2006).
11. David Harvey, *A Brief History of Neoliberalism* (Oxford: Oxford University Press, 2005), 7.
12. Pierre Bourdieu, "Utopia of Endless Exploitation: The Essence of Neoliberalism," *Le Monde Diplomatique*, December 1998, http://mondediplo.com/1998/12/08bourdieu (accessed January 15, 2008).
13. John Abraham and Graham Lewis, "Citizenship, Medical Expertise and the Capitalist Regulatory State in Europe," *Sociology* 36 (2002): 67–88.

14. See the Emerging Biopharmaceutical Enterprises Web site, http://www.ebe-biopharma.org/ (accessed March 13, 2008).
15. Mark Goodale, "Ethics, Human Rights, and Anthropology," *American Anthropologist* 108, no. 1 (2006): 26.
16. Karl Marx, and Friedrich Engels, *Manifesto of the Communist Party* (1848; Chicago: Encyclopedia Britannica, 1952), 421.
17. Thomas H. Marshall, "Citizenship and Social Class," in *Citizenship and Social Class*, ed. Thomas H. Marshall and Tom Bottomore (1949; London: Pluto, 1991).
18. The history of corporations is *also* a history of corporate welfare. The world's first welfare housing estate, the Fuggerei in Augsburg (Bavaria, Germany), was founded in 1521 by the head of the Fugger bank and still exists today. So it is not a new phenomenon that businesspeople hand out money for social welfare. What is new about GCC is the integration of "doing good" into daily business procedures and a systematic blurring of the boundaries between corporate "gifts" and "commodities"; see Stefan Ecks, "Global Pharmaceutical Markets and Corporate Citizenship: The Case of Novartis' Anti-cancer Drug Glivec," *BioSocieties* 3, no. 2 (2008): 165–81.
19. Dirk Matten and Andrew Crane, "Corporate Citizenship: Towards an Extended Theoretical Conceptualization," Research Paper Series 4 (Nottingham: Nottingham University Business School, International Centre for Corporate Social Responsibility, 2003).
20. James Ferguson and Akhil Gupta, "Spatializing States: Towards a Study of Transnational Governmentality," *American Ethnologist* 24 (2002): 981–1002.
21. World Economic Forum and The Prince of Wales International Business Leaders Forum 2003, http://www.weforum.org/pdf/GCCI/Findings_of_CEO_survey_on_GCCI.pdf (accessed March 13, 2008).
22. Gautam Kumra, "One Business's Commitment to Society: An Interview with the President of the Novartis Foundation for Sustainable Development," *McKinsey Quarterly* 3 (2006). See http://www.mckinseyquarterly.com/article_abstract.aspx?ar=1820&L2=33&L3=117 (accessed March 13, 2008).
23. Ibid.
24. See Institute for Human Rights, Human Rights Compliance Assessment, https://hrca.humanrightsbusiness.org/ (accessed March 13, 2008).
25. Abraham and Lewis, "Citizenship, Medical Expertise and the Capitalist Regulatory State."
26. Aihwa Ong, *Neoliberalism as Exception: Mutations in Citizenship and Sovereignty* (Durham: Duke University Press 2006).
27. Ibid., 21.
28. Michel Foucault, *Naissance de la biopolitique: Cours au Collège de France, 1978–1979* (Paris: Gallimard/Seuil, 2004).
29. Thomas Lemke, "The Birth of Bio-Politics: Michael Foucault's Lectures at the Collège de France on Neo-Liberal Governmentality," *Economy and Society* 30 (2001): 190–207.

30. Foucault, *Naissance de la biopolitique*, 265 (my translation).
31. Ernst & Young [Ernst & Young Global Limited (EYG)], "Unveiling India's Pharmaceutical Future," *Health Sciences Industry Report 2005* (London: EYG, 2005), 6 and 9.
32. For an analysis of how marketers try to expand the reach of SSRI antidepressants in Japan, see Kalman Applbaum, *The Marketing Era: From Professional Practice to Global Provisioning* (New York: Routledge, 2004), 61–66.
33. World Mental Health Survey Consortium, "Prevalence, Severity, and Unmet Need for Treatment of Mental Disorders in the World Health Organization World Mental Health Surveys," *Journal of the American Medical Association* 291 (2004): 2581–90.
34. See, for example, Emily Martin, *Bipolar Expeditions: Mania and Depression in American Culture* (Princeton, N.J.: Princeton University Press 2007).
35. Indian doctors' "strategic ignorance" regarding the safety of antidepressants also echoes complex alliances between prescribers, companies, and regulatory agencies more generally. See Linsey McGoey, "On the Will to Ignorance in Bureaucracy," *Economy and Society* 36 (2007): 212–35.
36. For similar findings in Argentina, see Andrew Lakoff, "The Private Life of Numbers: Audit Firms and the Government of Expertise in Post-Welfare Argentina," in *Global Assemblages: Governmentality, Technology, Ethics*, ed. Aihwa Ong and Stephen J. Collier (Malden, Mass.: Blackwell, 2005).
37. For a further analysis of general practitioners' prescriptions of antidepressants in India, see Stefan Ecks, "Three Propositions for an Evidence-based Medical Anthropology," in "Objects of Evidence," ed. Matthew Engelke, special issue of *Journal of the Royal Anthropological Institute* (2008): S77–S92.

III

COMMUNITIES OF FATE

VINCANNE ADAMS, KATHLEEN ERWIN, AND PHUOC V. LE

Governing through Blood | BIOLOGY, DONATION, AND EXCHANGE IN URBAN CHINA

Imagine being offered a cash payment of up to 20 percent of your monthly salary and a week's paid vacation at a resort in exchange for a 200-to-400-milliliter blood donation that takes about thirty to sixty minutes? Now imagine that this compensation is paid for by your employer rather than by the blood bank where you make your donation. Imagine this, and you gain some sense of what occurs in urban Shanghai as a result of China's bold national effort to increase its supply of safe, transfusable blood. China has had much to overcome in this campaign. Traditional notions of blood as a vital essence tied to *qi* (spirit or energy), and publicity campaigns revealing the unfortunate spread of HIV by way of paid donation centers, have both worked against efforts to ensure an adequate supply of safe blood. Today, however, more and more people—particularly young urbanites—are convinced that donation is harmless to their health and, more important, an act of altruistic patriotism. The success of blood donation public health campaigns is interesting not simply because the campaigns reveal the process through which traditional cultural perceptions can be either transformed, ignored, or accommodated with behavioral change but also because they reveal forms of biopolitical governance that may be peculiar to China as it transforms itself from a planned socialist economy to a free market system. Donations of blood, and the goods and benefits that follow in the wake thereof, tell us much about China's sociopolitical transformations.

What, then, might be said of these transactions that compensate donors so generously for their sacrifice of a few hundred milliliters of blood? In this essay we argue that this transaction reveals a biopolitical logic; it offers a glimpse of the unique condition of modernity in China, in which reciprocal obligations between citizens and the state are managed in and through blood. It also articulates the problematic relationship between the privatization of the economy, exemplified in commercial blood donation practices that have been authorized by an emergent biotechnology sector, and citizens who are ambivalent about these transformations. Blood donation that is compensated, but not commercialized, is seen as the ideal form of citizen participation in a national program of modernization—in fact, a biotechnological and biopolitical triumph. At the same time, this "altruistic" and "patriotic" donation of blood is also, as we will see, richly compensated.

The first and most obvious way to understand this logic is for what it says about how the state—as manifest in the form of the *danwei*, or work unit—disciplines its subjects, by transforming suspicious citizens into willing donors of what they view as their "vital essence." Governance is made possible through this practice. But it also offers a unique way of reading the "other side" of biopolitics, in the inscriptive practices that transform a notion of blood in relation to family, lineage, spiritual essence, and life forces into a set of transactional contracts with the welfare state. This politicobiology—the scripting of biology by politics—works to ensure that citizen subjects are able to extract the promise of (the) return gift(s) from the state by way of the work unit (an institution of governmentality writ large). Our analysis suggests that biotechnological modernity can be enacted in many different forms, often peculiar to the political and social histories where it is emergent.

Biopolitics and History in China

Biopolitics, by now a widely understood concept thanks to the work of Michel Foucault and others identifying the key organization and institutional arrangements of modernity,[1] refers in our usage to the conditions of modernity that enable governance to devolve from institutions of police and the monarchial "state" to institutions that govern by way of tactical knowledge of the self. Through these discursive institutions—institutions that form the modern state as an "order of things"—people who aspire to "the good life" become the foundation for a disciplinary nexus that ties governance to regimes of desire rather than of coercion or force. The emergence of biopolitical forms of governance is generally associated with the rise of modernity and the simultaneous rise of two intersecting axes along which power manifests.[2] These axes, one biopolitical and the other anatamopolitical, attend to different aspects of modern life. The first concerns population-level interventions and conceptualizations of the social and is enacted through public policy, welfare programs, and the informational systems that are deployed from them. The second concerns new ways of conceptualizing and engaging the subject as an individual—subjectivizing processes that shape notions of the self and how one should want to behave. Foucault originally identified the two of them as operating together in a grid of "biopower." In this essay, we refer to this grid as the "biopolitical."

Scholars who write about the rise of a biopolitical sphere in China have been generally concerned with understanding how China offers unique insights about both modernity and the cultural specificity of subjectivity.[3] China's unique forms of communist-socialism provide interesting deployments of governmentality by way of the government-supported "work unit," which is in distinction to other forms of governmentality that, by definition, function outside the formal sphere of the state (in academic, medical, and scientific settings, for example). China's tumultuous history of effective engineering to create political economic reform—from the Maoist revolution, to the Great Leap Forward, the Cultural Revolution, and the current efforts to build a market-socialist political economy—make China's modernity different from the modernities of Europe and America in part because of the unique subjectivizing processes that these reforms have demanded and that have all invariably been tied to state practices and institutions. Nevertheless, even given these differences, it is possible to talk about modern forms of governance in China as "biopolitical."[4] In this essay, therefore, we mean to trace the meanings of the biopolitical in China, and its antecedent notions of a biological self, in the practices of blood donation.

We also note that the debates about blood donation in China are situated within larger international debates over blood donation, the social production of trust,[5] and the ethical problematics of reciprocity in commercial transactions involving bodily tissues as well as intellectual property.[6] In China, as we will see, commercial transactions involving blood were identified early on as a source of contamination and therefore a site for the production of suspicion and mistrust.[7] China's official response to this, the outlawing of commercial sale of blood in the case of whole blood used in transfusions, was an attempt to align Chinese blood donation practices with those recognized in the international community as the only "safe" way to produce uncontaminated blood—that is, through unpaid, voluntary, altruistic donations.[8] However, as we show below, this was only partially successful. The ways this policy has played out in practice among Shanghainese citizens, for example, is revealing in what it can tell us about forms of specific governmentality by way of the production of "trust."

Blood and Blood Donation in China

Consider for a moment some of the ways that contemporary Shanghainese talk about traditional ideas of blood:

> Female blood is given by God (laughs). Because traditional Chinese notions are deeply rooted that men are not to give blood, [because it] is seminal blood and precious. One old saying says that the male body is not to be given out or exchanged even for gold.[9]

> "One drop of semen equals ten drops of blood." Yes, I have heard of this saying. It is to warn males to control their desire, that it is bad to have an excessive sex life. It means that semen is precious. It takes ten drops of blood to make one drop of semen.[10]

> Semen is the vital essence of men, and so is blood. Both are too precious to lose much of. If you do, your health is impaired. Most emperors died at early ages. They had many concubines besides an official wife. This [early death] may be due to the high frequency of sex in their lives, which affects health and longevity. This is told and passed from generation to generation. I'm not sure if it's scientifically correct, but it is spread and accepted among Chinese.[11]

In an article on the subject, Kathleen Erwin presents a range of cultural concerns that influence contemporary Chinese notions of blood, and particularly the ways it is viewed as a vital bodily essence, similar to qi.[12] She notes that these concerns have shaped urbanites' willingness to consider blood donation, which has contributed to a general reluctance to donate it, even when blood donations are mandatory. Moreover, she notes, China's public health efforts to stem the spread of HIV, the rising incidence of which had been implicated in practices of blood selling, may also have influenced people's willingness to donate. Based on preliminary research, her work explores the contours of blood selling compared to voluntary yet compensated donation. Erwin focuses on how the commodification of blood, like other body parts and fluids, might be understood as a continuum, in which "selling blood" is at the extreme end rather than existing as a separate unit.

Our analysis here explores the ways in which exchanges in and around blood in China can provide insights into Chinese biopolitics, where forms of governance have shifted radically over two to three generations but constitute, as Erwin notes, a circulatory system of exchange to which blood flow can be likened. What is at stake in the giving and selling of blood, in this analysis, is not what it says about bodily commodification as an inevitable outcome of modernity, but rather what it can tell us about biopolitical governance in a rapidly transforming state. In this view, the question of what blood can do for the body, the family, and the larger community is replaced by the question of what blood can do for the citizen, the work unit, and the nation and, in turn, what they can do for the citizen. First, in order to set the stage for our discussion, we explore how blood is understood in this conceptualization, in relation to family, semen, lineage, and health.

Blood and the Family

In traditional Chinese medicine, blood is considered a vital essence, ensuring overall health of the body.[13] Its connection to the other vital essences such as qi or *jing* (semen) is well developed. Healthy blood is seen as contributing to the cultivation of healthy semen; healthy semen, in turn, ensures the longevity of the family. The medical anthropologist Arthur Kleinman links the fear of semen loss among urban Chinese to physiological stress, neurasthenia, and weakness.[14] One of our informants explained to us the connection between blood and semen: loss of either can lead to weakening of the vital essence: if a man emits too much semen, it depletes his body of energy, just as if he had lost blood. The traditional saying "Ten drops of blood equals one drop of semen" was explained by informants like this:

> This [saying] refers to the relationship of blood and semen. *Jing* may refer to the spirit of a person and it is linked with blood. We say, "A

> flourishing qi and blood make a person fit." [To call someone] a healthy person means that he or she has healthy blood, which leads to good semen. Taking blood out of the body can affect the semen.[15]

> It refers to the fact that semen and blood come from the kidney where *yuan qi* resides. Once taken away, human health is deeply impacted and cannot be regained. But, we know that scientifically this cannot be explained.[16]

Other informants tied blood weakness to seminal weakness in relation to traditional sociopolitical formations, as did the informant quoted earlier, who noted that most emperors died at early ages, perhaps due to the "high frequency of sex in their lives." She also noted:

> Now blood donation is encouraged. A normal and appropriate frequency of sex is fine. Excessively high or low is harmful to health. This is how ten drops of blood equals one drop of jing.[17]

Here, preservation of the family and the lineage, and the paternal concern for self-discipline in this process, reveal interesting links among conceptions of the role of semen in preserving not just individual but also social health by way of the family and the blood lineage. Blood strength requires conservation of the semen, and strength of the semen is tied directly to health of the blood.

Because of blood's importance to individual and family health, there is a large repertoire of nutritional and medicinal supplements known to boost blood: red bean paste, pig's liver, red dates, chicken or duck soup, *xue er* (a kind of albumin), lotus seeds, longan, walnut, black sesame, and a *jiao* (donkey skin) boiled with walnut and sesame. If the preservation of semen, and thus the lineage, is the responsibility of the father, then the replenishment of blood in order to make the semen strong is delegated to the mother. We found that informants talked about the maternal role of nurturing in this life-sustaining and regenerating effort as equally significant to the role of the father. Ideas about maternal nurturing are often couched in discussions of food preparation and particularly the preparation of replenishing foods that were specially bought and prepared for children who donated blood. Mothers cooked good foods for their husbands and children to ensure their strength. One informant talked about how she often bled excessively during her menstruation and her mother always prepared extra-nutritious and blood-replenishing foods during her periods to help her: red dates, chicken and duck soup, pig's liver.

In a culture that places such high value on the preciousness of blood, it is not surprising that efforts to generate voluntary donations of blood among the public have met with some resistance. In fact, the history of blood donation in China suggests that this resistance had to be actively managed and overcome. Citizens were not asked to donate voluntarily during the early days of the revolution and socialism; they were told to donate as a mandatory or compulsory requirement of the state. Citizens were asked to overcome their fears of blood donation and believe that donations of blood would keep the nation strong. They were asked to adopt a patriotic attitude about their obligatory blood donation and to set aside or erase their traditional fears and beliefs about blood. What was important, however, was that citizens felt the need to be rewarded for this sacrifice.

Our elderly informants talked about the early days, and what it used to be like:

> My parents didn't allow me to donate blood. They thought blood donation would injure qi. I saw people donate blood and they were fine, so I had no such thought. I am a party member, and I should donate blood actively. At that time, people went to donate blood by work number. They thought blood donation was a big deal, and could affect health. My parents cried when I went to donate blood. They thought of me as an unmarried girl. I lived in a convalescent home for one week after donating blood. You could choose to rest at home, but my parents were both workers and they had no time to look after me. They thought I worked hard in the textile mill and told me to have a good rest. During that time, they came to see me and brought me nutritious food. Some people got fat after blood donation, but it was not the fault of blood donation. They had eaten too much after donating blood.[18]

> During the Cultural Revolution, my work unit was organized to give blood regularly. The work unit was Food Shop of North Station. We got 50 yuan annually, donating blood once every two or three months. We donated quite frequently over a period of a year. We were organized to go traveling afterward for four to six days. The money was for compensation, but the holiday was to restore

health. . . . I managed the manufacturing, and I was the assistant of the workshop director. The workers went to donate blood based on their job number, but we could not just tell them to donate blood. We went first, [but] I was not qualified. . . . The factory prepared the tonics and money to pay the workers. We Ningbo people steam red dates, red beans, and walnuts [to replenish the body]. We cook soybean curd with a little steamed food [nutritional tonics]. The blood station gave a bottle of milk and two cakes. At the time nothing was compensated. Honestly, we had high morality. Nothing was compensated for us except for 300 renminbi [yuan]. We went to donate blood voluntarily, and we did not care about the money. . . . [However] even if you gave 300 renminbi, [some] people would not donate blood. Though 300 renminbi was not a small amount in the 1980s. Workers from textile mills were rich then. They did not think much of 300 renminbi; they thought 200 milliliters of blood was more valuable. [This informant also took three paid days of rest vacation.][19]

I was required to donate blood; I didn't propose it myself. The blood center assigned the quota to each unit, and people donated blood at a certain ratio. Most people didn't want to donate blood, so the unit leader took out the roster; you would go if it was your turn. If five persons were needed, then number 1 to number 5 would go. If the five persons were qualified, it was done; if two of them were unqualified, the next two would go until the number was enough. I donated blood because it was my turn. To tell you the truth, I was afraid of blood donation.

(What about compensation?)

Compensation? The blood station gave us a glass of milk, a cake, and a little money, not much, less than a hundred. The work unit gave me more, 400 renminbi for 200 milliliters of blood, and 800 renminbi for 400 milliliters blood. I donated 200 milliliters and got 400 renminbi. The vacation was also determined by the blood volume, generally seven to fourteen days. I rested for seven days. There was no food or drugs. When I rested at home, my work unit sent people to visit me, to check whether I was uncomfortable, how I was recovering. They bought fruits for me and told me to eat certain nutritious foods. There was no traveling just after blood donation,

> but after a period, if there was convalescence quota, they would choose you first. I went for convalescence after blood donation.[20]

The mechanisms used by the state to increase the blood supply were wrapped up in a complex set of sentiments about one's obligation to the state and what the state, in turn, was obligated to do for the donor. Early on, Mao called for citizens to donate blood as a patriotic act, which he did while using metaphors of blood as a vital essence for a healthy society.

> During the Cultural Revolution we believed in Chariman Mao, who said that Party disciplining was like blood circulating, needing to be metabolized. So, now I think taking a few hundred milliliters of blood is just fine.[21]

At the same time, it was understood that citizens should be compensated for their blood donation. The act of donating was scripted as an act that enabled one to fulfill an extraordinary obligation demanded by society, but it was also an act that enabled the donor to gain symbolic rewards by being patriotic. The fact that the donors were compensated with money and leave time was not, we were told by our informants, what motivated donors. The true compensation was a way of ensuring health, of replenishing those who sacrificed for the good of the nation. These patriotic gestures were thus different from those that Richard Titmuss observed among British or American blood donors, whose acts of donation to the complete stranger were, for him, true gifts given with no expectation of any return. Referring to the British and American voluntary blood donors, he writes, "As individuals they were, it may be said, taking part in the creation of a greater good transcending the good of self-love. To 'love' themselves, they recognized the need to 'love' strangers."[22] He noted, however, that such altruism was only possible in a state, such as the United Kingdom, that had institutional means of caring for the welfare of all. The National Health Service played an important role in ensuring altruistic donations that were considered valuable only if they were uncompensated. Lawrence Cohen also notes this for India, in the case of organ donation, in which the exchange of body parts reveals the ethical reinforcement of social ties between people.[23] People show their care for one another, and the success of the social unit, by way of altruistic giving.

In China, notions of "the gift" are almost always explicitly embedded in expectations of reciprocity, whether the gift is given to a known individual, or to the greater society. And while uncompensated donation is held as an ideal form of patriotic generosity by the government itself (whose policies strive to achieve an entirely uncompensated donation system), we found that compensation—or what is understood as the state's obligatory reciprocation of this valuable gift—is inextricably woven into donation, largely because this is how notions of citizenship are and have been defined in China.[24] The best kind of blood donation is a willing fulfillment of an obligation that will rightfully be reciprocated through, in this case, some form of compensation.

The obligation to give blood by way of the work unit in China creates the cultural space within which citizens are able to give, not "altruistically" in the sense used by Titmuss, but "patriotically." Compensations that follow in the wake of this patriotic giving are thus best seen as a form of reciprocation between citizen and the state. Reciprocation by way of blood donation should, in other words, be understood not as a coercive form of socialist governmental control over its citizen-subjects, but as an expected fulfillment of the state's obligation—as well as caring—for its subjects (or in the case of the work unit, its workers). This is how nearly all informants saw it:

> Blood donation is a personal matter. It's voluntary and obligatory with no payment, instead of being duty. Once a person is forced to do something, he will never do that again in a lifetime. To promote voluntary blood donation and set up positive notions are key issues to benefit the society and [foster] social harmony.
>
> (Should donors be compensated?)
>
> I think it's necessary. It shows care and concern for employees and their welfare on the part of the company. The significance is valuable, compared to its actual worth. Donors get social respect.
>
> (What compensation is appropriate?)
>
> All sound good. It's great to get each. One week for rest, a trip to a near place. As for money, it's different in each company—1,000 yuan in a working unit, 100 to 200 in a school; if the unit is financially strong, 3,000 to 4,000 is also possible.[25]

Embedded in this type of donation are foundational ideas about what it means to be a good citizen, and this, we feel, achieves a sort of biopolitical perfection. The citizen sees this service to the nation as what defines his/her patriotic citizenship. Compensation, however, is often a focus for donors, even when there is vocal opposition to the idea that compensation could be the motivation for giving. That is, money and leave time are not seen in any way as gestures meant to "pay" donors for their blood. "Blood selling," we were told, is entirely different. Compensated, obligatory, yet altruistic donations are understood as a means through which the state or work unit expresses its caring and reciprocal obligation to its citizens for their contributions to meeting society's need (for, in this case, blood).

> If you lived at home, you would get more money. For example I got 100 renminbi, and our unit also gave the convalescent home 100 renminbi, which was to cover my meal fees. If you lived at home, you could get 200 renminbi. My unit would pay the bed fee and service charge. We had free travel, and I have been to Mogan Mountain for a period of time after giving blood. These are not compensations. It is promoted that blood donation should be voluntary. These are prizes for the donor; it would be different if they were called compensations. I think caring is important, when leaders and colleagues come to see you. It is a kind of spiritual consolation. I don't donate blood for compensations. I go when I am needed.[26]

> A relatively longer rest allowance plus financial compensation are appropriate. The longest official holiday is seven days in our country, so the rest allowance can be doubled to fourteen days. Donors can use the compensation money to travel. Work units stand for the country. Donors would feel happy being cared for by the country. If donors are only allowed to take two days leave from work with as little as 100 yuan [in compensation], they may refuse to donate again and tell others not to do so. All in all, good compensation would ensure a better achievement for blood donations.[27]

The type of transaction these informants described for us is an embodiment of the socialist state, where governance is organized as a reciprocal exchange between citizen and state, by way of the work unit. As one informant told us about the act of blood donation, "It is a civilian obligation. Everyone is I and I am everyone."[28]

The Shanghainese we spoke with frequently pronounced that giving blood was an act that enabled them to be even better citizens.[29] The fact that blood was considered valuable and that one is put at risk by donating only made this act even more significant as a way to show extraordinary patriotism. Some people talked about going out of their way in order to donate, even when they were offered a chance to avoid doing so. It was an act of "glorious" patriotism. Sometimes, this zeal to be a patriotic donor was expressed in relation to the idea that compensation was not necessary, even though recognition for one's generous act was.

> Rich people do charity. I'm not that rich, so blood donation is my way of making a contribution of kindness. I understand the slogan on the blood vans saying "Donate blood from your heart." I wanted to donate blood in spring 2006, when I passed a blood van on my way to work as an hourly household attendant. I was wearing a mask over my mouth on that chilly day, so the doctor asked me if I had a cold. I said, "A little." So I was refused. But the idea had been haunting me until I saw another van later, on my way to work. When I was off duty, the van was gone. I asked the community committee where it was. The lady made a phone call. Soon a motor tricycle came to pick me up [to transport her to the mobile donation van].[30]

> When I was in college, after the donation, the blood stand gave me a pack of milk and cookies, and a plastic kettle with the Red Cross logo on it as a souvenir—nothing else. Later, when I worked, the working unit gave me several hundred yuan. The leader also consoled us with some food as a gift, and we took two days off for rest. I don't think this is payment. It is not much payment for 200 milliliters of blood. They [the compensations] are not important to me. Instead, the care from the leaders is more important. At least to me, I feel it is much more important that we are not forgotten as donors. As long as my physical condition allows, I'd go for blood donation. But I don't do it because of reciprocals.[31]

The perception of a need for compensation is high and untroubled by the idea that it might be seen as a kind of "payment for blood."

> In the work unit, they are compensated with money and food. Besides taking a few days off, donors are also sponsored with a paid resort vacation. But most of them don't know about the discount on

future blood policy [in which donor family members were given free emergency transfusion blood equal to the amount donated]. In my unit, this influenced those who decided to donate. For example, two colleagues went to donate blood after they were assured with positive answers about the payment, the resort vacation.

(What if people refuse to donate even if it is their turn?)

The leader would persuade them and assure them that the payment would be 3,500 yuan, with resort and two weeks paid off.

(3,500 yuan cash, are you sure?)

Usually it is 3,500 yuan or so. Part of it is donated by the colleagues unit, 10 yuan each. The administrative department and the worker's union pay for the rest. We have a large number of employees who are easily called upon for collection of the money for relatively fewer donors. It is not payment. Because blood collected under donation policy is an obligation and not for any return. And the money is collected from supporters of common people instead of the government, hospitals, or blood collection organizations. The money is encouragement and reciprocal to donors who are recognized by the society, citizens are the working units. And it is necessary. And the vacation is much more welcome than the money, as it's a good chance for relaxation.[32]

More generally, however, we found that there was a sense in which donations that were uncompensated were somehow incomplete, that they suggested the failure of the system, not its greatest achievement. It is taken as a sign of failure if the loss of blood is not attended to, either by the family or by the work unit. That would be a sort of "uncompensated blood donation."

Compensation is fine. It doesn't have to be much to show the humane side of government policy. The working unit is a collective organization; a government stands for the country. Laws and policies are the raw image of a government. As a necessary component of the country, a working unit knows its employees better and should show more caring. Compensation doesn't have to be in cash. The unit leader can pay a visit to donors after blood donation. The salary is paid during rest. The working unit and government should do everything to encourage kindness and to make it flourish.[33]

Obligatory, compensated blood donations in China tell us a story about the ideal (or idealized) relationship between citizen and state (as manifest through the work unit). It emerges as a form of exchange in which biological essence is compensated for by way of welfare from the socialist state. The relationship also functions within the context of two extremely important socioeconomic programs, namely, those set in motion by the socialist revolution and then by the reforms toward open market liberalism. But the idealized story, in which the state is seen to fulfill a reciprocal obligation to its patriotic donor-citizens, is in fact a way for the state to distinguish voluntary donation from corrupt forms of mercenary donation that have emerged with economic reform and liberalization—specifically, the crisis that emerged from for-profit blood buying and selling during the first half of the 1990s. Indeed, it is critical to the maintenance of these current compensation practices that the distinction between selling blood—motivated by a desperate need for money by the poor, backward peasants—and donating blood for "free" be maintained. While the first is seen as an uncaring, purely instrumental economic exchange, the latter is seen as a manifestation of caring between a patriotic ("country-loving," or *ai-guo*) donor, and a reciprocally caring state or work unit.

Obligatory, compensated blood donation is a means by which the work unit (standing in, as noted earlier, for the state) expresses itself as a provider of welfare, fulfilling an obligation it set forth with the founding of the People's Republic. Indeed, the Chinese Communist Party defined its policies in the first decades after liberation as eradicating feudal patriarchy and setting up in its place a paternalistic state, on which citizens came to rely for what had previously been provided through the family.[34] This process underscores an important accomplishment of the socialist state in regards to blood donation specifically: it has established a discourse about blood that not only generates donors who give despite their reluctance to part with vital bodily essence, but it has done so in a way that has rescripted the meaning of blood itself, turning what was once the trope signifying family lineage into a trope for the successful and—like the family—care-giving welfare state, as expressed by the reciprocities and generosities of the work unit.

In order to be seen as patriotic service to the nation, however, compensated blood donation has to also defend itself against the accusation that compensation is, in some sense, another form of "paying for blood." Informants were very clear that this was not the case, as they walked delicately through the terrain of compensation used to "inspire donation" and payment used to buy blood. Despite the superficial similarities, they insisted that being compensated for blood donation would not be like "selling one's blood," since the work unit must care for those who have sacrificed on the society's behalf.

> Payment is symbolic. . . . It is not money-oriented as is blood selling. If they do, the benefits are there for them to do so. If not, they feel less motivated. Proper compensation may provoke initiatives for potential donors from employees. It's more likely to show caring from the working unit and make a harmonious atmosphere around the company for a better working relationship.[35]

Reciprocal, obligatory, compensated blood donation is made possible as a cultural form, a success of socialism, in part because it can be distinguished from the crude commodification of blood that is found in "blood selling." This distinction was accomplished, or was hastened, by the fact that blood selling was demonized early on in public health campaigns, which suggested that risk of HIV from blood donation was causally tied to "blood selling." The logic of distinguishing between "payment" and "compensation" had to be navigated very carefully for some:

> I think it's not appropriate to give payment for volunteer blood donation. It is too complicated. If we are not ready for voluntary blood donations, alternatives may be adopted. Compensations, such as vacation time, may show humane caring and give donors a chance to travel from the official angle. It's a way of supporting and encouraging others. Actually, I am quite interested in this. Something is established on the basis of economy. With the development of our economy and citizen awareness, people would finally accept the notion that blood donation is harmless to health.[36]

The emergence of the market economy in China poses several concerns to the risky business of compensating people for donating blood but not actually paying them for their blood. Selling blood was seen as a most degraded form of giving blood, unworthy of any of the glory that came from voluntary (albeit well-compensated) contributions. Why?

Perhaps blood sellers, their mere presence in society, and the trauma of what they do, efface the possibility of the successful welfare state. Selling one's blood in China, just as in places like the United States, is considered undesirable not just because it is associated with risk of contamination (and it is important to remember that in the case of China's donors, it was not the donors but the processes used that put donors at higher risk), but because blood sellers represent a kind of failure of the politicoeconomy. These people are seen as being so poor that they must sell their vital essence. If Marx recognized alienation at selling the fruits of one's labor—being separated from the profits of one's hard labor by way of disenfranchisement as he noted, they have only their labor power, which they must sell—then this is even worse; their labor power is the "selling" of their life's essence. Selling is without reciprocity or caring, not to mention that it is seen as exploitative.[37] Selling blood is purely instrumental, rather than emotional. Whereas a patriotic (*ai-guo*) act by its very definition is an act of "love" for society, a love that it reciprocated by social welfare, selling blood (as a commodity) constitutes a transaction that has no social or emotional obligation between citizen and state built into it.

The weight of cultural trauma associated with this predicament—in well-developed socialist communism—is not just ironic, it is unbearable, in that it represents the failure of the socialist state in a way that can't be accounted for as it can under a free market system (which builds in poverty as a likely outcome). Thus we found that people were not only ready to distinguish obligatory, compensated donation from blood selling but that they did so in a way that demonized blood selling and the blood sellers. Sellers were not patriotic—in fact, they were seen as motivated by desperation—not by love.

That the market economy was seen as a reason to compensate donors had to be negotiated against the possibility that this would lead, in the end, to a situation of commodification of blood. It had to be carefully scripted as "not selling" in order to avoid the pitfalls of the growing effects of free markets in a well-established socialist milieu.

Of the various kinds of blood donation in urban Shanghai—uncompensated, obligatory donation; blood selling; uncompensated, nonobligatory donation; and obligatory, compensated donation—only the last is unproblematic in that it has been most consistently successful in meeting the needs of both public health and society and the donors. Donors who give blood but are not compensated well for it fail to obtain the state's reciprocity, thereby weakening the "caring" relationship between citizen and state. Donors who sell their blood for payment represent a failure of the socialist welfare state as well because their poverty is a troubling beacon of socialism's increasing economic disparities. At a time when market economies demand that compensation be given to donors who give blood, it is important to sustain a point of comparison against which compensations can be seen as "nonpayment" but, rather, as symbolic caregiving on the part of the successful state. "Selling blood," although in truth another way of receiving compensation, serves as that point of comparison, and so is denied the patriotic praise that is heaped on compensated donors in work units.

Compensated, obligatory donations of blood, as noted, demonstrate citizens' loyalty to the state (and its manifestation through the work unit). It is important to citizens, however, that they do not think of this as simply fulfilling an obligation set forth by the state. Blood donors in the work unit may indeed be fulfilling a quota, but they do so voluntarily, out of a will to be generous to their society (in some cases) or out of a desire to be a good citizen (in others). This is not giving with an explicit expectation of return, even though, in the end, it is only blood donation that is compensated and that meets cultural expectations for success. The incentive provided by the work unit in actual benefits should not, in this sense, be construed as providing a motivation for them to give. That donors receive the ample rewards of the state, strengthens, rather than weakens, the bonds between them and the state and affirms that donation is an act of noncoercion and free choice, free of the contaminating stigma of commodification. It allows the state to fulfill its obligations to its citizens (who need blood for modern medical care), and it allows donors to express their caring for Chinese (socialist) modernization through the contribution of their vital essence. Incentivizing blood donation like this is costly, but it achieves a great deal for everyone involved: it is a biopolitical triumph.

Conclusion

It is very much like a credit system for blood donation, by which the overall morality of citizens is shown. Since citizens have made social

> contributions, there should be an equivalent policy, which doesn't have to be financial, to contribute to them in return. Most donors are attracted by vacation and stipends. It's a relaxation and adjustment for them as long as it doesn't harm health. Cash is most favored. Rest is more necessary than traveling. A rest allowance is preferred with additional financial compensation, which makes donors feel much more comfortable.[38]

If biopolitics entails governance through disciplines of body, making politics work through medical sites and new subjectivizing regimes, then this process also entails an inscription process that might be called politicobiology. In China, the recognition of the body as an object—a process that is seen as a hallmark of Western regimes of modernity and the rise of the welfare state—is not required in the instance of blood donation and China's welfare state. The transfer of welfare from family to the work unit has been accomplished without having to erase traditional notions of blood as a sacred and vital essence. The body is not made biological, neutrally scientific, or objective. The Chinese body remains laden with the sociopolitical requirements of Chinese social life. The reciprocal exchange that must occur for the bodily essence to be infused with national glory is, in this case, the creation of a system that compensates a donor's voluntary sacrifice (within the frame of obligatory giving) in ways that the family previously might have. Blood in some sense, and for many in Shanghai, still means the same things it used to, and it is still a vital essence. That it is still considered a vital essence is all the more significant, given how many Shanghainese convince themselves to donate. But the meaning of the body's blood is also rescripted in this process.[39]

Blood is and always has been a site for political concerns that were tied to lineage, virility, and family, and now it can affirm a nation's successful modernization. China is deeply embroiled in economies of blood. First, the blood products industry, which procures blood and resells it in the blood products market (where it is bought for use in pharmaceutical and research industries), is large in China. Second, China's effort to successfully increase its internal supplies of safe whole blood for use in clinical settings is unprecedented, considering both existing sentiments against donation and the loss of blood as well as fears of contamination through blood. Moreover, as China marketizes, citizens grow increasingly worried about their social welfare and about the state's retreat from ensuring long-term social and medical care. Blood donation transactions in China reveal how the state, and citizens, are managing these dual economies of blood and assuaging their fears of social change.

Rescripting blood in a way that affirms old reciprocal notions of caring and welfare with new institutional forms for this caring (the work unit) both authorizes new kinds of social relationships and reinscribes old familiar relationships. Blood is a locus for inscribing national sentiment and responsibilities to give and be cared for. "We don't have an obligation to give. Donors are given rest allowance from work," donors say. Blood is scripted as a political substance that circulates through the body the way that resources of money, rest days, and vacation supply the working citizen with nourishment. "The work unit," we were told, "is like the family for those who work there." This politicobiology that takes old meanings of blood as a "precious vital essence" in the logic of the old empire and gives them new meanings in the logic of the modern socialist marketizing state makes sense; blood does the work of shifting responsibilities for social welfare from the family to the work unit, while also substituting concerns about longevity of the family lineage to those of the health and survival of the nation. It does so at a time and in a way that assuages fears of both loss of one's own blood and loss of state protections. This politicobiology affirms that Chinese citizens are indeed modern, uncoerced, self-disciplined subject citizens, but it also affirms that the particular nexus of meanings and institutional forms of biopolitics, in general, are not universal across modern nations.

China's unique cultural, political, and socioeconomic history shapes its modernities in distinctive ways,[40] along with its particular relationships of modern governance. Studies of the unique subjectivities of Chinese moderns,[41] suggest that idealized notions of the self—as defined in a corporeal way—have been conscripted in processes of state making. Just as notions of a biological blood circulate in Western societies and contribute to conceptions of what it means to "give blood," so too do notions of this bodily fluid in China shape notions of what it means to give it up in the act of "donation." In China, giving one's blood becomes a way of giving one's self, but this has to happen in the careful rescripting of what is, in fact, actually demanded by the state.

The state requires work units to meet quotas for blood donation. Donors in work units are thus responding to a demand placed on them, often because they're simply "the next in line." However, the act of donation is consistently rescripted not as a forced event, not as a mandatory act but rather as an act of self-sacrifice and altruism. Many could give, but those who do, do so for patriotic reasons. Moreover, giving blood only achieves successful cultural status when accompanied by hefty remunerations provided by the work unit. But again, only by being carefully scripted as nonpayment, and thus not as "selling" one's blood. These forms of bodily engagement are not forced—they are part of the self-disciplinary regime that makes up modern China and reiterates the contours of socialism's achievements for each citizen but especially those who sacrifice their blood for the welfare of all. In turn, such citizens are rewarded grandly and in a manner that lavishly pronounces the value of such self-discipline.

Biopolitics works through this scripting and tells us about what it means to be a modern Chinese subject nested in webs of self-disciplinarity and unique state apparatuses. Analyses of biopolitics foreground the way that states configure behavioral norms and in so doing exert a politics through bodies. What we see here is perhaps a politicobiology in which blood has to be scripted as first and foremost a political site before it can be of value in circulation, but then demands a politics of its own in return. Politics works to make biology real, and then biology—that is, blood—calls for a return favor. Blood becomes a vital essence for not just the individual but for the state itself, being rescripted as something that can only keep the individual healthy if it carries the weight of socialist achievement, and this means making sure blood and bodies that lose it are replenished. This mandate becomes more and more important to modern Shanghainese as fears of the dismantling of socialist state reign become increasingly common in the minds of citizens. So, if politics inscribe the value of blood in circulation through work units, then blood itself speaks back to the state in its demands to be replenished by whatever excess the work unit can afford. The unique forms of biopolitics that the modern Chinese state present to us through blood donation practices are perhaps as interesting as the fact that these practices suggest that we think about how blood (or bodies or biologies) also work as a locus of power in the biopolitical nexus.

Notes

The data on which this analysis is based come from two years of research in Shanghai, drawn primarily from interviews that were conducted in collaboration with colleagues at the Shanghai Academy of Social Sciences between 2005 and 2007. The original grant funding, NIH R21 MH073415, was awarded to Kathleen Erwin and subsequently transferred to Vincanne Adams, who has held principal investigator responsibilities since 2005. Phuoc V. Le worked as a coresearcher on the award from 2005. All three worked collectively on data collection and analysis. We wish to acknowledge the funding from the NIH, as well as our generous colleagues at the Shanghai Academy of Social Sciences, Dr. Xu Anqi and Dr. Li Yihai.

1. Michel Foucault, *History of Sexuality, Volume 1* (New York: Vintage Books 1981); Paul Rabinow, ed., *The Foucault Reader* (New York: Pantheon Books 1984); Paul Rabinow, *Essays on the Anthropology of Reason* (Princeton: Princeton University Press, 1996); Jacques Donzelot, *The Policing of Families* (New York: Random House, 1997); Nicholas Rose, *The Politics of Life Itself: Biomedicine, Power and Subjectivity in the 21st Century* (Princeton, N.J.: Princeton University Press, 2006).
2. Foucault, *History of Sexuality, Volume 1.*
3. Ann Anagnost, *National Past-Times: Narrative, Representation and Power in Modern China* (Durham: Duke University Press, 1997); Aihwa Ong, *Flexible Citizenship: The Cultural Politics of Transnationality* (Durham: Duke University Press, 1998); Judith Farquhar, *Appetites: Food and Sex in Post-Socialist China* (Durham: Duke University Press, 2002); Matthew Kohrman, *Bodies of Difference: Experiences of Disability and Institutional Advocacy in the Making of Modern China* (Berkeley: University of California Press, 2005); Lisa Rofel, *Desiring China: Experiments in Neoliberalism, Sexuality and Public Culture* (Durham: Duke University Press, 2007); Susan Greenhalgh, *Just One Child: Science and Policy in Deng's China* (Berkeley: University of California Press, 2008); Mayfair Mei-Hui Yang, *Gifts, Favors and Banquets: The Art of Social Relationships in China* (Ithaca, N.Y.: Cornell University Press, 1994).
4. Scholars have discussed the applicability of notions of biopolitics and biopower, as developed by Foucault for European modern societies, to analyses of socialist and postsocialist China. Foucault provided a coherent explanation for the self-disciplinary governance that defined modernity, in which people chose to follow behavioral norms designated by medical, psychological, political, and economic regimes of knowledge as opposed to being forced into behavioral regimes under a police incarceration model of control. In the case of China, explorations of these kinds of modern governance have focused on economy and exchange (Yang, *Gifts, Favors and Banquets*; Rofel, *Desiring China*; Ong, *Flexible Citizenship*), population and reproductive behavior (Anagnost, *National Past-Times*), and regimes of governmentality (Kohrman, *Bodies of Difference*). In some sense, all of these analyses have argued that

things are to some extent the same as those found elsewhere insofar as they are modern and rely on a kind of self-discipline, but also that they are different in China.

5. Richard M. Titmuss, *The Gift Relationship: From Human Blood to Social Policy*, ed. Anne Oakley and John Ashton (1970; New York: Free Press, 1987); David Archard, "Selling Yourself: Titmuss's Argument against a Market in Blood," *Journal of Ethics* 6 (2002): 87–103; Abdallah S. Daar, "Rewarded Giving," *Transplantation Proceedings* 24 (1992): 2207–11.
6. Lawrence Cohen, "Where It Hurts: Indian Material for an Ethics of Organ Transplantation," *Daedelus* 128, no. 4 (1999): 135–65; "Operability, Bioavailability, and Exception," in *Global Assemblages: Technology, Politics, and Ethics as Anthropological Problems*, edited by Aihwa Ong and Stephen J. Collier. Malden, Mass.: Blackwell, 2005; Cori Hayden, "Taking as Giving: Bioscience, Exchange, and the Politics of Benefit-Sharing," *Social Studies of Science* 37, no. 5 (2007): 729–58; G. Whyte, "Ethical Aspects of Blood and Organ Donation," *Internal Medical Journal* 33 (2003): 362–64; Patricia A. Marshall and Abdallah S. Daar, "Cultural and Psychological Dimensions of Organ Transplantation," *Annals of Transplantation* 3, no. 2 (1998): 7–11.
7. N. Zaller, K. E. Nelso, P. Ness, G. Wen, X. Bai, and H. Shan, "Knowledge, Attitude and Practice Survey Regarding Blood Donation in a Northwestern Chinese City," *Transfusion Medicine* 15 (2005): 277–86; Nickolas Zaller, Kenrad E. Nelson, Paul Ness, Guoxing Wen, Turgun Dewir, Xuhua Bai, and Hua Shan, "Demographic Characteristics and Risks for Transfusion-Transmissible Infection among Blood Donors in Xinjiang Autonomous Region, People's Republic of China," *Transfusion* 46 (2006): 265–71; Hua Shan, Jing-Xing Wang, Fu-Rong Ren, Yuan-Zhi Zhang, Hai-Yan Zhao, Guo-Jing Gao, Yang Ji, Paul M. Ness, "Blood Banking in China," *Lancet* 360 (2002): 1770–75; Timothy D. Mastro and Ray Yip, "The Legacy of Unhygienic Plasma Collection in China," *AIDS* 20, no. 10 (2006): 1451–52; Kathleen Erwin, "The Circulatory System: Blood Procurement, AIDS, and the Social Body in China," *Medical Anthropology Quarterly* 20, no. 2 (2006): 139–59.
8. Titmuss, *The Gift Relationship*.
9. Interview no. 26, female, forty-two years old.
10. Interview no. 38, female, forty-seven years old.
11. Interview no. 14, female, thirty-four years old.
12. Erwin, "The Circulatory System."
13. Shigehisa Kuriyama, *The Expressiveness of the Body and the Divergence of Greek and Chinese Medicine* (New York: Zone Books, 2002); Ted Kaptchuk, *The Web That Has No Weaver: Understanding Chinese Medicine*, 2nd ed. (New York: McGraw-Hill, 2000).
14. Arthur Kleinman, *Patients and Healers in the Context of Culture* (Berkeley: University of California Press, 1981).
15. Interview no. 1, male, fifty-seven years old.
16. Interview no. 32, male, fifty-four years old.

17. Interview no. 14, female, thirty-four years old.
18. Interview no. 38, female, forty-seven years old.
19. Interview no. 1, male, fifty-seven years old.
20. Interview no. 37, female, fifty-three years old.
21. Interview no. 30, male, fifty-eight years old.
22. Titmuss *The Gift Relationship*, 307.
23. Cohen, "Where It Hurts."
24. Yang, *Gifts, Favors and Banquets*; Li Zhang and Aihwa Ong, *Privatizing China: Socialism from Afar* (Ithaca, N.Y.: Cornell University Press, 2008).
25. Interview no. 12, female, twenty-five years old.
26. Interview no. 38, female, forty-seven years old.
27. Interview no. 30, male, fifty-eight years old.
28. Interview no. 36, female, eighteen years old.
29. The data and research here are limited to Shanghai and we do not make claims about floating or rural populations of Chinese donors, as they are not necessarily connected to work units in the same ways as the individuals we discuss here (see Shao Jing, "Fluid Labor and Blood Money: The Economy of HIV/AIDS in Rural Central China," *Cultural Anthropology* 21, no. 4 [2006]: 535–69, for a good analysis of one rural area's experience with donation, and Zaller et al., "Knowledge, Attitude and Practice Survey," for other data on rural donation trends).
30. Interview no. 24, female, forty-six years old.
31. Interview no. 8, male, twenty-six years old.
32. Interview no. 2, male, fifty-three years old.
33. Interview no. 14, female, thirty-four years old.
34. Emily Honig and Gail Herschatter, *Personal Voices: Chinese Women in the 1980's* (Stanford, Calif.: Stanford University Press, 1988); Anagnost, *National Past-Times*.
35. Interview no. 26, female, forty-two years old.
36. Ibid.
37. Shao, "Fluid Labor and Blood Money."
38. Interview no. 33, male, twenty-three years old.
39. For more on the success of the public health and government programs to increase donations, see V. Adams, K. Erwin, and P. V. Le, "Public Health Works: Blood Donation in Urban China," *Social Science and Medicine* 68, no. 3 (2009): 410–18.
40. Lisa Rofel, *Other Modernities: Gendered Yearnings in China after Socialism* (Berkeley: University of California Press, 1999).
41. Tani Barlow, Formations of Colonial Modernity in East Asia (Durham: Duke University Press, 1997); Anagnost, *National Past-Times*; Farquhar, *Appetites*; Ong, *Flexible Citizenship*.

AIHWA ONG

Lifelines | THE ETHICS OF BLOOD BANKING FOR FAMILY AND BEYOND

In March 2006, at Sotheby's New York salesroom, a Singaporean collector unfamiliar to Asian art dealers paid nearly one million dollars for the painting of a dazed-looking Chinese man. The painting brought the highest price at New York's first auction of Asian contemporary art. Much of the art sold was politically charged, referring to Mao Zedong, Tiananmen, and consumer culture.

But the painting in question seems decidedly apolitical, part of the "Bloodline Series" of portraits by the Chinese painter Zhang Xiaogang. Zhang has since become one of the most sought-after contemporary Chinese artists in global art markets, and his works are shown by the gallery PaceWildenstein in New York City (which opened a branch gallery, Pace Beijing, in China in 2008).

Like other pictures in the "Bloodline Series," *Comrade no. 120* is based on passport shots; but, projected as they are onto large canvases, each one takes on the monumental aspect of Chinese ancestor portraits. American art critics frequently note the blank expressions and stiff formality of Zhang's figures, many of them clad in proletarian fatigues, as an indication (indictment) of the oppressive degree of uniformity imposed by Mao's authoritarian regime. A description in the Sotheby's catalogue notes, as the "eyes of the sitters stare out at us like glistening black pearls, there is a tangible sense of catharsis for the suffering they have endured."[1] Such well-intentioned misreadings rob the authority of the paintings and undercut their intended messages. To me, Zhang's paintings seem to capture the fleeting moments of remembering and forgetting in the turbulent family histories of modern China. Zhang has said of his "Big Family Series," which seem in-

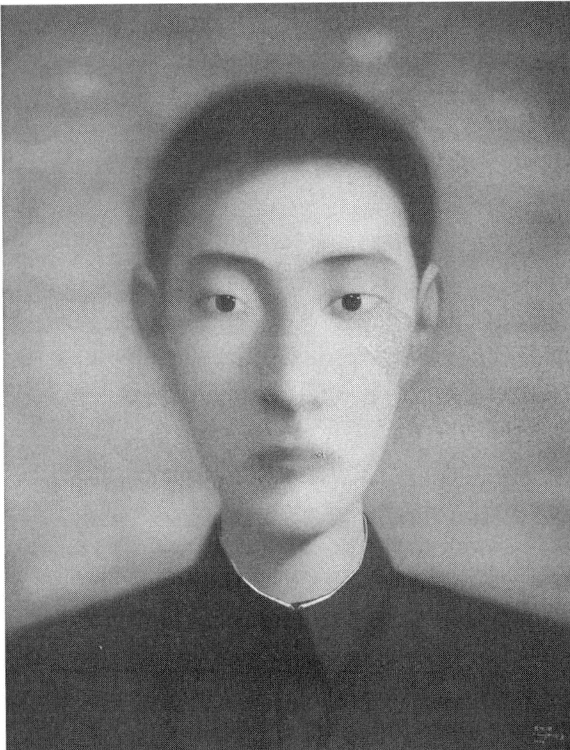

Figure 1 "Bloodline Series": *Comrade No. 120*, by Zhang Xiaogang (1988). COURTESY OF SOTHEBY'S.

spired by outmoded genres of photographic family portraits, that "we are mutually restricted and interdependent."[2] The power of the "Bloodline" paintings lies in the intertwining material and immaterial elements of Chinese sociality. The red traceries linking members in family group images indicate that biological matter is always already constituted by kinship.

Given the degree of symbolism in Zhang's oeuvre, I am interested in the purchase of this portrait of a young man by the wealthy Singaporean. Besides the bloodline motif in this series, there is almost always a translucent mark on the otherwise unblemished faces of his subjects. Is this patch a clue of the suppressed self, as some Western observers have suggested? Or is the blemish a kind of DNA marker, or even the imprint of medical procedure, a cry for healing invisible wounds? Is the Singaporean's purchase of *Comrade no. 120* an act of reclaiming Chinese ancestry, a tracing of family bloodlines back to the mainland? Or can one read the desire for Zhang's works as a search for a new umbilical cord that can sustain the contemporary Chinese family in the face of biological damage?

This essay tracks the boom in blood banking in Singapore and the surrounding region as an ethical process of fashioning new lifelines for overseas Chinese navigating biological risks and the pathos of family ruptures. Recent health threats (SARS, avian flu, dengue fever) in Singapore have fueled a sense of renewed biological vulnerability in the midst of modern affluence and have spurred investment in technoscientific methods as tools of biosecurity. This turn to biomedical procedures opens a window onto the articulation of ethical dispositions at the intersection of the family unit and nation, and rejuvenates an old ethnic/racial solidarity. Indeed, the rise of private blood banking for potential stem cell therapy in the case of future illnesses in the family is predicated on the Chinese belief that kinship is grounded in a material "shared essence" (i.e., blood), which goes beyond the individual or family to include ethnic kinship (see the essays on China in this volume). This being so, we should understand the ethics involved in the use of such biomedical techniques as also not reducible to an individual or family scale, or indeed any single scale, but as engaging different levels of valuation and projection surrounding blood.

A novel configuration of biotech, ethical, and aesthetic elements in Singapore sets the parameters within which blood and its value are constituted. I propose in this essay to track the many registers and scales that can be discerned in the valuation of blood, and to do so will draw links among official tissue networks, the private banking of cord blood, the promissory marketing of blood banks, and representations such as Zhang Xiaogang's paintings. The first of these, the storage of human tissues by the state, is legitimized in terms of securing citizens' future needs, and the embrace of biomedical knowledge and practices is becoming a norm of responsible citizenship. At the same time, private companies advertising cord blood banking boosts the promissory value of stem cells, prompting parents to bank the umbilical cord blood of their infants. Among young educated parents, this biomedical procedure has become what enlightened ethical subjects do. The convergence of these different circuits of blood creates a biomedical and ethical network that resuscitates folk beliefs in fixed ethnic essences. The enriched possibilities of blood seem to be echoed in the blood symbolism of the lively market in contemporary Chinese art, giving an aesthetic figuration to the projection of diasporic yearnings for material and symbolic connections with the ancestral homeland and emergent world power.

Bioethics and Other Ethical Regimes

The scholarship on emerging economies of human organs has focused on the ethical problems involved when the use of human body parts becomes contaminated by commerce. A popular view of human tissue collection is the fear that even when commercialized organs banks are regulated, they still harbor seeds of social injustice. In their book, *Tissue Economies*, Catherine Waldby and Robert Mitchell warn that the globalization of markets in human organs, as well as recent legal thinking, has blurred any strict lines separating donations from market activity and values.[3] While Waldby and Mitchell decry the exclusion of the poor from expensive biomedical treatments, they also maintain that the production of biovalue can be for the ethical good, for example, in shaping potential biocommons.[4] When we go further, taking a broader range of intersecting regimes—bioethical, communal, and political—into account, we can see the extent to which regulatory systems interact with biotechnologies and cultural values in shaping ethical practices.

Bioethics is currently focused on the subject of clinical treatment and experimentation. First, bioethics is concerned specifically with the ethical treatment of living human tissues, patients, and research subjects in a formalized domain such as the clinic or the laboratory. Second, bioethics looks at the human rights of individuals, and the protections drawn up by bioethicists have become universal standards for conducting biomedical research. Only recently has bioethics started to question the assumption that the moral agent or victim is always an individual; this narrow scale has been expanded by anthropologists concerned about entire ethnic groups, for example, aboriginal populations who are perceived to be powerless against predatory pharmaceutical companies.[5] But the bioethics regime associated with pharmaceutical and clinical practices is only one among many diverse ethical regimes that already operate in the political-cultural spaces of biotechnology.

A useful way to capture the multiple and intersecting scales that are brought together in ethical decision making use what I call a situated approach. I use "ethics" and "ethical" not in the sense of normative morality, that is, to ascribe the values "good" or "bad" according to some abstract universalizing ethical order. Instead, I follow to an extent the thinking of Foucault, for whom "ethics" refers to the self-constituting practices of subjectivity and thus the formation of political sensibility. Instead of ethics as obedience to an established moral order, we have ethics as a critical activity of self-questioning and decision making about truth and the exercise of freedom. Foucault acknowledges some reference to others in the act of ethical self-constitution, but his focus on the care of the self is ultimately concerned with oneself as the ethical substance at stake in one's action.[6]

While I agree that ethical self-determination is always situated within a shifting field of power relationships, I differ from Foucault by noting that what is at stake in individual moral reasoning is the ethical constitution of the social network in which the moral subject is embedded. Whereas Foucault is tightly focused on the ethical scale of the self-caring subject, my approach locates ethical work in the management of relationships between an individual and overlapping circles of attachments. By situating moral reasoning at the intersection of multiple ethical scales, I hold that individual self-formation is ultimately concerned about weighing the ethical stakes of one's action for the various collectivities in which one is enmeshed.

I do not reduce my analysis of the ethics of biomedical procedures to the scale of the individual patient or donor, but consider how individual decision is invariably colored by broader contexts of social obligations and collective interests. Whereas bioethics is still very concerned with voluntary choice and informed consent in biomedical procedures, other ethical regimes governing kinship and collective interests (e.g., religion, communalism, nationalism) are in play, influencing an individual's decision to undergo a biomedical procedure. My concept of situated ethics thus defines the ethical configuration as the space that brings into tension freedom, self-determination, and informed consent, on the one hand, and the moral claims of the family, community, and large collectivities, on the other.[7] However, in certain biomedical situations, ethical decision making formed at the nexus of multiple affiliations may raise skepticism in the "West."

Singapore's Ethical Configuration

This complex ethical configuration at multiple scales is missed by Western observers anxious about the rise of Asian biotech capacities. Francis Fukuyama has charged that the shift of stem cell research overseas is a form of "ethical arbitrage" whereby research institutes relocate to "ethics-free" Asian environments. He mentions Singapore as an example of a place with "a more favorable regulatory climate."[8] But picking on Singapore, Fukuyama could not be more off target. The island-state is well known as one of world centers for enforcing international best practices in business, research, and manufacturing. Indeed, every effort is made in Singapore to make visible adherence to international norms and establishing forms of ethical consensus. Indeed, without strict bioethical guidelines in place, the Biopolis hub could not have taken off as an international site of commercial scientific research. The growing centrality of biomedical genomics has cast ethical ripples across the social landscape, as voluntary biomedical decisions enroll broader ethics of collective rejuvenation.

Biomedical genomics in Singapore is working in tandem with a mode of governmentality I call vitalist politics, that is, governing through a pragmatic and ethicalized investment in the vital processes of the total living situation. In the island-nation, vitalist politics is perhaps most visibly realized through the expansion of public repositories of human tissues for the "public good," defining Singaporeans as a biological public freely sharing a common pool of "Asian" genomic resources. Organ banks and biomedical insurance help configure an emerging space where medical consumers are encouraged to donate and collect human tissues as an ethical necessity for saving and/or extending Asian lives. Public repositories of "Asian" tissues provide a new biosecurity infrastructure for the nation, and new blood technologies suggest a lifeline cast to future generations, and potentially a kind of umbilical cord to vulnerable coethnics beyond the immediate family.

What is the particular set of conditions that have prompted tiny Singapore to become one of the world's most efficient collectors of human tissues? The most important condition is, precisely, cord blood[9] banking, which has emerged as a powerful, pragmatic, and symbolic practice that supports the goal of the government to collect human tissues and stem cells that are compatible with local populations, for example, in the treatment of leukemia, which is widely perceived as an "Asian" cancer. This small city-state is ahead of the United States in this regard, where only a few state governments, among them California, have set up public cord blood banks; moreover, in the United States, the number of cord blood transplants is still small, and public awareness of cord blood as a treatment is still low.[10]

Another factor favoring Singapore is its attention to ethics. The collection and research use of human tissues have of course been at the center of bioethical debates for decades. In the light of its ambition to be Asia's foremost biomedical hub, Singapore has been careful in shaping ethical policies. Singapore models its research standards and consent procedures after Britain, which legalized therapeutic cloning in 2001. The following year, Singapore approved therapeutic cloning and established the Bioethics Advisory Committee (BAC). As in Britain, ethical debates were conducted without much fanfare, and ethical concerns, while raised, were muted. An official was quoted as saying that the government had considered issues calmly and did not want to draw attention to its "liberal" attitude toward stem cell research in case it risked igniting religious passions.[11] BAC "recognized the need to moderate extreme views at the outset." A poll of religious leaders found the main religious groups of Buddhists and Muslims (a combined estimate of 67 percent of the total population) to be "for therapeutic cloning."[12] Thus, the bioethics board was a means to build ethical consensus among diverse religious communities. BAC describes its ethical position as "just" and "sustainable." The claim that it is "just" refers to its "obligation to respect the common good, particularly in the sharing of the costs and benefits"; "sustainable" refers to its goal to extend the horizon of social obligation "to respect the needs of generations yet unborn."[13] Under the law, BAC approved therapeutic cloning to produce stem cells, as well as taking stem cells from aborted fetuses or surplus embryos from fertility treatment. BAC's sustainable ethics justified the building of a nation-wide system of tissue repositories, a vital infrastructure that makes visible the ethical premises of genomic research. Indeed, as Kaushik Sunder Rajan notes in his contribution to this volume, regulatory structures and human infrastructure work hand in hand in new experiments for making ethical subjects. Singapore is a tentative experiment that enrolls cord blood donation as an ethical practice beyond the consideration of mere bioethics in the clinic.

The larger background of Singapore's biotech ambition is a deep-rooted sense of political and environmental insecurity. The term used in international relations studies for this phenomenon is "securitization," which occurs when a state claims an existential threat, recognizing a condition of danger that then becomes constitutive of state identity. Critics have argued that this kind of emergency mode of governance should be rejected in favor of a calculative mode focused on diffusing risks through biopolitical interventions.[14] One example of such a calculative logic is the development of "vital security systems" that have the capacity to mitigate threats to the infrastructure.[15] In Southeast Asian contexts, where national crises tend to be precipitated by financial, epidemic, and environmental threats, vital security processes are infrastructural, biopolitical, and ethically framed.

In recent decades, Asian milieus have been poised on the edge of biological disasters: the spread of the HIV virus, the SARS epidemic, and the avian flu. Complex adaptations to health crises and other disasters (the 1997–98 financial crisis, the tsunami of 2005) have created a climate of hypersecurity where new problematizations of nation and population are shaped by discourses of population risks and sustainable ethics. Hypervigilance by the state includes the buildup of biotechnological and biomedical systems in order to securitize the life of the nation. Alongside biotech development, a vitalist politics primes the population to take up novel biomedical practices to mitigate threats to wealth, health, and the future.

Risk-adverse Singapore and Singaporeans are more security-conscious than other Southeast Asians about the assorted challenges and disasters always looming on the horizon. Biotechnology as industry has become the solution to the threat of economic irrelevance in the face of China's emergence as a manufacturing giant. Becoming Asia's Biopolis seems to be the new way to redefine Singapore's distinctive identity.[16] But contrary to Western perceptions, biomedical genomics in Singapore is never simply a commercial undertaking. Its emergence as a center of biotechnology in Asia facilitated its role as a key combatant against the SARS epidemic, as it deployed an array of techniques, from screening arrivals in ports to treating SARS patients in state-of-the-art hospitals. Elsewhere I describe the confluence of biomedicine, surveillance of body heat, and other high-tech surveillance of individuals exposed to SARS.[17] Fear of body heat transmuted into a kind of political fever, a hypervigilance that primed the population to face future health epidemics. Singapore prides itself as being more ready to face biological risks than, say, mainland China and other Asian sites, where interventions have been slow or spotty. In the midst of regular outbreaks of infectious diseases, the adaptive mechanisms in Singapore are of a more complex order.

This is the emerging complex of governing that I call vitalist politics. Foucault's concept of biopolitics, whereby governing is very much about the well-being of the population at the collective level, has mutated into interventions at an ever more intimate level of biological existence. The term "vitalist politics" refers to the ensemble of biosecurity systems and ethical discourses that are directly and indirectly oriented toward safeguarding the vital elements for securing life in a risky environment. In Singapore, governing is increasingly focused on technical and ethical investments in the total living situation, that is, necessary social practices for people living in the tropics. The growing importance of genetic material in modes of governing and self-governing is crystallizing a notion of citizenship centered on such vitalism. Thus, biotech development in response to perceived risks becomes inseparable from practices of sustainable ethics that make visible Asian populations as vulnerable ethnobiological communities.

This vitalist thrust of biotech rule to secure the anxious present is wedded to a neoliberal calculation to tame future unknowns. The very nature of human stem cell research, of which Singapore is very proud, and now cord blood technology, is based on future probabilities of cures for a spectrum of diseases from cancers to spinal cord injuries. The tension between measures instituted to provide biomedical security and the biomedical speculation they generate creates risks in many areas of investments, whether in infrastructure or in private tissue banking. In security-conscious Singapore, the hype of biotech shares and added-value health insurance seems to encourage risk calculations that speculate on the unknown future.

Public Blood Banking: "National Life-Saving Resource"

A discourse of genetics, it has been observed, is increasingly used to describe the human condition, clotting everyday consciousness with thoughts about genetically inherited diseases, the screening technologies to detect them, and the need for forms of genetic capital and genetic therapies. Such biomedical instrumentalization alters understandings and frames "the ways in which life itself can be owned, capitalized, and patented."[18] However, in this Asian milieu, biomedical genomics is viewed as an activity beyond potential commercial gains. In many Asian cultures, body parts and genetic materials have particular resonance for the survival and sense of distinctiveness of nations and peoples. At the same time, biomedical science represents cutting-edge modernity. In the public imagination there is growing belief that biobanking is "a life-saving gift," an unavoidable, even ethical necessity for ensuring collective vitality. This belief in the ethical weight of the bioeconomy is constitutive of new relationships between biomedical knowledge and ethical reasoning at multiple scales.

Leading experts, education campaigns, and biomedical consumers anticipate biorisky scenarios and the biosecurity measures promised by the life sciences. An array of government inducements has increased enrollment in all levels of science education, and youngsters are increasingly switching from seeking jobs in multinational corporations to training as scientists who may end up working in well-funded laboratories. As a term of praise, the phrase "scientists as heroes" was first heard in the combat against SARS (which killed some medical workers), but more recent school campaigns cast leading scientists as rock stars, with their own comic book images. Edison Liu, the head of the Genome Institute is widely recognized as the nation's top science hero. Official and corporate discourses in Singapore stress the centrality of the life sciences, not only for the economy, but also for "the public good." A major aspect of making Singapore a science park is to have citizens make voluntary contributions to the ever-growing repository for human organs.

Singapore is one of the earliest Asian sites to collect cord blood, and the public bank has collected over one thousand units, but has a goal of ten thousand units in order to reach the 80 percent match for the patients who need it.[19] Cord blood is a vital source of haematopoietic stem cells (HSC) that are extremely versatile in generating other cells, and are thus a source of potential treatment of heart disease, diabetes, Parkinson's, Alzheimer's, and spinal cord injury, among others. Donations are entirely voluntary, and donors sign consent forms. Singapore's strict bioethical regulations give citizens confidence that the use of human materials is ethical and medically sound. As an informant notes, Singapore is focused on biotechnical application for its own population. The accumulation of human organs is "quite pragmatic: these donations are made only to citizens. It bypasses the need for the sale of organs, which is criminalized."[20] The sale of human tissues and organs is strictly forbidden.

In establishing a reputation for transparent and ethical regulation in biomedical research, Singapore has sharply distinguished itself from rival Asian countries such as South Korea, which has been criticized by Western observers as lacking "an adequate system of science governance."[21] Furthermore, the well-regulated Singapore tissue banks are an object lesson for preventing the kind of health situation that occurs in China, where HIV and other infectious risks have arisen because of poor regulation of blood transfusions. As Kathleen Erwin notes, rampant illegal sales of blood in China have transformed the "gift of life" into a "commodity of death."[22] Singapore's clean reputation is clearly part of a bid to become a significant global player; and rigorous ethical standards must begin at home.

Appeals to both national and private interests spur voluntary contribution to a public cord blood bank. "Parents-to-be will play a vital role in successfully building up our national life-saving resource," said the director of the facility. "The more donated umbilical cord bloods we collect and store, the higher the chance of patients finding a match at the Singapore Cord Blood Bank. Hence, we'd like to encourage more parents to donate their baby's umbilical cord blood, which would otherwise be discarded after childbirth." Furthermore, there is an appeal to self-interest that articulates ethnicity. The cord blood bank director notes that because "of their unique ethnic immune genotypes, 65%–80% of Asians worldwide currently are unable to find a match" in blood stem cells, a distinct disadvantage should they need stem cell transplants.[23] Such claims about the need for intra-Asian blood collections were borne out in 2005 when a Singaporean leukemia patient received cord blood from the Shanghai Stem Cell Bank, which has the largest collection in China. The patient's family had contacted stem cell banks in Singapore, Taiwan, and the Chinese mainland for a genetic match.[24]

The majority of Singaporean Chinese are descended from dialect groups (e.g., Hokkien, Teochew, Cantonese, and Hakka) that at one time collectively identified themselves as *Tangren* (people of the Tang dynasty, not Han) from southern China. Since the 1970s, language policies have reconstituted the dialect groups as a single Mandarin-proficient (but largely English-speaking) ethnic Chinese population.[25] The new biomedical technologies now add a scientific heft to historical, cultural, and ethnic affiliations, thus further drawing disparate Chinese ethnicities in Southeast Asia, China, and Taiwan into a diffuse "racial" collectivity (see essays by Jennifer Liu and Wen-ching Sung). The promise of blood transfusion for leukemia has stirred a new kind of altruism as overseas Chinese receive scientific evidence of their long-held belief in a single Chinese race. Thus in Singapore and other Asian sites, the biovalue of tissue repositories goes beyond the commercial gains, becoming the expression of a new moral bioeconomy to treat race-specific problems in a transnational realm.

As elsewhere, tissue donation is a new practice of the affluent and educated classes, which in Singapore tend to follow ethnic lines. The Singaporean population (approximately 4.5 million) is dominated by ethnic Chinese, with small proportions of ethnic Indians and Muslim Malays. There is a human organ transplant act (HOTA 2004) that allows for the removal of organs—liver, heart, and corneas, all for transplant after death—from citizens and permanent residents, unless they have previously made objections. Opting out is not just a biomedical option, but a mechanism that separates those who contribute and those who do not to the nation's "pragmatic" approach to biosecurity.

Attempts to register organ donors by ethnic group have proceeded steadily as the authorities seek to have proportionate organ donations by each group in order to balance their ethnic representation on wait-lists for organs. Widespread complaints that Malays lagged in organs donation resulted in the overturning of Muslim religious prohibitions, and the pressure is toward enforcing proportionality in organ donations as a mark of common citizenship. The discourses of bioresponsibility are mapping ethnic and racial communities as more or less amenable to the life sciences, as well as contributing to the production of the national store of banked human tissues.

The Singapore example of a state-driven opting-out program for harvesting organs (now being copied by Great Britain) is a clear alternative to the situation envisaged by Waldby and Mitchell, in which privatized blood banking becomes the prerogative of the wealthy and a threat to an emerging biomedical commons.[26] The Singapore case further complicates the conventional picture because it demonstrates that the establishment of a public tissue network need not reduce privatized blood banking, but could in fact indirectly stimulate it, as a private investment in speculative biosecurity, that is, a new kind of biological insurance that shapes a reimagination of the shared essence of a bionation.

Private Blood Banking

SPECULATIVE AND INSURABLE VALUES

As interest in Singapore's biomedical future heats up, new parents are induced to become more knowledgeable about technology by anticipating biorisky scenarios and the biosecurity promises offered by the life sciences. In newspaper articles, expectant couples are encouraged to consider a new kind of biological responsibility. Besides finding a name and a nanny for their new baby, young couples must now ponder "the option of taking 'biological insurance,'" that is, consider storing their baby's cord blood. They must throw their infant a "lifeline" for future medical emergencies.[27] The news media churn out hopeful stories of potential cures for "Asian" diseases, and the "life-saving" value of their newborn's blood as a source of stem cells. Writing from the redoubt of Harvard University, a state-employed Singapore scientist first acknowledges that it is difficult to dismiss fears that the biomedical sciences may be used in a way that violates the autonomy of the child, as, say, by seeking the creation of "designer babies." He then offers an alternative view, that "expanding mankind's control over human reproduction is nothing more than an extension of the parental responsibility to care for one's offspring."[28] Such expressions of biomedical hope and new parental responsibilities instill a sense of need for private blood banking. Because genomic cures are still in the future, there is a speculative dimension to claims about the curative power of stem cells, but the promise of anticipated scientific miracles speaks to the anxiety of people eager to be modern and "techno-savvy" parents.

Beyond media reports, the commercial stimulus behind such beliefs comes from the company CordLife, the first "fee-for-service" tissue storage facility in Southeast Asia to be accredited by the American

Association of Blood Banks. Founded in Singapore in 2001, CordlLife has been praised by the Singapore government for contributing to the island's growth as a hub for world-class health care services. The founder is Steven Fang, a British-trained Singaporean engineer who has had experiences working with pharmaceutical companies in the United States. Believing that bioentrepreneurship is the new thing, Fang uses technologies developed at Harvard and the Massachusetts Institute of Technology for stem cell procedures in order to set up commercial blood banking throughout the Asia-Pacific region. For this achievement, the company was named a "Technology Pioneer" by the World Economic Forum in 2007, a recognition that gives Fang access to the global venture capitalists who gather in Davos. Fang himself was given a "Young Entrepreneur" award. He talks to me about the chief motivation behind his business: "The pharmaceuticals business is established with the view to save lives. Changing life is greater than making money. Stem cell technology must be made available to the masses, i.e., Asians."[29] The parent company of CordLife, CyGenics Ltd., is registered on the Australian Stock Exchange. CordLife is the only private blood bank to have AABB accreditation in Singapore, and although it is now extending its reach to North America, it is still mainly focused on providing facilities for storing cord blood in Asia (it has facilities throughout Southeast Asia, and has recently expanded into North Asia, India, and Australia). According to Fang, the company's ambition is to build up the blood inventory in order to catch up to current world leaders in stem cell therapy within a decade.

This articulation between biocapital, bioethics, and technological advancement is driven home in a variety of educational programs. Fang describes CordLife as the "caretaker of the client's blood, like a commercial bank with safety boxes, ensuring the quality [and] usability" of what is banked, and the company's liability (contracts specify a term of twenty-one years, which is renewable). Fang notes that because CordLife is the first company in the field, it has been "easy to convince everyone" of the need for its services, which it has done by selling "through fear," that is, by presenting troubling data on childhood and teenage vulnerabilities, and by advising that "parental safeguards are needed" to protect their children.[30] On its Web site, CordLife urged Asian parents: "Storing your child's precious cord blood stem cells provides you with peace of mind. It can be your child's future key to treatment of more than 80 diseases."[31] Family cord blood banking will not only secure a private source for potential autologous transplants (where the donor and recipient are the same individual), but also bypass risky sources of allogenic (donated) tissues in the few public repositories throughout Asia. Responsible parents wishing to protect their children against genetic risks by investing in potential cures have no choice but to bank the cord blood (see figure 2). The emphasis is on a new way of delivering cures, and on engendering a new kind of parental responsibility to invest in what is still an uncertain form of therapy.

The various reports and statements of the industry and its commentators make it clear that blood banking compares itself to the money market, using terms such as "banking," "insurance," "value," "capital," and "investment in the future." There is much "hype" surrounding publicly traded biotech firms and their dependence on "promissory biocapitalist futures" to increase their economic value, as Sunder Rajan notes in connection with firms in Silicon Valley.[32] Capital operates within speculative markets "in which prices [values] move in response to the balance of opinion regarding the future movement of prices," as another study notes.[33] But the speculative stories surrounding biotechnology markets also contribute to the production of other kinds of values, especially the ethics of responsible health practices. Privatized blood banking can be compared to a speculative market where the opinions of doctors, politicians, and bioentrepreneurs drive the growth of economic and ethical values of family investment in the technology. Cord blood banking operates within speculations about the future movement of biomedical value in response to stories of hope (instead of the balance of actual cures created or available). By raising awareness of genetic information, predictions of potential therapies add an ethical value to private investments in blood banking, which becomes a family treasure store of potential cures.

Indeed, the Singapore state is reinforcing such understandings by pushing bioinsurance. Parents who bank their newborn's blood with CordLife are now covered by NTUC Income, one of the largest state-controlled insurance companies in Singapore. The policy is called Medicord, and it has three plans of varying costs. The insurance is sold by speculations about the future: "As *more* treatments are discovered and cord blood stem cell therapy *becomes more* widely available, the number of such transplants using cord blood *is expected to rise* in the years

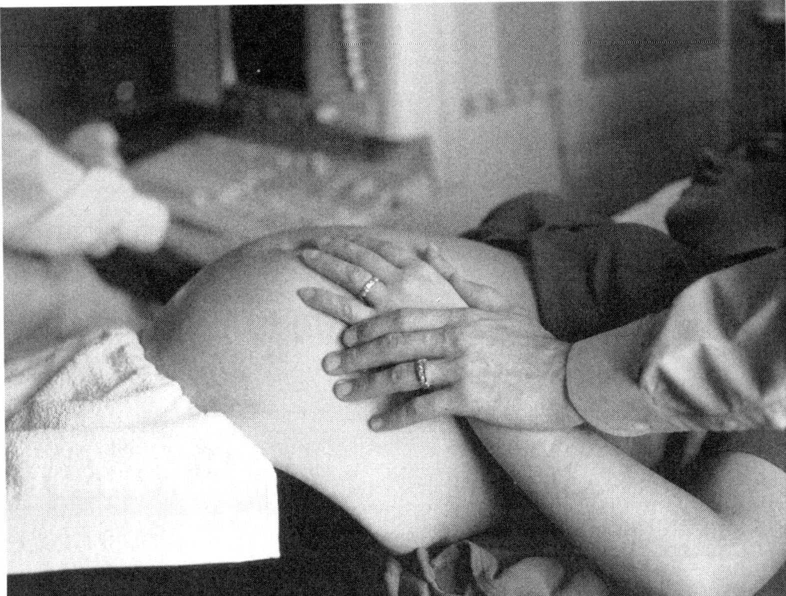

Figure 2 "Cord blood banking emphasizes the responsibility of expecting parents." COURTESY OF CYGENICS CORDLIFE, SINGAPORE.

ahead" (emphasis added).[34] Bioinsurance adds to the speculative nature of the tissue economy by adding an ethical value to the practice of family blood banking.

BIOSUBJECTIVIZATION

The hothouse atmosphere of scientific Singapore raises speculative and insurable values in cord blood banking, thus creating a realm of what we may call biosubjectivization. The flood of information on genetic illnesses primes family anxieties and brings about two kinds of subjectifying effects: the normalization of hedging biological risks, and the interweaving of biomedical practice and ethnic thinking.

Company handouts and articles that appear in the media at the rate of one to two a week aim to change family thinking about ethnicity. Fang agrees that the overall effect is to "strengthen ethnic identity" because of the linking of family blood to the delivery of cures for illness in the family. He gives an example of a mixed-race family who, he said, should not draw on donated blood for fear that it might be incompatible and rejected by their bodies. The private storage of blood from one's children as a means of potential cure will increase the belief in and feeling of a family's ethnic identity.[35] Questions about whether stored stem cells will be useful as therapies in the long term, or in the case of genetically inherited diseases, are not publicly discussed.

The convergence of biocapitalist and family interests promotes blood banking as a form of self-governing practice that anticipates and plans for biological possibilities in the family's future. The notion of hedging against hazardous biological futures is spreading among ordinary citizens, regardless of whether they have members of the family who can benefit from such practices in the present. Indeed, the private banking of cord blood requires thinking in the present about possibilities of future interventions using stem cell therapy, and such thinking fosters responsibility among parents to hedge against risks in their children's future. This new economic and ethical configuration of the parental role goes beyond standard healthy child-rearing norms such as the immunization of infants. The effect of biotech information is to relocate an older parental obligation toward children in a new site of possible insurance for a child's future. This new responsibility to participate in what is still a speculative biomedical market for the sake of the imagined future vulnerabilities of one's child may be too demanding an ethics of biosecurity.

Nevertheless, at a CordLife fair I attended in Singapore, many young expectant couples were drawn to the booth for baby gifts and brochures urging them to sign up right away for cord blood storage to the tune of about $1,000 local dollars the first year, and a smaller fee in subsequent years. It appears that cord blood banking is becoming normalized among the younger generation of parents. Newspaper reports about parents having a new baby in order to provide stem cells for a sick older sibling[36] further reinforce the sense that the expenses are worthwhile because they can secure the health of more than one family member. The growth of public tissue banking is never enough, or is beside the point, to parents caught up in the need to invest in this hedge fund to profit their children's biological future. At a global level, Waldby and Mitchell note that cord blood has acquired a "speculative value" that partakes of the dream of regeneration, "the dream that every biological loss can be repaired."[37] The dream of hedging your bets in the realm of biological risks to children is spreading among a new generation of affluent parents, who come to consider cord blood banking as yet another medical responsibility when a child is born.

In 2003, CordLife acquired Cytomatrix, a Boston stem cell company, thus gaining expanded research facilities to produce human T cells, a critical component of the immune system.[38] Now with a United States base, CordLife is promoting the practice of storing cord blood in America, at least among parents on the East Coast. In 2006, an American friend of mine who gave birth in a New York hospital was advised to store her infant's blood with CordLife. She and other mothers in the ward agreed to bank their babies' cord blood, as yet another area opens up for hedging bets in these anxious times. My New York friend sent me the CordLife materials for Americans, and I note that there are no pictures of pregnant Asian parents (as there are in figure 2), but a key image is of a female Caucasian toddler looking at her navel.

In Singapore, the ethics of this form of health management for the affluent is different from the ethical strategies adopted by patient advocate groups who network in the interest of sick loved ones.[39] Rather, the ethics of investing in cord blood as a possible therapy in the child's future is an extension of the ethics of management of risks to which the family group may be exposed in the unknown future, that is, a kind of entrepreneurial preemptive action to bank against the possibilities of biological risks for their children. Cord blood insurance is becoming one more element—besides insurance of the family home, car, laptop, and so on—in an ethicomaterialist ensemble that knowledgeable Singaporeans must invest in. The commercial manipulation of bioanxieties among the newly affluent appears to be limitless, promoting a kind of vitalist citizenship that attempts to control any foreseeable biological risks.

Recoding Ethnokinship

The link between blood banking and the expansion of parental responsibility strikes a deep resonance especially among the ethnic Chinese. Singaporean Chinese, no matter how Westernized in education, continue to view blood as the substance and symbol of kinship and filial piety. There is such profound, unquestionable belief in blood connections that kinship ethics cannot be separated from the continuity of family bloodlines. These cultural beliefs provide an interesting comparison to the British situation described by Marilyn Strathern. In her study, genetic material is transferred but has no kinship value; she cites the case of egg donors who feel no biological or moral connections to the eggs that they provide to childless couples.[40] Similarly, in Chinese beliefs, embryos do not have kinship status per se. But in the Chinese case this is because only the baby born into the family is a social person; embryos not used or discarded by the family are nonhuman and never had kin value to begin with. There is thus in Chinese beliefs a sharper separation between what is considered family tissue and what is judged to be unwanted biological material, which has no symbolic meaning. Not only is there no possibility of moral connection to rejected reproductive tissues, but they are considered part of "hospital waste." At a Singapore fertility clinic, a patient told me that her surplus eggs are just "waste matter" that the government is free to collect for "scientific research." Genetic materials such as blood only have symbolic investment when they are part of the originating family, or useful for safeguarding its health. Blood is meaningful only when it circulates within the kinship network.

The perception of the individual as a cluster of blood cells in a larger configuration of blood is powerfully suggested in painting 16 of Zhang's "Bloodlines," *The Big Family*, which depicts a red baby emerging from a family unit composed of figures linked by bloodlines. The notion of family bloodlines is common in many cultural regimes, but the Chinese have long considered the giving of blood the most powerful expression of interconnectivity and loyalty. Kinship links between the family of origin and the family of procreation depend in a material way on the flow of female blood. Female blood carries strong emotional resonance because of its association with life-giving and life-sustaining capacities. In the old days, female blood as a symbol of health and filial love found expression in a daughter's drawing of her own blood to make soup for a sick parent or parent-in-law. As life-givers, women are very powerful, but this power to cross life and symbol borders is obscured by pollution beliefs about the "uncleanliness" of female blood. Menstrual and birth blood are "out of place," that is, they are symbolically unclean—not because they lack value but because such bleeding is a forceful reminder of female power and its threat to male authority.[41] As "outsiders" in a still-patrilineal culture in Singapore, ethnic Chinese women rely on the birth of sons to anchor themselves in the male-oriented kinship system.

Whether these beliefs percolate in the heads of young couples as they eagerly peruse documents at the CordLife fair, I could not say. But their easy embrace of this technology, just one more really scientific thing to do in preparation for the baby's future, gives new meaning to the material and symbolic links between mother and the newborn. When I asked the expecting couples why they were interested in cord banking, my question drew blank stares: "Of course, we will do anything to protect the health of our baby!" To these couples, the question seemed silly. By becoming a biomedical tool, birth blood (contained in the placenta and usually thrown away at the hospital) now enhances the mother's status as the producer of new biovalues and endorses the technomodernity of parents who wish to protect their child against unknown kinds of future bioinsecurity.

The combination of blood bonds and blood-storing mechanisms promises to give new vitality to ethnic Chinese family values, reexpressing traditional beliefs but also rejuvenating and manifesting them in new ways. Folk beliefs in the regenerative capacities of blood are now confirmed by the life sciences, further reinforcing the concept of blood as a transnational biovalue that Chinese people share, no matter where they are located in the world. The possibility of storing this blood for use at a later time and in a different space, by one's own child or other children, bolsters beliefs in biological sameness and vulnerabilities.

The project of collecting blood as a life-saving resource, at both the public and the private level, is giving a modern visibility to the ethnos as a blood-sharing community. Attempts to sort Asian blood donations by ethnicity in public blood collection drives for leukemia treatments strengthen traditional beliefs in the potency of shared biological essence. The beneficiaries of these public blood drives are not known by the donors. Cord blood banking, by contrast, is a private practice, and donations benefit family members. The family benefit, while paramount for donors, is not the only advantage of private cord blood banking, for the commercial storage of blood preserves genetic materials that could be made available to a wider collectivity.

Private cord blood banking can be an important supplementary storage system that expands the public tissue network, perhaps increasing the availability of distinctive strands of Asian DNA materials for private or public uses. This complementary relationship of public and private blood banking broadens the circle of blood sharing beyond the family to the community and the cross-border collectivity of Asian patients needing stem cell therapy. The cumulative effect of giving blood in private arrangements and in public collection drives creates a biomedical code for deep-seated beliefs in a shared material essence among Chinese people at large.

Descriptions of tissue economies depend on strict binary oppositions between private and public, autologous and allogenic tissues, restrictive and collective repositories. Such perspectives cannot capture the complex interactions and ethical decision making that occur at the intersection of bioethics and other ethical regimes, that is, in the space of a particular ethical assemblage.

Southeast Asia and sites beyond it are haunted by social upheavals and recurring biological disasters, which have marked modern times. Beneath the glittering urban scene, the fate of peoples and nations is still precarious. Added to this complexity, we find techniques of biosecurity and bioinsurability that raise other ethical issues, giving rise to a vitalist politics that seems to sharpen ethnic differences, and a bioeconomy that is based on an ambiguous projection of future demographic differences and needs. It is clear that bioethics must move beyond the clinic to consider moral decisions and dilemmas linked by overlapping scales of risk and ethics.

Among the privileged ethnic Chinese of Singapore, the embrace of blood banking can be situated within a transnational network of inherited culture and health dilemmas. Such practices point to a new coding of genetic substances as signifying a kinship that extends beyond the immediate family to a tentative biosociality emerging out of shared diseases, genetic materials, and bioscience practices.[42] New genetic technologies thus suggest new ways for engaging in a kind of social autoproduction that already proceeds on other fronts.

As Sarah Franklin and Susan McKinnon have noted, "The substantial-codings that might signify kinship include a diverse range of phenomena—including genetic disease syndromes, the 'informatics' of computer programming, and family photography."[43] In Singapore, cord blood banking may be the "substantial-coding" that signifies an expanding ethnokinship. The mobilization and concentration of new genetic information in blood banking stirs an old imaginary of an ethnos that is both historically rooted in shared essence and transnational in scale.

Contemporary harnessing of blood, prompted by pharmaceutical interest, stirred by biopolitical risks, and produced by biotechniques, animates and ramifies a rich kinship symbolism that reverberates across science and commerce. Overseas Chinese have long placed great importance on photographic ancestral portraits, a form that inspires Zhang's paintings, as a means for registering and tracking kinship connections across time and space. In this light, the acquisition of Zhang Xiaogang's *Comrade no. 120* by a wealthy Singaporean becomes a poignant emblem of acts by overseas Chinese that "re-member" China, by reconnecting family bloodlines to mainland ancestor figures. This purchase of an anonymous "ancestor" seems a symbolic substitution for the dwindling practice of ancestor worship, especially when Chinese in diaspora are separated from the graves of ancestors on the mainland and from the rich soil of cultural China. Now, thanks to private blood banking, the act of preserving bloodlines can be extended literally, into the distant future and across transnational space. The banking of an infant's blood, like the collecting of ancestral ghosts, is a new practice among affluent Chinese who link the ethical decisions they make to safeguard their children's health with re-membering the umbilical cord that connects them back to the motherland.

This desire to be linked materially and symbolically to the motherland gains symbolic resonance as well from Zhang Xiaogang's global prominence in the contemporary art world. The aesthetic figuration of modern "Chinese" experiences and essences in the paintings that circulate in global art markets articulates the emerging status of modern Chinese subjects who have the means to perform the ethical role of owning and protecting works fraught with "Chinese" symbolic value. In an interview broadcast on CNN, Zhang said that he paints his black-and-white faces in order to depict "cloned people, as if dreaming." The faces are poised between amnesia and memory of emotional connections to family members once lost but now recoverable. In his "Bloodline Series," the faint marks, like scars, that we see on each face form a recurring motif that connects the individual pictures. One painting depicts a baby's face already marked by some genetic defect, as if signaling the need for biomedical vigilance and intervention by his loved ones. The "scar" is both a trace of the elusive memory and the imprint of flowing bloodlines. These reflections on the Chinese "big family," Zhang confides, is crucial to an "understanding of life itself."[44]

Notes

This essay draws on intensive interviews with officials, scientists, journalists, bioethicists, bioentrepreneurs, and citizens in Singapore and elsewhere from 2002 to 2008. I thank Andy Hao, Catherine Waldby, and Charles Briggs for helpful comments on earlier versions.

1. Sotheby's Contemporary Art Evening Auction, sale L08020, London, New Bond Street; session 1, February 27, 2008, http://www.sothebys.com/app/live/lot/LotDetail.jsp?lot_id=159430431.
2. Quoted in http://www.operagallery.com/artist/ZHANG+Xiao+Gang_659;0;0.aspx (accessed December 2009).
3. Catherine Waldby and Robert Mitchell, *Tissue Economies: Blood, Organs, and Cell Lines in Late Capitalism* (Durham: Duke University Press, 2006).
4. Ibid., 158–59.
5. Cori Hayden, "Benefit-sharing: Experiments in Governance," paper presented at the Social Science Research Council Workshop "Intellectual Property, Markets, and Cultural Flows," New York, October 24–25, 2003. Hayden has argued for a notion of "benefit-sharing" of native bioresources as a matter of justice for encouraging a more equitable distribution of values among sourced communities and bioprospecting and biomedical entities.
6. Michel Foucault, *Ethics: Subjectivity and Truth*, vol. 1 of *Essential Works of Foucault, 1954–1984*, ed. Paul Rabinow, trans. Robert Hurley and others (New York: New Press, 1997), xxxiii–xxxiv.
7. A related but different concept is Michael Fischer's "ethical plateaus" or domains of ethical challenge engendered by the workings of biotechnologies, information technologies, and environmental sciences that elicit, shape, or help constitute embedded subjectivities. See Michael M. J. Fischer, *Emergent Forms of Life and the Anthropological Voice* (Durham: Duke University Press, 2003).
8. See Joseph E. Davis, "An Interview with Francis Fukuyama," *[Paleopsych] Hedgehog*, October 19, 2004, http://lists.extropy.org/pipermail/paleopsych/2004-October/000710.html.
9. I use "cord blood" (instead of "cordial blood") because it is a branded term that codes this new practice in Southeast Asia and beyond.
10. Elizabeth Fernandez, "Legislators Touched by Leukemia Push to Save Umbilical Cord Blood," *San Francisco Chronicle*, August 13, 2007, A1, A10.
11. Lim Say Boon, "Economics and Science at Stake over Stem-Cell Research Debate," *South China Morning Post*, September 8, 2002, 4.
12. "Singapore Relaxes Jail Penalty for Human Cloning," *International Herald Tribune*, May 12, 2004.
13. Sylvia Lim and Calvin Ho, "The Ethical Position of Singapore on Embryonic Stem Cell Research," *SMA News* (Singapore Medical Association) 35, no. 6 (June 2003): 22–23.

14. Claudia Aradau, "Beyond Good and Evil: Ethics and Securitization/Desecuritization Techniques," *Rubikon E-journal* (December 2001).
15. Stephen J. Collier and Andrew Lakoff, "The Vulnerability of Vital Systems: How 'Critical Infrastructure' Became a Security Problem," in *Securing "the Homeland,"* ed. Myriam Anna Dunn and Kristian Søby Kristensen (New York: Routledge, 2007).
16. Aihwa Ong, "Baroque Ecology, Effervescent Citizenship," in *Neoliberalism as Exception: Mutations in Citizenship and Sovereignty* (Durham: Duke University Press, 2006).
17. Aihwa Ong, "Assembling around SARS: Technology, Body Heat, and Political Fever in Risk Society," in *Ulrich Becks: Kosmopolitisches Projekt*, ed. Angelika Pferl and Natan Szaider (Badan-Baden: Nomos Verlagsgesellschaft, 2004).
18. Sarah Franklin, "Life Itself: Global Nature and the Genetic Imaginary," in *Global Nature, Global Culture*, ed. Sarah Franklin, Celia Lury, and Jackie Stacey (London: Sage, 2000).
19. Leong Chin, "A Life-Saving Gift," *Straits Times* (Singapore), September 25, 2005.
20. Interview with a professional, Singapore, June 16, 2004.
21. See Herbert Gottweis and Robert Triendl, "South Korean Policy Failure and the Hwang Debacle," Commentary, *Nature Biotechnology* 24, no. 2 (February 2006): 141–43.
22. See Kathleen Erwin, "The Circulatory System: Blood Procurement, AIDS, and the Social Body in China," *Medical Anthropology Quarterly* 20, no. 2 (2006): 139–59.
23. Quote by the Children's Cancer Foundation (Singapore), on the Cord Blood Bank of Singapore Web site, "Strategic Alliances," http://www.ccf.org.sg/train_research/cord_blood_bank.html (accessed December 2009); the author of this unsigned article is Dr. Fidah Alsagoff, executive director of the Children's Cancer Foundation.
24. "Umbilical cord blood headed from China to Singapore," *Stem Cell Research Blog*, August 21, 2005, http://stemcell.taragana.net/ (article no longer available).
25. As China emerges as a global economic powerhouse, Mandarin proficiency has spread throughout the Asia-Pacific region, and not only among ethnic Chinese communities.
26. Waldby and Mitchell, *Tissue Economies*, 130.
27. "Life Line," *Business Times* (Singapore), September 24, 2005.
28. Koh Buck Song, "Perfect People's Fears," *Today* (Singapore), April 14, 2004.
29. Interview with Steven Fang, January 27, 2007, World Economic Forum, Davos, Switzerland.
30. Ibid.
31. Quotation from http://www.CordLife.com/ (accessed March 19, 2006).

32. See Kaushik Sunder Rajan, *Biocapital: the Constitution of Postgenomic Life* (Durham: Duke University Press, 2006), chap 3.
33. Susan Strange, *Casino Capitalism* (Manchester: Manchester University Press, 1997), 111.
34. Tan Kin Lian, quoted in "Leading Singapore Insurer, NTUC Income, to Provide Insurance for CordLife Customers," press release from CordLife's parent company, CyGenics Ltd. (Australia), n.d.
35. Interview with Steven Fang.
36. Chang Ai-lien, "Parents Save Son by Having Another Baby," *Straits Times* (Singapore), August 6, 2004.
37. Waldby and Mitchell, *Tissue Economies*, 120.
38. CordLife, "Singapore-based CordLife acquires U.S.-based Cytomatrix," press release, April 29, 2003.
39. Nikolas Rose and Carlos Novas, "Biological Citizenship," in *Global Assemblages Technology, Politics, and Ethics as Anthropological Problems,* ed. Aihwa Ong and Stephen J. Collier (Malden, Mass.: Blackwell, 2005).
40. Marilyn Strathern, "Emergent Properties," in *Kinship, Law, and the Unexpected* (Cambridge: Cambridge University Press, 2005), 76–77.
41. For practices in rural Taiwan, see Emily M. Ahern, "The Power and Pollution of Chinese Women," in *Women in Chinese Society*, ed. M. Wolf and R. Witke (Stanford, Calif.: Stanford University Press, 1975), 193–214.
42. Paul Rabinow, *Essays on the Anthropology of Reason* (Princeton, N.J.: Princeton University Press, 1999), 99.
43. Sarah Franklin and Susan McKinnon, "Introduction: Relative Values: Reconfiguring Kinship Studies," in *Relative Values: Reconfiguring Kinship Studies*, ed. Sarah Franklin and Susan McKinnon (Durham: Duke University Press, 2001), 11.
44. "Talk Asia," with Anjali Roa, *CNN TV News*, viewed in Shanghai, July 15, 2007.

MARGARET SLEEBOOM-FAULKNER

Embryo Controversies and Governing Stem Cell Research in Japan | HOW TO REGULATE REGENERATIVE FUTURES

Human embryonic stem cell research is controversial in many societies partly because it makes use of human oocytes and human embryos, which usually die in the experimental process, and partly because of the ways in which these biomaterials are acquired. This creates difficulties for research. Despite the fact that now over 1 percent of Japanese newborns are conceived through IVF (in vitro fertilization), which co-generates "supernumerary" embryos, and despite the fact that in Japan approximately fifty thousand oocytes are discarded per year, researchers have trouble obtaining them.[1]

The national discussion on human embryonic stem cell research in Japan is said to be hardly alive,[2] and cannot be expected to inform policy makers on the subject. Public discussion in the context of civil society takes place in a social space between state and society.[3] It is thought that as no religious or cultural canons forbid human embryonic stem cell research in Japan, any national debate on the normative status of the embryo would be uncontroversial. Paradoxically, according to most of the fifty people I interviewed over two years from April 2006 to April 2008—including scientists, regulators, monks, and housewives—debate on human embryonic stem cell research is considered to be very important to science policy making. But regulators and scientists argue repeatedly that the debate is monopolized by the voices of a few minorities. Of the forty scientists and regulators that I interviewed, thirty declared that the public in Japan is not really interested in human embryonic stem cell research, apart from a few minority groups whose special interests range from eugenics to spinal cord injuries and religious beliefs.

In Japan, perhaps because discussions on genomics and stem cell research are largely orchestrated by the government, the term "national discussion" (*kokuminteki giron*) is used to refer to debates on these subjects rather than "public debate" (*kooshu tooron*). In this essay, therefore, I make a distinction between "national discussion" and "public debate." The former refers to a discussion that is held or promoted on a national basis, involving active participants and stakeholders from any administrative and socioeconomic part of society. The latter aims to involve people who do not have direct interests in the debate (the "general public") but who are thought to have a right to know and understand the issues concerned, and to express their views on it. I argue that, in Japan, a national discussion may have been held on human embryonic stem cell research, but not a public debate,[4] and that most direct stakeholders in human embryonic stem cell research perceive a public debate as something bothersome and even un-Japanese. But at the same time, stakeholder groups regard it as necessary and useful, for different reasons. Thus, scientists expect the public to support them once their intentions and the research purpose is understood; regulators believe debate encourages the acceptance of regulation; while social movements believed debate would raise awareness of the problems involved in this kind of research.

It should be pointed out here that these terms are relative, as becomes immediately clear when one tries to apply them to human embryonic stem cell debates in China and South Korea, countries that were quick to enter this scientifically advanced field. In South Korea, especially after the scandal involving the stem cell scientist Hwang Woo-Suk, the debate on the bioethics of human embryonic stem cell research was held in a context of nationalist ideology. Although this debate could also be referred to as a "national discussion," the nationalist tone that the debate took in South Korea is virtually absent from the discussion that has taken place in Japan. In China, meanwhile, the term "national discussion" seems to be entirely out of place, as the debate is confined to narrow circles of scientists and intellectuals on the Web and in some specialist journals. In fact, debate on the value of the embryo seems to be suppressed rather than encouraged.[5] Furthermore, the reasons for the authorities to encourage debate and the circumstances in which the debates are held vary substantially between China and Japan. Although both countries have only research guidelines for stem cell research—that is, no legislation—the guidelines in Japan are far more restricting and, indeed, are a source of despair to many scientists involved in human embryonic stem cell research. In China, regulation for stem cell research is rather loose. The Chinese state then, if it can be said to encourage debate at all, aims at persuading scientists to stick to internationally acknowledged guidelines, such as those published by the International Society for Stem Cell Science. In Japan, by contrast, debate aims to persuade the public to trust the work of stem cell scientists, rather than to make those scientists comply with international guidelines.

Despite, their limited applicatory value, I use the distinction between national discussion and public debate to discuss the relevant views of the three "minority voices" in the light of their needs, hopes, and fears and the expectations they have of the role of human embryonic stem cell research in their lives and in society. Their claims have come to play an important role in the Japanese national discussion on stem cell research. In the first section of this essay, I explain the relationship between regulation and the perceived need for national debate. In the next two sections, I describe the views of three minority voices on human embryonic stem cell research and how in the national discussion they are amplified and used by regulators and scientists. In the final section, I discuss how the national discussion, based on expectations of science, perceived risks, and doubts about the future of human embryonic stem cell research, is shaped into official policies.

Regulatory Difficulties and the National Discussion on Human Embryonic Stem Cell Research in Japan

When President Bush in 2001 declared a moratorium on federal funding for human embryonic stem cell research,[6] scientists and liberal bioethicists were indignant. In Asia generally, the reactions of scientists, media, and policy makers to these bioethical scruples have an overtone of scorn and, in many cases, disbelief. In Japan, the discussion on human embryonic stem cell research can hardly be compared to the heated debates sparked by the use of embryos in research in the United States and Europe.[7] In the words of the developmental biologist Kazuto Kato, leader of Genomics Square, a platform for discussion between scientists and the general public in Japan, the question whether human embryonic stem cell research should be allowed is "no longer a big issue."[8] He explains, "It is assumed that since there are no cultural canons prohibiting abortion in Japan, the use of embryos for research, including [human embryonic stem cell research], is not a matter for great dispute. Some Japanese thinkers claim that Japanese Buddhism would place more emphasis on issues related to death, rather than on birth."[9] Consequently, in this view a debate on the status of the embryo in the Japanese context could hardly be considered relevant.

Compared to Europe and the United States, then, Japan has little public discussion on human embryonic stem cell research.[10] The cultural background of Japan is widely held to explain the scant bioethical concern about embryo research in Japan, which has facilitated the Japanese government's great efforts to promote such research. Among the government's incentives for genomics in general, and embryo research in particular, have been the building of a research infrastructure, financial support of research projects and the Millennium Project,[11] and the establishment of various national and governmental bioethics committees and strategies to devise and facilitate research and bioethical regulation. On November 30, 2000, the Japanese Parliament enacted the Human Cloning Regulation Act, creating ample allowance for in vitro human embryo research, and in September 2001, the Koizumi government approved the use of embryonic stem cell lines for basic research.[12] With the subsequent issue of "Guidelines for Derivation and Utilization of Human Embryonic Stem Cells" (2001) by three ministries,[13] Japan became one of few countries that officially permitted research on human embryonic stem cells.

Those who believe that in Japan the status of the embryo is unimportant might be surprised to hear that the status of the embryo in Japan is a matter of concern after all. Although the 2001 guidelines allowed the destruction of embryos, they also emphasize that it is necessary for the researchers to express "respect" for stem cells and the embryo. They must obtain informed consent from the donors, and permit donors to withdraw that consent if they wish.[14] Each research application must be double-checked, first by the "local" institutional review board (IRB) and then by the committee of the Expert Group on Bioethics (Seimei Rinri Senmon Chooshakai) of the Cabinet's Council for Science and Technology Policy (CSTP, Kagaku Soogoo Kenkyuukai), formally headed by the prime minister, on a governmental level.[15] The cell lines in question may only be used for basic research, and fertilized eggs can only be obtained from married couples after written consent and without compensation. From these guidelines it can be surmised that not only the moral status of the embryo but also that of oocytes is a matter of great concern to regulators. In short, researchers are expected to adjust their emotional and moral faculties and behavior to the guidelines.

In a next step on the road to the full regulation of human embryonic stem cell research, on June 23, 2004, Japan's highest-ranking organization for science and technology policy making, the Cabinet's Council for Science and Technology Policy (CSTP), opened the door to the cloning of human embryos.[16] Shortly thereafter, on July 1, 2004, the Expert Group on Bioethics of the Council voted unanimously to allow the use of stem cells from aborted fetuses in clinical research.[17] In line with the Cloning Restriction Law passed in June 2001, for the purpose of banning human cloning, the council was asked to deal with such matters as the handling of cloned embryos. After three years of debate, the Expert Group on Bioethics of the Council reached a decision in favor of embryo cloning for the use of medical research and regenerative medicine,[18] that is, the science and technology built around stem cells' regenerative capacity. Nevertheless, critics contested the decision, not only for failing to allow for sufficient public debate but also because there had been insufficient parliamentary debate.[19] Despite these major organizational and financial efforts to stimulate the life sciences, however, in 2006 Japan still had not been able to set up full regulations for embryo cloning, making it difficult for the science community to proceed with human embryo cloning and embryo research. Moreover, only a few scientists concentrate on human embryonic stem cells, and research groups interested in human embryo cloning are hard to find.

Minority Voices and the Debate on Reproductive Resources

If in Japan the broad public is not aware of the debates around human embryonic stem cell research, who then are the critics of this research? Why are provisions made in the regulations for human embryonic stem cell research, and why have embryo cloning and the procurement of oocytes become issues? As I noted at the start of this essay, many scientists claim that, apart from some patient groups that fervently encourage research into stem cell therapies, and with the exception of a few religious groups that oppose it, the majority of the population is not interested in stem cells. The existing national discussion, considered crucial to science policy making, is, they claim, monopolized by the voices of only a few groups, notably the Anti-Eugenics Network (Yuusei Shisoo wo Too Netto-uuku), an advocacy group for feminists and the disabled, the Japan Spinal Cord Foundation (JSCF), and a few radical religious sects, among which are the Shinto Oomoto sect and the Buddhist Seichoo no Ie.

Japanese religiocultural concepts of "life" are of great relevance to the ways in which various groups of people express their agreement or opposition to embryo and/or oocyte donation. The Bioethics Committee of the Council for Science and Technology Policy officially defined the embryo as the "germ of life" (*seimei no myooga*). This view is regarded by many researchers as typically Japanese, contrasting greatly with what is regarded as the Western religious dogma, that the embryo is conceived by the grace of God, which leads to the view that induced abortion is evil. The view of the embryo as the germ of life, according to Professor Ida Ryuuichi, means that its destruction equals killing a potential human. But at the same time, as a nonreligious view, it does allow the argument that the use of embryos left over after IVF treatment (supernumerary embryos) could actually lead to something positive, such as new therapies to cure disease.[20] This view is widespread in regulatory circles, and is echoed by most stem cell researchers. This does not mean, however, that Japan has no opponents of current induced abortion practices or of human embryonic stem cell research. The Shinto Oomoto sect and the Buddhist Seichoo no Ie sect both oppose abortion induced for economic reasons and reject any form of embryo research. The Oomoto sect proclaims that the human soul enters a gamete at the time of fertilization, although it acquires its full human status only gradually in later stages of growth. For this reason, according to the sects, the human embryo should not be used for research, including embryonic stem cell research.[21] The Oomoto sect tries to spread its message both to governmental committees and the general public in a variety of ways, including making public comments on the draft guidelines for human embryonic stem cell research. Nevertheless, according to Kato, it is probably fair to say that the main direction of the stem cell debate in Japan is not strongly influenced by recognized religious groups.[22]

Some of the staunchest supporters of human embryonic stem cell research are found among the members of the Japan Spinal Cord Foundation. Especially young people with recent spinal injuries and people with severely debilitating forms of spinal cord injury place great hopes on stem cell therapies, which have been among the targets of large amounts of government research funding. Until recently, the bleak prognosis for effective treatment and for restoring the loss of function in patients suffering from spinal cord injury caused the government and local communities to focus on long-term care services. However, since the early 1990s, the regeneration of central nervous system tissue became regarded as a possibility, and high hopes were placed on effective treatment.[23] Nevertheless, there is also a modest amount of cynicism about the promises of science research. This is partly due to the disappointing experience of several Japanese patients, who traveled to Beijing and South Korea for treatment, where they were disillusioned by the unrealized promises of scientists such as Huang Hongyun in Beijing and Hwang Woo-Suk in South Korea. I asked the president of the Japan Spinal Cord Foundation about the opponents of human embryonic stem cell research. He explained:

> I don't know them directly. There are those who want fast cures and others who do not. Most are waiting for a cure. We are now waiting for the discussion about "the dignity of man [*ningen no songen*]" to be resolved. Especially people that suffer from ALS [amyotrophic lateral sclerosis] are desperate. It is really necessary to respect the spinal cord injury people. ALS people are really just waiting for therapy. They would do anything to get a cure. They hold on to a straw.[24]

Evidently, "respecting humans" here means helping those who are crippled, in pain, and desperate. The reference to the "straw" indicates that there exists awareness about the bioethics of expectation and disappointment. On the other hand, the bioethical questions surrounding donating reproductive material have not been touched upon in the group. I was the first person to raise the issue, causing some confusion about its relevance to finding a cure for spinal cord injuries. To this group of patients, human embryonic stem cell research means the quest for a cure for spinal cord injuries.

Among the opponents of human embryonic stem cell research are members of the Anti-Eugenics Network. One member of the network, Mrs. B, explained the mission of the organization as reflecting upon and dealing with issues of discrimination and living in relation to the new life sciences, from the point of view of women and handicapped people.[25] The Anti-Eugenics Network opposes human embryonic stem cell research for various reasons. One is that this research has gone ahead even though there has not been a thorough public debate on its merits, risks, and ethicality. Another concern is the provision of oocytes necessary for the cloning of embryos; the Anti-Eugenics Network is of the opinion that women cannot make a judgment about such a gift without first knowing what they really want, independent from the pressure of the medical establishment and independent of the interests of others surrounding them. This, the network argues, should be organized first, before women are asked to give away their oocytes to organizations that are going to profit from their "gift" in the long run. Many women feel anxious about oocyte and embryo donation, especially as it places a claim on them for the provision of reproductive materials, often under circumstances that are not conducive to making rational decisions, for example, after hormone treatment in an IVF clinic, just after becoming pregnant, or after the failure of an IVF cycle.[26]

Among the organizations for the disabled in Japan there is much scepticism about the ability of science to deliver on its promises. The constant announcement of scientific discoveries and expectations for the future has generated a situation for handicapped people in which high hopes and disappointment have become a bottomless well of exhaustion and frustration. Furthermore, the enormous financial support for genomics research, according to many handicapped people, should be spent on other needs and facilities for handicapped people in general, not just for the few that could benefit from stem cell therapy. This point is especially emphasized since uncertainty existed about the Japanese government's plans in early 2006 for the care of handicapped children.[27]

This brief description of minority voices in Japan's national debate about human embryonic stem cell research can be summarized in terms of claims on the future. The Oomoto sect demands a society in which reproductive materials are respected as part of nature. The opposition of the Anti-Eugenics Network is linked to the interests of women, from where embryos and oocytes are thought to derive, and the interests of handicapped people, who are not expected to benefit from human embryonic stem cell research as a whole; the network wants gender equality and recognition for the disabled and unborn. Members of the Japan Spinal Cord Foundation, however, are strongly in favor of such research, so that patients can reclaim their lives through the advancement of science; its support for research, however, is highly personal, and issues of embryo and oocyte donation hardly play a role in discussions held at the foundation.

Minority Voices and the Views of Academics, Scientists, and Regulators

Although "Japanese culture" plays an important role in the way political discourse around the regulation of human embryonic stem cell research is formulated, the views summarized above show clearly that it is incorrect to presume the existence of some kind of Japanese essence responsible for the Japanese indifference toward the normative status of the embryo. However, neither is it correct to consider the three minority voices in the debate as the main carriers of this debate in Japan. These minority groups may be regarded as radicals in society by a large proportion of scientists and regulators, but at the same time, they represent views of women's groups, various groups of disabled people, and religious groups as well. The main aims of these groups, however, are linked to quests other than establishing an opinion about human embryonic stem cell research. One of the reasons that we do not hear the voices of other groups is because the debate does not link with the purposes of other organizations. Another reason may be that they are not "interesting" enough for the people responsible for discussing the ethical nature of human embryonic stem cell research: members of official committees, people close to the media, and members of the Japanese Diet. The views of some of the "minority" voices are loud and clear, not so much because they are powerful groups in Japanese political life, but rather because their views have been quoted, manipulated, and hijacked by politicians and academics for their own ends.

The interviews conducted with people who have a stake in the debate on human embryonic stem cell research indicate a great need for such a debate in Japan. There are various reasons for this, most of which are not shared by the different interest groups involved, as will become clear below.

Professor G from the University of Tokyo and a member of the Expert Group on Bioethics of the CSTP, was one of the main opponents to the final recommendation of the committee to allow embryo cloning in Japan. At a time when scientists pointed out Hwang Woo-Suk's success in Korea, and the South Korean government followed their advice to further research efforts in this area of research, Professor G had already commented that there "was something wrong." As so many oocytes had been collected for the research, he believed that the oocytes had been acquired by unethical means. He also knew many watchers in the Anti-Eugenics Network who were angry about the government's plans to go ahead with research in the absence of proper debate.[28]

There is also a need for a global debate, Professor G argued: if China and India go ahead with stem cell research, it means an unfair (*fusei*) situation in scientific development.[29] Another problematic matter, according to Professor G, is that the Japanese can go abroad for organ transplants while transplants are severely restricted in Japan.[30] We clearly need common standards. Professor G points out that even within Japan, Joodo Shinshu (Pure Land Shin Buddhism) has a strict position on abortion,[31] based on its concept of the importance of life (*inochi no taisetsusa*)—though he suspects that Joodo Shinshu's ulterior motive for stimulating Japanese birth is related to colonial expansionism. Professor G claims that the modern state wants to control reproduction, and he is interested in studying how religion is related to this function. Referring to Sooshiren, the largest Japanese women's movement, which also supports the rights of the disabled,[32] and the Anti-Eugenics Network, Professor G defines his stance as follows:

> Feminists oppose state control over reproduction, and some religious movements do so too. And I support them. I am close to the views of the Oomoto sect on cloning embryos, and I agree with their views on abortion—but they are not as strict as Catholics are.[33]

Here, various ethical positions, from religious groups and feminists, are cited as part of the public orientation of a member of a prestigious committee, who has attracted attention as an opponent of human embryonic stem cell research and as a troublemaker for science. Various people who have sat with Professor G on committees have been annoyed by his "unscientific attitude" and his explanations of the values of Japanese society, with reference to feminists, Japanese religious sects, and the disability movement.[34] Although all these groups have called for public debate, complaints continue to be vented about the scant involvement of the public. Professor G's citation of the minority voices seems to make more public engagement difficult. Instead of quoting the views of people from various walks of life, the philosophies and political stances of minorities are used in public statements by individuals like this committee member, which seem to obscure the debate on human embryonic stem cell research.

Other regulators, such as Professor H, consider the Anti-Eugenics Network as their backbenchers. Professor H, a strong voice against voluntary donation, served as a member of the Committee for Human (somatic) Cloning in a Clinical Setting for the Ministry of Health, Labor, and Welfare. Professor H said that in this committee he was "hated by all" (*mina ni kirawareta*) for obstructing regulation for embryo use in a clinical setting.[35] Professor H explains some of the difficulties faced by the committee. In the summer of 2004, it became known that two fetuses had been discovered in the waste bin of Yokohama City Hospital (Yokohama Shinai Byooin), although procedure rules stipulate that the fetuses should go to a special furnace for destruction. Afterward, surveys indicated that the Yokohama City Hospital incident was not an isolated case, a matter that turned the incident into a public scandal. All the committee members realized that it would be difficult for quite some time to regulate embryo/fetal research in a clinical setting. Furthermore, other bioethical problems had compounded the regulation of this research. For instance, if embryo research were to be allowed for medical purposes, a range of medical applications might come under that rubric: the committee might also have to regulate the production of cosmetics. The lack of knowledge about stem cells would complicate any established research protocol, and some highly placed science leaders expressed their fears of uncontrolled experimentation, for example, injecting embryo cells into people's brains.[36] Referring to the Anti-Eugenics Network, Professor H expressed doubts about embryonic cloning: "It is all in support of regenerative medicine, but as yet regenerative medicine is not advanced enough." Besides, Professor H wants donors to ask themselves for what reason they should donate their embryos. They may not know whether it is truly for the benefit of science, or donate just to please the physician, or others around them. Professor H is convinced that there has not been sufficient public discussion on cloning embryos. In Japan, according to Professor H, the people who recommended human embryonic stem cell research were in charge of the discussion on the subject. Instead, he believes, consensus on a societal level should be required before allowing it. In fact, Professor H is calling for a discussion that involves the public.

In Japan support groups and charity organizations receive very few financial donations. Fiscally, financial donations, including those to science and medical research, are discouraged. Patient organizations derive their main financial support from the state and from relatives and friends of patients. In this situation patient organizations can hardly afford to support medical research, which in the case of human embryonic stem cell research in Japan is financed mainly by the government. It is not surprising then that scientific leaders and principle investigators of research centers refer to the needs of patient groups such as the Japan Spinal Cord Foundation to attract research funding. Some well-known principal investigators and science leaders, such as Okano Hideyuki from Keio University, Nakatsuji Norio from Kyoto University, and Nishikawa Shinichi from the RIKEN Center for Development Biology in Kobe, are regularly invited by patient organizations to give public lectures to explain why human embryonic stem cell research is necessary. Moreover, there is no doubt that these scientists genuinely hope to help the patients.

The Japan Spinal Cord Foundation therefore feels supported by scientists and has faith in scientific developments, not least because its scientific allies are both fundraisers and members of committees that regulate stem cell research. Mr. C from the foundation explains:

> As a patient organization we want to make information about scientific research known. We organize meetings and invite scientists to speak so that patients can ask questions about safety, risk, benefit, and the state of the art. In Japan there are quite a few researchers, and we have three particular connections [with well-known scientists].[37]

The mobilization of this group in support of a balanced discussion on human embryonic stem cell research in another context, however, can be regarded as strategic. A genetic counselor, Dr. D, described the final meeting of the bioethics committee of the Council for Science and Technology Policy, before the completion of their report of recommendation on whether to allow human embryonic stem cell research in Japan:

> In the summer of 2004 there was a public hearing. The discussion was aimed at consensus in Japan. There were several people with spinal cord injuries present. The chair, [Professor I], pointed to them and asked the representative to say something. It was almost as if these people were invited to put pressure onto the committee. It came across like an argument and seemed to make opponents of human embryonic stem cell research look like villains.[38] It seems that the voice of the Japan Stem Cell Foundation would hardly be heard at all, if political and scientific stakeholders had not amplified it.

Other leaders in the discussion on bioethics, however, refer to bureaucratic hurdles, blaming both bureaucrats and foreign concepts of bioethics for the poor regulation of human embryonic stem cell research. Professor J, who occupies an important position in the Medical Ethics Committee of the Faculty of Medicine, University of Tokyo, denies the relevance of any Japanese concept of "respect for the embryo." Professor J asserts that Japanese culture has never regarded abortion as a problem before, and has no reason to start worrying about it now.[39] The embryo is not regarded as a full human being. The reason Japan started applying the *foreign* concept of respecting the "dignity of man" to the embryo in its regulations, argues Professor J, is that Japan feels compelled to follow the example of the West. In fact, Professor J experiences the current administrative guidelines as a hindrance to human embryonic stem cell research in a clinical setting. His frustration with the guidelines is related to the complexity of Japanese regulation, which is responsible for the lack of clear standards for the evaluation of embryonic research.[40] Instead, Professor J aspires to facilitate such research in his efforts to develop science and help patients:

> In my position I would like to show the people that using science and technology and doing research is OK. Convincing people of that is my work—in order to facilitate the development of science.[41]

Bioethical discussions in Professor J's view are not helpful:

> The Anti-Eugenics Network has sent me many letters. They always refer to *hito no songen* [human dignity], but they never come up with a better justification for not helping patients than that.[42]

Although the views of the Anti-Eugenics Network on human dignity may have been misread, it is evident that the complexity of current regulations and the inconsistency of the application of concepts such as human dignity form an obstruction to both public debate and scientific practice. At the same time, however, even though the regulators and leaders of bioethics discussed here are in favor of a public debate in Japan, their quotation of the wishes, quests, and ethical problems of small publics in society defeats its purpose. If the broader public cannot identify with the minority voices of small groups of patients, referring to these rather than addressing the problems raised by opponents in the debate may be counterproductive.

Facilitating the Future of Human Embryonic Stem Cell Research

In this last section I try to elucidate how the way is gradually being paved for the facilitation of human embryonic stem cell research in Japan, through the deliberation of bioethics committees and the organization of a "national discussion," and by proceeding in small steps. I will argue that although this process is sensitive to international developments and the views of various stakeholders at home, nearly all of my interviewees expressed dissatisfaction about the lack of public debate on human embryonic stem cell research in Japan. The "national discussion" may result in the political acceptance of this research and provide adjusted guidelines for it, but the general sentiment is that a more engaging "public discussion" would be required to successfully persuade a large proportion of the population to cooperate as oocyte and embryo donors and facilitators of research.

It is evident that both opaque regulation and an apparent lack of concern among the public do not encourage the donation of embryos and oocytes. The current, rather untransparent, regulations do not inspire confidence. Unlike regulatory measures in other technologically advanced societies, much of the regulation prepared in Japanese organizations is self-imposed and without penal provisions; it has no legal authority and is extremely complicated.[43] Furthermore, according to research by Yonemoto Shoohei and Nudeshima Jiro, the organizations in charge apply guidelines with different degrees of rigor, depending on the case in question. For this reason, leading bioethicists have pointed out that embryos, donors, and research subjects lack legal protection.[44]

Clear regulation of human embryonic stem cell research would make the work of scientists in the field less problematic, for reasons related to the need for reproductive materials, funding, and good reputation. Science leaders and principal investigators in Japan have pointed out the need to make embryos and oocytes more easily available to aid the progress of regenerative medicine, developmental biology, and stem cell science. The slow rate of the advance of Japanese human embryonic stem cell research compared, for instance, to mouse genomics is put forward as proof of Japan's comparative handicap in the international arena.[45] In Japan, embryos for stem cell research and oocytes for therapeutic cloning can only be obtained by following strict procedure. Embryos are supplied free through IVF hospitals, but procedures are in place to guarantee informed consent from donors and the application of bioethical guidelines on a case-by-case basis.

Better regulation and the organization of national discussion constitute the official answer to the question of how to stimulate human embryonic stem cell research in Japan. It is in this light that the regulation of human cloning and embryo cloning can be explained as a step forward in the direction of facilitating research. Thus, when in June 2001, legislation was introduced to strictly prohibit human cloning (regulation via legislation in Japan in itself is a rarity), it created at the same time the possibility for embryo cloning in the future. After all, the "ban" on human cloning only meant that scientists were allowed to clone "specified embryos," but prohibited to grow them into human clones.[46] In a way, it sanctioned the step toward embryo cloning, a direction enabled by the success of Hwang Woo-Suk in South Korea in early 2004. Not even half a year later, in July 2004, the Expert Group on Bioethics decided to allow embryonic cloning, after the creation of adequate regulation for oocyte donation and the construction of a solid scientific basis for cloning. Even though regulating the donation of oocytes would take some time, supporters of human embryonic stem cell research regarded it as a step forward. But the cloning scandal around Hwang Woo-Suk in December 2005, and the little progress made internationally, meant a setback to the advancement of the regulation. In May 2006, the Council for Science and Technology Policy decided that although embryo cloning would be allowed, it could only actually take place after sufficient experimentation on primates. And although some scientists complained that this was tantamount to prohibiting human embryo cloning, as the cloning of monkey embryos is regarded as very difficult, others argued that the current regulation has prepared Japan for sudden international advances in human embryo cloning. It enables the Japanese embryo research community to go ahead directly whenever an international breakthrough occurs in the field.

At the same time, the efforts at creating regulations for oocyte donation moved ahead. Couples were allowed to volunteer spare eggs, left over after IVF treatment, for the purpose of embryonic stem cell research. To this purpose, the Expert Committee for Science and Technology decided to appoint a coordinator to negotiate between researcher/hospital and volunteers. According to Professor G, these moves were entirely in agreement with the two strict conditions formulated in July 2004, under which human embryo cloning would be allowed: first, that the bioethical risks around oocyte donation be contained, and second, that a solid scientific basis for research be in place (i.e., ample animal experimentation). Similarly, Professor H regards the regulation permitting oocyte donation as a preparation for the next phase of human embryo cloning, as the government does not want to risk falling behind on global scientific development.

This attempt at regulating for future research purposes may have advantages for scientists with the ambition to engage in therapeutic cloning, but it is not at all clear that stem cell research will head in that direction. Some stem cell researchers believe such research is unlikely ever to be very successful; others believe that if it is successfully applied to diseases such as diabetes and Parkinson's disease, the number of oocytes required would be enormous. To remedy this, some hope to make use of the oocytes of animals, such as rabbits and cows, to facilitate at least basic research in this area. Other researchers, as publicly stated by Dr. Yamanaka Shinya, feel a distaste for using oocytes, although they do not dismiss their use for serious diseases, such as spinal cord injury.[47] Yamanaka over the last few years has developed a method to generate so-called induced pluripotent stem cells (iPS), reprogramming adult cells from ordinary human tissue such as skin. This method does not need oocytes or embryos, except perhaps for reasons of comparison. But even in this case, research regulation is unlikely to keep up with scientific developments, and certainly not with the public imagination. Although Kyoto University is still exploring whether the new cells are subject to Japan's restrictive law on human embryonic stem cell research, current regulations may already be outdated: pluripotent stem cells could, without using special laboratory equipment, easily generate oocytes and sperm that could be used for cloning. However, it is not clear whether induced pluripotent stem cells have the same capacity as human embryonic stem cells. And the clinical application of induced pluripotent stem cells is just as problematic as human embryonic stem cell therapy. Yamanaka pointed out that Japan's regulators would do well to be prepared to create new regulations.[48]

The national discussion on human embryonic stem cell research in Japan, as elsewhere in the world, was based on great expectations. From the outset, perceived risks and doubts about the future of stem cell research were accommodated for in official policies and they became part of a nation-wide discussion, which had followed substantial government investment.[49] In fact, some regulators of guidelines and observers of developments in human embryonic stem cell research believe that the outcome of the debate on such research in Japan had been favorable before it had even started. The government supported the research and regarded it as a good investment in the late 1990s. According to Dr. E,[50] the question put to people in government campaigns was "Shall we allow human embryonic stem cell research?" while listing its potential in the area of regenerative medicine. The lack of public response was interpreted as general agreement. If the question had been "Shall we prohibit human embryonic stem cell research?" a lack of response would not have meant support for the prohibition of research; a negative response also would not have meant such research should be crossed off the agenda. In this way, according to Dr. E, public opinion could be twisted into whatever policy the government wants to support.

Nevertheless, it is important to scientists, regulators, feminists, and religious groups that a wider public take a stance in the debate on human embryonic stem cell research. Each group has its own reasons, related to the claims it makes about the future role of stem cell research in society. In the debates that have occurred scientists and regulators refer only to a few: to demands by the disabled for a future without disability, and by women for a society in which they and their role in reproduction is respected and taken seriously; demands from people of religion, which rise from their discomfort with (post-)modern society and their desire for a simpler, "natural" way of life; and the demand, from scientists and regulators themselves, for international guidelines for human embryonic stem cell research. As long as the discussion is limited to notions of "the Japanese cultural attitude" or statements from minority-interest groups listed above, the stance of people from all the various socioeconomic and cultural backgrounds in Japan will remain unclear.

Given that until now discussion has been limited to the selective quotation of opinions from minority groups pursuing their own narrow agendas, nearly all stakeholders are now calling for a wider public debate. Although a national discussion on human embryonic stem cell research has been held in Japan, most of my interviewees were dissatisfied with its impact, and called for more public debate, as *wide public* engagement with the debate is seen as a condition for the success of stem cell research. This will mean not only the expression of conflicting views but also negotiation through debate among those different views. As has been the case in other areas of biomedical research in Japan, such as organ transplantation and biobanking,[51] insufficient involvement of the public may lead to public mistrust of scientists and the government, a questioning of the reasons for their undertakings, and also, an unwillingness to cooperate, donate, and participate when called upon. Such public debate, perhaps, could also address the anxieties and psychological burdens that accompany the separation of a disenchanted, scientistic worldview and the socioculturally and religiously informed bioethics of everyday life, which according to some bioethicists underlies the current opposition.[52]

Notes

The research on which this chapter is based was funded as part of an Economic and Social Research Council (ESRC) Fellowship under the Stem Cell Initiative (RES-350-27-0002) and an ESRC grant (RES-062-23-0215) for the joint-research project of Cambridge, Durham, and Sussex Universities entitled International Science and Bioethics Collaborations. A different version of this essay appeared in *Science as Culture* 17, no. 1 (March 2008), and I would like to thank the journal for the permission to reuse it.

1. Interview with Professor H, RIKEN (Rikagaku Kenkyuusho) Center for Developmental Biology, Kobe, May 8, 2006. (As this essay aims to discuss the dynamics of public discussion, and not persons, the interviewees in this article have been made anonymous. It was agreed with interviewees not to draw attention to their views as individual persons. Views that they have expressed at other occasions in public or in publications are of course fully attributed.) Also, see Yukiko Nakajo et al., "Physical and Mental Development of Children after *in vitro* Fertilization and Embryo Transfer," *Reproductive Medicine and Biology* 3 (2004): 63.
2. Kazuto Kato, "The Ethical and Political Discussions on Stem Cell Research in Japan," in *Grenzüberschreitungen* [Crossing Borders], ed. W. Bender et al. (Münster: Agenda Verlag, 2005).
3. Brian J. McVeigh, *The Nature of the Japanese State* (London: Routledge, 1998), 46.
4. Note that I do not claim that other countries, such as the United Kingdom or the United States, have experienced a public debate in the sense that the general public has been involved in a manner satisfactory to all interested parties.
5. Jing-Bao Nie, *Behind the Silence: Chinese Voices on Abortion* (Lanham, Md.: Rowman and Littlefield, 2005).
6. "President Discusses Stem Cell Research," August 9, 2001, http://www.whitehouse.gov/ (accessed February 30, 2008; no longer available).
7. See Suzanne Holland, Karen Lebacqz, and Laurie Zoloth, *The Human Embryonic Stem Cell Debate* (Cambridge, Mass.: MIT Press, 2001).
8. Kato, "The Ethical and Political Discussions," 369–79.
9. Ibid., 374–75.
10. Ibid., 369–79.
11. The Millennium Project, set up under Prime Minister Keizo Obuchi, included more than twenty universities and several foundations, consortia, and public and private research institutions in an initiative to develop the life sciences. It was sponsored jointly by the Science and Technology Agency (STA); the Ministry of Education, Sports, Science and Technology (MEXT); the Ministry of Health, Labor, and Welfare (MOHLW); and the Ministry of Economy, Trade, and Industry (METI).
12. Jiro Nudeshima, "Human Cloning Legislation in Japan," *Eubios Journal of Asian and International Bioethics* 11, no. 1 (2001), see http://www.eubios.info/EJ111/EJ111B.htm (accessed January 20, 2010); Masahiro Morioka, "The Ethics of Human Cloning and the Sprout of Human Life," in *Cross-Cultural Issues in Bioethics: The Example of Human Cloning*, ed. Heiner Roetz (Amsterdam: Rodopi, 2006).
13. The three ministries that issued the guidelines were the MEXT, the MOHLW, and the METI.
14. Ryuuichi Ida, "Ethical Questions of the Human Embryonic Stem Cells Research," *Rinsho Shinkeigaku* (Clinical Neurology) 42, no. 11 (November 2002): 1147–48.

15. Researchers must explain the prospect and nature of their research proposal, prove their proficiency and experience in using stem cells from other species, name the principal researchers, and regularly submit reports on their progress. Furthermore, applicants must identify those in charge of the internal ethical review, who judge the criteria governing the distribution and handling of fertilized eggs and the cell lines created from them. See Sara Harris, "Asian Pragmatism," *EMBO Reports* 3, no. 9 (2002), 816–17, http://www.nature.com/cgi-taf/DynaPage.taf?file=/embor/journal/v3/n9/full/embor069.html (accessed January 20, 2010).
16. "Government Council Okays Human Embryo Cloning for Basic Research," Foreign Press Center, July 6, 2004, http://www.fpcj.jp/e/shiryo/jb/0427.html (accessed February 30, 2008; no longer available).
17. David Cyranoski, "Japan Sets Rules for Stem Cell Research," *Nature Medicine* 10 (2004): 763.
18. "Government Council Okays Human Embryo Cloning for Basic Research."
19. Cyranoski, "Japan Sets Rules," 763.
20. Lecture by Ida Ryuuichi on bioethics, law, and stem cell research, Kyoto University, April 31, 2006. Professor Ida kindly provided me with his PowerPoint presentation.
21. For the Oomoto sect's view on HESR, see http://www.oomoto.or.jp/English/enBiet/escells.html (accessed January 20, 2010).
22. Kato, "The Ethical and Political Discussions," 374–75.
23. For a review of treatment possibilities, see the Web site of the ICCP (International Campaign for Cures of Spinal Cord Injuries Paralysis), http://www.campaignforcure.org (accessed January 20, 2010).
24. Interview with president of the Japan Spinal Cord Foundation, June 1, 2006 (the translation is mine).
25. The views of the Anti-Eugenics Network were published at http://cat.zero.ad.jp/yunet/index.html (accessed February 30, 2008; no longer available).
26. Interview with Professor H, June 8, 2006.
27. These views derive from the Web site of the Anti-Eugenics Network (http://www.cat.zero.ad.jp/yunet/sentan2.html); the page with documents submitted to various stem cell research institutes and the MEXT was at http://www.cat.zero.ad.jp/yunet/sentansiryoes.html (accessed February 30, 2008; no longer available). Shortly after, the government White Paper announced a measure that could improve the care of disabled children. See http://www8.cao.go.jp/youth/english/whitepaper/2007/pdf/2-3.pdf (accessed January 20, 2010).
28. Interview with Professor G, May 30, 2006.
29. Ibid.
30. This statement refers to various issues. One is the prohibition for children to donate their organs; as a consequence, children in need of a transplant go to the United States. A second problem is the extremely low number of available

organs for transplantation in Japan. Many Japanese are thought to go to China to receive kidney transplants (Clifford Coonan and David McNeill, "Japan's Rich Buy Organs from Executed Chinese Prisoners," *Independent*, March 21, 2006).

31. Pure Land Shin Buddhism is a branch of Pure Land Buddhism, which in turn is a branch of Mahayana Buddhism. The Pure Land sect (Joodo Shinshu) is practiced mainly in Japan (Shimazono Susumu, "Why Must We Be Prudent in Research Using Human Embryos: Differing Views of Human Dignity," in *Dark Medicine*, ed. William R. La Fleur, Gernot Boehme, and Shimazono Susumu [Bloomington: Indiana University Press, 2008]).
32. See Sandra Buckley, *Broken Science: Voices of Japanese Feminism* (Berkeley: University of California Press, 1997); Tiana Norgren, *Abortion before Birth Control: The Politics of Reproduction in Postwar Japan* (Princeton, N.J.: Princeton University Press, 2001); Azumi Tsuge, "How Japanese Women Describe Their Experiences of Prenatal Testing," *Frameworks of Choice: Predictive and Genetic Testing in Asia*, ed. Margaret Sleeboom-Faulkner (Amsterdam: Amsterdam University Press, 2010).
33. Interview with Professor G, May 30, 2006 (translation mine).
34. Interview with Dr. F, Science Council, May 31, 2006.
35. Interview with Professor H, June 8, 2006.
36. Interview Professor K, June 20, 2006.
37. "Particular connections" refers to scientists. Interview with patient group Japan Spinal Cord Foundation, June 1, 2006 (translation mine).
38. Interview with Dr. D, June 4, 2006.
39. Interview with Professor J, June 5, 2006.
40. Brian T. Slingby, Noriko Nagao, and Akira Akabayashi, "Administrative Legislation in Japan: Guidelines on Scientific and Ethical Standards," *Cambridge Quarterly of Healthcare Ethics* 13 (2004): 245–53.
41. Interview with Professor J, June 5, 2006 (translation mine).
42. Ibid.
43. Slingby, Nagao, and Akabayashi, "Administrative Legislation in Japan."
44. Shoohei Yonemoto and Jiro Nudeshima, "Science Policy Perspectives on Advanced Medical Technologies and Biomedical Research in Industrialized Countries," Mitsubishi Kagaku Institute of Life Sciences annual report 2004, http://www.mitils.co.jp/ann_report/pdf/pdf01/40-yonemoto.PDF (accessed January 2010).
45. According to a well-known human embryonic stem cell researcher, Professor L (interview, May 1, 2006), the damaging effect of regulation is expressed in the fact that internationally Japan publishes one out of three articles on mouse embryonic stem cell research, but none at all on human embryonic stem cell research (see *Biotechnology*, April 2006).
46. Morioka, "The Ethics of Human Cloning and the Sprout of Human Life," 1–16.

47. Shinya Yamanaka, "Scientists at Work," *New York Times*, December 11, 2007.
48. "Japanese Scientist Says Regulations Needed for Non-embryo Stem Cells to Avoid Abuse," *International Herald Tribune*, January 9, 2008.
49. Junji Kayukawa, *Kuroun Ningen* (Human Cloning) (Tokyo: Koubunsha Shinsho, 2003).
50. Interview with Dr. D, University of Tokyo, June 5, 2006.
51. Masayuki Yoshida, "Reconsidering the Japanese Negative Attitude toward Brain Death and Organ Transplantation," *Eubios Journal of Asian and International Bioethics* 14 (2004): 91–95; Tohru Masui, "Cultivating Trust and Motivation in Human Experiments: The Process of Creating Biobanks," in *Human Genetic Biobanks in Asia*, ed. Margaret Sleeboom-Faulkner (London: Routledge, 2008).
52. See the International Network for Life Studies Web site, http://www.lifestudies.org (accessed February 30, 2008).

IV

BIOSOVEREIGNTY | *Mappings of Chineseness*

JENNIFER A. LIU

Making Taiwanese (Stem Cells) | IDENTITY, GENETICS, AND HYBRIDITY

A prominent stem cell researcher announced that the aim of his study was to establish human embryonic stem cell "lines with genetic characteristics of the Taiwanese."[1] In producing uniquely Taiwanese stem cell lines he is simultaneously participating in the discursive production of a uniquely Taiwanese identity founded in genetic claims to difference. Contemporary social science literatures suggest that identity is a contingent and shifting abstraction. For some in Taiwan's elite scientific circles as well as in the popular media, however, genomic science is used to claim a material and historical basis for a unique Taiwanese identity. Following Latour that "science is politics by other means,"[2] making "Taiwanese" as a scientific category can be viewed as supporting an oppositional political claim toward both Taiwan's Kuomintang (KMT) party and the mainland's Chinese Communist Party (CCP).

Appeals to genomic science to know the truth about identity render identity as an irreducible material essence, granting science epistemological privilege and erasing the myriad cultural, imagined, agentive, and affective components of identity formation. In this way, identity becomes an object of scientific knowledge, and is constituted as a "field of truth."[3] In this chapter, I track one such identity-making discourse circulating in Taiwan. It suggests that the Taiwanese (*Taiwan ren*) represent a genetically distinct population from the Chinese (*Huaren*). I argue that both this strand of Taiwanese identity making and the making of Taiwanese stem cells rely on a series of discourses and practices of purification and hybridization that result in the production of populations understood as natural kinds, and constituted as biopolitical objects.

Genetic Nationalism

It is into highly charged discourses about Taiwanese nationalism that a strand of genomic science inserts a claim, via population genetics, to authenticate a uniquely "Taiwanese" identity.[4] There is nothing particularly new about using genetic knowledge to buttress or deny claims about ancestry or identity,[5] and a substantial literature addresses new forms of subjectification, sociality, and citizenship that emerge in light of advances in genomic science.[6] Paul Rabinow shows how DNA samples in a French biobank were reframed as a "national patrimony" in an effort to resist their commercialization.[7] French DNA was thus reconceptualized as something more than a biological object and made into an entity invested with value in both an economic and a moral sense. In this volume, Wen-Ching Sung shows how Chinese DNA is similarly viewed as a multivalent national resource in need of protection from foreign exploitation. Not only the materials of knowledge production, but genomic knowledge itself can take on nationalistic valences. Joan Fujimura shows that the material continuity between all forms of life inferred from shared DNA can be used to bolster a sense of national pride, when a prominent genomic researcher suggests that new genomic sciences will substantiate a Japanese view of the world in which ideas about continuity and animism figure prominently.[8]

In these accounts, claims made through genomic science in relation to nationalist projects require an essentialization of what it means to be French, Chinese, or Japanese. Similarly, Taiwanese identity claims made in relation to genomic knowledge require a specific conceptualization of what it means to be Taiwanese. The construction of a Taiwanese identity based in claims about genetic ancestry offers a unique example of how knowledge production in the biological sciences is taken up in projects of identity making and nation building.

Situating "Taiwaneseness"

Taiwan's recent history includes a series of foreign occupations including seventeenth-century settlements by the Dutch and Spanish, followed by an influx of Minnan and Hakka from southern China. Fifty years of colonial Japanese rule ended in 1945 when, in contested treaties, Taiwan was ceded to the Nationalist KMT government. Claiming to be the true representatives of China, the KMT invoked martial law until 1987, effectively creating minority rule over the Minnan and Hakka majority already living on the island.[9] Following a period of reform and transition, full electoral democracy was established in 1996. Although Taiwan currently operates an autonomous democratic government, Beijing's "One-China" policy claims Taiwan and its people as part of China.

Former president Chen Shui-bian was reelected in 2004 in a divisive, contested, and close election. In his election campaigns he ran on a strongly proindependence platform. Both his proindependence stance and his presidency were subsequently weakened by a loss of public support in the midst of an economic downturn and a series of scandals involving the first family. Nonetheless, his party, the Democratic Progressive Party (DPP)[10] remains involved in a deliberate project of building a national identity. The proindependence project articulates with various alternative modes of identity building, including divisive ethnicity-based discourses, educational reform, and the "new Taiwanese" movement of the 1990s. The "new Taiwanese" (*xin Taiwanren*) advocate a more inclusive approach to "Taiwaneseness" measured as a level of attachment and commitment rather than a specific ethnic origin.[11] Lowell Dittmer succinctly captures the tension and variability in mobilizing ethnicity in Taiwanese identity making:

> The focus has heretofore been on the impact of ethnic origins on national identity. True, after 30 years in which ethnicity was coercively "constructed" by the ruling KMT in support of a superimposed Chinese cultural heritage, the ethnic (or subethnic) cleavage seems to have reemerged in essentially primordial form (viz., *benshengren* vs. *waishengren*), in which capacity it functions as a potent mobilizational weapon in the tactical armory of the DPP in its electoral struggle in pursuit of "creeping independence." But the rise of the "New Taiwanese" since 1996 shows that ethnicity still has constructivist, as well as primordial, features, with ethnic identification subject to variation on both calculations of material or strategic advantages and idealistic emotional appeals.[12]

Scholarly analysis of Taiwan's contemporary identity focuses on a moving target, as Dittmer points out. It is in this dense, variable, and richly contested terrain of identity and nation building that genetic science is used to make truth claims about what it means to be Taiwanese.

On "Chineseness"

Narratives of identity are made in contradistinction to other ways of being. In Taiwan, multiple and at times contradictory discourses circulate on what it means to be Taiwanese, and these are most frequently shaped in constitutive tension with what it means to be Chinese. Narratives of "Taiwaneseness" and Taiwanese modernity, however, are refracted off multiple others. As for diasporic or overseas Chinese[13] more generally, the Taiwanese "face many directions at once—toward China, other Asian countries, and the West—with multiple perspectives on modernities."[14] I am interested here, however, in a particular argument that seeks to create a Taiwanese identity that disarticulates itself from a Chinese identity.

An argument to be not Chinese requires an examination of what it might mean to be Chinese. An emergent literature addresses itself to the multiple ways of constituting "Chineseness" in contingent configurations that are simultaneously local and transnational. While much of this literature is concerned with generating explanations to account for the apparent exceptionalism of Chinese transnational capitalist networks,[15] more subtle accounts attend to the new kinds of subjectivities, imaginaries, discourses, and cultural practices that emerge alongside new conceptualizations and lived realities of "being Chinese."[16] Less common still are accounts of those who seek actively to disarticulate themselves from their ascribed identities as Chinese.

The standard historiography of the Chinese, generally promoted by both the Chinese Communist Party (CCP) on the mainland as well as the KMT, supports a common origin for all ethnic Chinese. In this story, a common ancestry is traceable back to Huang Di, the Yellow Emperor, and spatialized on the Central Plains of northern China. This account links all ethnic Chinese to a common ancestral, territorial, and cultural origin,[17] and it had been the official story taught in Taiwan since KMT rule began in 1945. Tu Weiming explains:

> The question of Chineseness, as it first emerged in the "axial age" half a millennium prior to the birth of Confucius in 551 B.C., entails

> both geopolitical and cultural dimensions. While the place of China has substantially expanded over time, the idea of a cultural core area first located in the Wei River Valley, a tributary of the Yellow River, and later encompassing parts of the Yangtze River has remained potent and continuous in the Chinese consciousness. Educated Chinese know reflexively what China proper refers to. . . . They know for sure that the center of China . . . is in the north near the Yellow River.[18]

In this way, China, and consequently "Chineseness," are spatialized to an originary location not far from China's contemporary capital of Beijing. Additionally, this spatialized origin is linked to an ancestral origin in Huang Di. While, as Tu articulates, civilizational and cultural references, rather than ethnic references, are often prominent in discussions and definitions of "Chineseness," Huang Di denotes an ancestral and ethnic origin, and is often evocative of continuity and ethnic pride among the Chinese.[19] Certainly there is no single "Chinese consciousness," and ways of being Chinese exceed static models based on national, territorial, ethnic, and cultural configurations.[20] The idea of some kind of Chinese essence is nonetheless mobilized to specific ends, including those of entrepreneurial capitalist alliances based on shared Chinese ethnic identity,[21] and those underwriting triumphalist narratives of Chinese capitalism and ethnic chauvinism among the elites of this capitalism.[22]

In contradistinction to this singular narrative, however, "Chineseness" is constituted, imagined, and lived in a multiplicity of ways. Moving away from the idea of "Chineseness" as an essentialized identity rooted in cultural, ancestral, or geographic narratives of commonality, (so-called) diasporic, migrant, transnational, residual, and mainland (People's Republic of China) Chinese are enacting and resisting "Chineseness" in new, contingent, and fluid ways.[23]

Chinese not territorialized upon the PRC nation-state have been named in multiple ways, most commonly as *Huaqiao* (overseas Chinese) or *haiwai Huaren* (Chinese living overseas). Some accounts highlight nativist attachments to, or longings for, an ancestral homeland; some focus on displacement and (non)assimilation, or even on second-wave remigrations to more affluent countries.[24] In nearly all such accounts, Taiwanese are glossed unproblematically as constituting part of this group of overseas Chinese. Some accounts even position them as the penultimate keepers of a residual authentic Chinese culture unspoiled by the perceived communist excesses on the mainland.

Such culturalist discourses generally position the Taiwanese as being more authentically Confucian, which in turn is strongly linked with Han identity, and then equated with "Chineseness." This position claims the Taiwanese as more culturally Han, and therefore as more Chinese than those living in China under the radical changes of the last century.[25] Counterdiscourses, of course, exist to disrupt these narratives by citing Taiwanese cultural uniqueness and cultural distance from the Chinese.[26] Whether claiming the Taiwanese as culturally distinct from the Chinese, or as more culturally Chinese than those contemporaries living on the mainland, both discourses rely on essentialist constructions of what it means to be Chinese. Any such claims are complicated by the contested political claim that Taiwan is part of China. Thus the question as to whether and how Taiwanese are Chinese draws on multiple narrative and political strands that may be alternately evocative of citizenship status, cultural status, territorial politics, or ethnicity.

Being Taiwanese

"Taiwanese," like "Chinese," is not a stable signifier. Marie Lin et al. (hereafter referred to as Lin) and Melissa Brown take this category to include the Hoklo or Minnan and the Hakka ethnic groups. Brown uses the term "Hoklo" to refer to those Taiwanese who speak the Minnan dialect (or "Taiwanese," *Taiyu* or *Taiwanhua*),[27] while Lin refers to these same people as Minnan.[28] Both the Hoklo/Minnan and the Hakka mainly began immigrating to Taiwan in the "first wave" of Chinese immigration from the southeastern provinces of China during the 1600s. However, many of the so-called Mainlanders (*waishengren*) who came to Taiwan as the communists took over China call themselves Taiwanese, as do their descendants who were born and raised in Taiwan.[29]

Additionally, many people, Minnan, Hakka, and Mainlanders alike, consider themselves to be both Chinese and Taiwanese. A set of excerpts from my field notes illustrates some of the complexity involved in these naming practices:[30]

> I handed [the researcher] my name card, printed in English on one side and Chinese on the other. She looked at it for a moment, then looked up at me and asked, "So, are you Chinese or Taiwanese?
>
> I asked R. and C. [both from Yilan county] if they considered themselves to be Taiwanese or Chinese or both. R. immediately and emphatically replied that they were Taiwanese, "of course!" But a few minutes later, he came over to me and said, "Well, actually, I think I am Chinese, too."
>
> E. told me that she is both Taiwanese and Chinese. She went further to say that she thinks this question will become obsolete. "I think it's a question because of the current political situation. I think in ten years or so, we will be either Taiwanese or Chinese, depending on the politics then."
>
> I asked L., a junior stem cell researcher, if she considers herself as Taiwanese or Chinese. Her parents are both *waishengren*, but she was born here, so I expected her to say both. But she immediately specified the complexity of the situation: "It depends on what you mean by the question. Do you mean nationally, culturally, or ethnically?" She makes a distinction between Aborigine and Han, and specifies that in referring to the Taiwanese she means Han. She does not make a distinction between Han and Taiwanese.

I use these examples to illustrate the flexibility and importance of context in these naming practices in Taiwan. In the second excerpt, R.'s distinction is one made between ethnic identity and national identity, while in the third excerpt, E. views Taiwanese and Chinese as principally political designations. Finally, for the stem cell researcher, there is no ethnic distinction between Taiwanese and Chinese; hers is a national distinction.

A series of public surveys addresses these questions of self-identification by attending more closely to naming practices such as what it means when one says "my country" (*wo guo*) or "my people" (*wo guo ren*).[31] These survey results suggest that the distinction between "Taiwaneseness" and "Chineseness" is more flexible and more slippery than is represented in most political discourses, and furthermore that public attitudes toward the question of Taiwan independence rely more heavily on practical and contextual circumstances than on ideological stances.[32]

Making Categories

A series of studies and papers conducted and published by Marie Lin and colleagues from the Mackay Memorial Hospital in Taipei County form the core genetic foundation for claims that differentiate a Taiwanese population from the Han Chinese. They define "Taiwanese" as comprising the Minnan and Hakka ethnic groups. Using population genetics techniques of human leukocyte antigen (HLA) allele counting, they disarticulate the "Taiwanese" lineage from the Huang Di origin story, and thereby delink them from the Han Chinese.[33]

Summarizing the origin story, Lin and colleagues write: "Taiwanese have been told that their ancestors originated from the Central Plains of North China but migrated to the southeast coastal area sometime after the Han Dynasty. . . . Hence they are assumed to be descendants of 'pure' northern Han Chinese from the Central Plains and thus belong to the great tradition of Han."[34]

Lin's HLA studies, however, suggest that the Minnan and Hakka Taiwanese come from a genetically distinct population whose ancestors are thought to be the ancient Yueh, indigenous to the southeastern coast of China, and ancestors also to the Singapore and Thai Chinese. These studies thus link the "Taiwanese" as genetically close to contemporary "Singapore Chinese" and "Thai-Chinese." It would seem, therefore, that it is not specifically being Chinese that this narrative seeks to disrupt, but being northern Han Chinese, with its attendant history of singular ancestry for all Chinese. In fact, the genetic data is used to substantiate a new historical narrative:

> The Minnan (Min) were one of the ethnic groups among the Yueh who lived in Fuchien. . . . The present-day Minnan are descendants of indigenous Minnan peoples although probably limited gene flow from the northern Han occurred. . . . The barbarian status of the Yueh gradually disappeared and they were finally given Han status in history, thus probably resulting in *misinterpretation and erroneous self-assertion* of present-day Minnan as "pure" descendants of the northern Han. In Chinese history, many ethnic minorities adopted Han culture, and many peoples from within these ethnic groups

> often announced that they were Han, most likely because the Han culture was more dominant at that time and so being a member of a Han ethnic group was both beneficial and a source of pride in the past.[35]

This narrative shows the flexibility that inheres in identity making, and recognizes that ethnic categories are made in relation to specific contextual factors. However, it reasserts genetic science as the true way to reckon descent and ethnic identity, rendering claims based on cultural or historical factors as "misinterpretation" or "erroneous self-assertion."

The scientific categories themselves, however, require examination since, as Foucault, Hacking, Bowker and Starr, and others in the science studies literature have shown, categories are consequential, and category making is an instantiation of power/knowledge.[36] Contrary to the perception that categories simply reflect real distinctions between groups, categories are reflective, rather, of present interests and available technologies.[37]

The category of southern Han is particularly illustrative of the work that goes into category making, as well as of the work that categories do. Lin places the "Taiwanese" (Hakka and Minnan) as closer to a distinct southern Han population. Writing on haplotype testing among Taiwan Aborigines, she gives the following comparative results: "All these haplotypes were also shared by other Asian populations . . . including Maori, PNG Highlanders, Orochons, Mongolians, Inuit, Japanese, Man, Buryat, Tlingit, Tibetans, Thai Chinese, Yakut, Thais, Javanese, Timor, Buyi, Miao, Singapore Chinese and 'Taiwanese.' However, no haplotypes were found to be shared by the indigenous groups and either Northern or Southern Han."[38]

This passage contains a noteworthy rhetorical move. As with any classificatory system, the logics of classification are obscured by the reified categories themselves. By inserting them into an accepted classificatory system of distinct groups, Lin reifies a distinction between southern and northern Han.[39] She creates an additional distinction, however, since by listing separate categories for "Taiwanese" and both the northern and southern Han, she effectively makes "Taiwanese" a separate and non-Han category. A subsequent paper iterates this schema, reporting that for "Taiwanese" three separate analyses suggest that "Minnan and Hakka clustered together with other southern Asian populations including southern Han, Singapore Chinese and Thai-Chinese. Northern Han formed a cluster with Koreans as well as Man and Hui populations."[40]

In this way, by naming categories of northern Han, southern Han, and Taiwanese in population genetics, these groups are made to appear as naturally occurring populations.[41] "Southern Han" is itself a category that emerges from a set of culturally particular and historically situated naming practices. When I asked a population geneticist close to these studies to clarify the relationship between the "Taiwanese" and the southern Han, she explained in this way: "Southern Han is just the people who migrated from the North. But most of the people in the south of the Yangtze are indigenous to that area, and actually most are ethnically Yueh. . . . They just put all the people including any ethnic mixture as southern Han; the Han culture became southern Han because they were defined by culture."[42]

This geneticist further explained that southern Han is therefore made up of both northern migrants and southern indigenous groups. This explication of the making of the category of southern Han—as a mixed group sharing an identity based on specific historical factors and cultural naming practices—underscores the situated character of categories in both identity making and population genetics. The rest of the argument, however, renders these kinds of naming practices and identity-making practices as inauthentic. The "Taiwanese" who imagine themselves as Han could be said to be engaging in a similarly situated practice of identity making, but instead are positioned as misrecognizing because, like the nonmigratory southern Han, they don't know the truth about their origins. It is through science, and specifically through population genetics, that these authors "hope to clarify the truth about the origin of 'Taiwanese.'"[43] The truth of identity origins is thus viewed as available through science and implies that cultural, historical, and other ways of reckoning identity are invalid.

What genomic science tells us about groups and relations, however, is determined largely by the project with which it is involved. Political discourses that use Lin's scientific findings to support a distinction between Chinese and Taiwanese rely on a conflation of Chinese with Han; they presuppose a singular kind of "Chineseness." Alternate modes of constructing Han or Chinese as a cultural identity exist.[44] A Confucian culturalist narrative, for instance, would claim the Taiwanese as Han, even in light of genetic discontinuity.[45] Thus an interest in supporting the conventional historiography and in constructing "Taiwaneseness" as compatible with "Chineseness" could apply a cultural categorical schema in making these identities, as Wen-Ching Sung shows in her chapter in this volume.

As Sung shows, Chinese genome projects are used on the one hand to articulate an ethnic *diversity* among China's fifty-six recognized ethnic groups that is also viewed as a resource for biotech development. On the other hand, narratives of genetic *unity* are used to buttress territorial claims over both Tibet and Taiwan. Specifically, the genetic relationship between the Han and the national minorities residing in the North and the South is respectively very close, while more significant differences exist between southern and northern Han populations.[46] In any of these accounts, whether arguing for a distinct Taiwanese genetics or an inclusive Chinese genetics, there is room for interpretive maneuvering. Thus even as Taiwanese studies seem to substantiate a material and scientific basis for a unique identity, Sung shows that genomic studies from mainland China make national unity out of ethnic multiplicity and continue to claim the Taiwanese as Chinese. This underscores the continual slippage that occurs between Taiwanese and Chinese as ethnic categories and as political categories.

Aboriginal Admixtures

While the scientific narratives of "Taiwaneseness" that I discuss operate principally by establishing the Minnan and Hakka as having links to the indigenous Yueh population of southeastern coastal China, a second narrative strand links these Taiwanese to indigenous populations in Taiwan. The "Taiwanese" are further distinguished by Lin's observation that 13 percent of the "Taiwanese" HLA-A, -B, and -C three-locus haplotypes appear to be of Aboriginal origin, and thus are presumed to result from several hundred years of interbreeding between the "Taiwanese" and the Aborigines.[47] While Lin notes that this indicates a relatively small Aboriginal contribution to the "Taiwanese" genome, this admixture is nonetheless seen to contribute to genetic distinctness and has been taken up in both popular and expert imaginations as further distinguishing the people of Taiwan from the Chinese. A pair of fieldnote excerpts captures a sense of how this information is taken up:

> When I initially expressed doubt about the uniqueness of the Taiwanese genome, and suggested to my colleague that this surely was a tactical political construction, she told me that I should look into it. That, in fact, the Taiwanese were genetically thirteen percent Aborigine.

> A genetic researcher, familiar with Lin's work, identified herself as Minnan Taiwanese. She recounted a story in which she visited a Maori tribe in New Zealand and a Maori man became excited upon learning that she was from Taiwan, because they shared an ancestral lineage. She was deeply touched, but said, "Of course he couldn't tell that I'm not Aboriginal, . . . (I am) Yueh and Aboriginal, probably a mix."

Taiwan is thought to be the originary site of the Austronesian language family, and the Aborigines of Taiwan have been linked genetically and linguistically with New Zealand Maori (among others) and are thought to be of Austronesian origin. This linkage is of particular importance since it posits a separate origin for these Aborigines, where mainland Chinese studies have tended to suggest that they migrated originally from China.

The significance of the Aboriginal contribution to the "Taiwanese" genome is further enhanced by the suggestion that "Taiwan's indigenous tribes are probably the most homogeneous (the 'purest') population in the world."[48] Since "purity" in population genetics is understood as a result of isolation from other populations, the Aboriginal contribution enhances the uniqueness of the "Taiwanese" genome. By linking with the autochthonous Yueh of southeastern China, contemporary "Taiwanese" can make an ancestral claim to a region on the mainland. By linking through centuries of interbreeding, even if to a relatively small degree, to the Taiwanese Aborigines, these "Taiwanese" can simultaneously make an attenuated claim to indigeneity on the island. These dual genetic narratives serve to authenticate a uniquely Taiwanese genetic identity, buttressed by claims of both Aboriginal purity and specific admixture.

Taiwanese Stem Cells

Population genetics relies on the production of categories of people in a comparative frame. By comparing genomic markers using techniques of HLA typing, mitochondrial DNA, and Y-chromosome testing, scientists infer degrees of relatedness between groups. HLA markers are also used in determining relative degrees of histocompatibility between individuals, and are critical in discussions of organ, bone marrow, and stem cell transplantation. In general, it is thought that the more closely related individuals are genetically, the more closely compatible they will be as biological material donors and recipients. Thus, population genetics and medical science suggest that individuals within a population are more likely to be histocompatible than individuals from different populations.

Current stem cell–based therapies, such as bone marrow and umbilical cord blood transplantation, rely on finding histocompatible sources, and a specific promise of stem cell therapies draws on the potential to create stem cell lines with a patient specific DNA. Furthermore, medical science points to differential incidences of genetic diseases in different populations.[49] Stem cells with "Taiwanese genetic characteristics" insert themselves into these discussions of population difference and therapeutic hope. At his talk, a Taiwanese clinician and stem cell researcher discussed the characteristics of the five human embryonic stem (hES) cell lines he had derived from thirty "discarded blastocysts" left over from in vitro fertilization (IVF) treatments. He described his research aims in a series of slides stating:

> It is necessary to establish hES cell lines with the genetic characteristics of the Taiwanese.
>
> The aim of this study is to establish hES cell lines from discarded and donated IVF embryos derived from Taiwanese.
>
> . . . to establish hES cell lines with genetic characteristics of the Taiwanese.[50]

When I asked him to clarify the importance of producing human embryonic stem cell lines with specifically Taiwanese genetic characteristics, he replied, "because people in the race—different populations have different genetics." In an anticipatory mode, he envisions a promissory future of foreseeable treatments and "spare body parts for tomorrow" and is "very optimistic that [stem cell scientists] can convert hopes to realities in the near future."[51] His project, therefore, is to ensure that the Taiwanese are included in the therapeutic promise of stem cell research by conducting research on that genetically distinct population, and their stem cells. Simultaneously, his rhetoric and his research represent the Taiwanese genome as unique, and thereby support the construction of a uniquely Taiwanese identity.[52] This researcher conducts his research in the frame of a populational therapeutics based in notions of shared heritable diseases and relative measures of histocompatibility.[53]

In this volume, Aihwa Ong invokes the notion of "communities of fate" as "the network of collectivities that become connected as a result of diverse ethical decisions and affects associated with the benefits of biotech innovations. Different forms of biotechnology can be used to manipulate corporeal and affective interests that reinforce a sense of community and shared fate, for instance by activating traditional values of family, ethnicity, and the nation in the course of ethical decision-making." Genetics is seen to bolster these corporeal and affective ties as ethnic groups are configured as therapeutic communities in which each individual serves as a potential therapeutic source for the other, while the group also shares perceived potential biological fates. In deriving "Taiwanese" stem cell lines, I suggest this researcher is working on both the ethnic group and the nation. Other narratives are also at play in stem cell fields. For instance, umbilical cord blood contains therapeutically useful stem cells, and Taipei's Sun Yat-Sen Cord Blood Bank, founded in 1998, suggests that its next aim "will focus on balancing the tilted donor-search for ethnic minorities in Taiwan,"[54] understood to suggest a focus on Aboriginal groups. In these stem cell narratives, new genetically inflected modes of identity and belonging overlay themselves upon older categories of ethnicity and nation; these modes presuppose a measurable genetic basis for ethnicity that is also expressed as biological similarity (i.e., histocompatibility).

Purity and Hybridity

Technologies of genetic identity making and technologies of making stem cells both rely on conceptual and technical processes of purification and hybridization. Stefan Sperling, invoking Mary Douglas, suggests that in the German context a concern with purity is expressed in relation to contamination fears in processes of importing both immigrant workers and human embryonic stem cell lines to regenerate the German *Volk*.[55] He shows that the same political rationalities are mobilized in Germany's policy discourses on immigration and human embryonic stem cell research, and processes of conceptual purification are required in order to ensure the suitability of both immigrants and stem cell lines for incorporation into the nation's body and body politic. In Taiwan, however, I suggest that a distinction is more aptly made between purity and hybridity, although contamination remains salient, in making both Taiwanese identities and Taiwanese stem cells.

In the space of the stem cell laboratory both purity and hybridity become multivalent. The technical requirements of the laboratory seem to require an intervallic switching between purposeful hybridity and necessary purity. Stem cell research elicits both imaginations and actualizations of self-replicating pure cell lines and pure therapies, yet it relies on a series of interplays between mixtures and pure forms. Human embryonic stem cell lines are immortalized through the production and ideally infinite reproduction of identical cells. Human stem cells cultured on animal feeder layers may not be therapeutically useful because of xenocontamination risks in vivo and many studies have been conducted on how to purify out the animal element. Murine models are commonplace in stem cell research, and they rely upon the production and maintenance of pure (i.e., genetically identical) strains of mice. But, for instance, the Jackson Laboratory, which conducts stem cell research and training, and produces and supplies strains of research mice, also advertises its "hybrid mice" as important research tools. These hybrid mice "are produced by crossing mice of two different inbred strains" (i.e., pure strains) and their usefulness as research instruments is buttressed by the purity of their hybrid strain. That is, "they are similar to inbred strains in that they are genetically and phenotypically uniform." In fact, this genetic and phenotypic uniformity is listed as the first of their characteristics that make them "particularly useful."[56]

Out of stem cell research laboratories has come a proliferation of previously unimaginable mixtures: embryos made from human nuclei placed within rabbit or cow eggs; and fish and pigs in Taiwanese laboratories with jellyfish genes such that they fluoresce green under black light, to name but a few. Purity in the stem cell laboratory comes to rely not only on a system that produces and catalogs contamination and hybridity conceptually, but on one that also technically produces these contaminants and hybrids. The lab-based dream of purity relies on the presence of the hybrid, conceptually and technically.

While the ultimate goal of stem cell research may be a therapeutics of pure self exemplified in the dream of autologous therapies, the production of stem cells with "Taiwanese genetic characteristics" is a therapeutics envisioned at the level of the population. Making the Taiwanese identity discussed here relies on mixing pure populations. Selves are made from hybridizations of others. That is, autochthonous populations are drawn on to produce a unique "Taiwanese" population that is necessarily hybrid. The techniques of measuring HLA haplotypes and alleles are countings of immunological markers used to infer historical degrees of relatedness.[57] And a subsequent rhetorical purification process serves to render this population as pure, in a sense. That is, there is a conceptual purification that goes along with the making of "Taiwanese" as a discrete category and a reified identity of its own. In this way, "Taiwanese" makes its uniqueness by claiming purity on the part of its genetic contributors.

Drawing on high levels of Aboriginal populational purity spatialized in Taiwan, and claiming "Taiwanese" descent from indigenous mainland ancestors, these geneticists contribute to a narrative of uniqueness made through genetic admixture, that is, through hybridization. Furthermore, population genetics understands purity to mean homogeneity, therefore even a population with an explicitly hybrid origin can be theoretically purified over time. Gene flow between populations is understood to stabilize in a convergence to common allele frequencies, which Alan Templeton explains as "the homogenizing force resulting from genetic interchange."[58] In this way, the conceptual purification is also supported by population genetics theory.

Purity and hybridity conceptually require the production of categories.[59] That is, neither the concepts of purification and hybridizaton, nor the populations themselves, exist outside of relational definitions and a categorical system. Similarly, the genomic science that seeks to authenticate a particular form of "Taiwaneseness" produces categories of people, understood as populations, and then places those populations in comparative tension to create readings or countings from which to infer degrees of relatedness, degrees of similarity and difference, degrees of purity and hybridity. Within this epistemological frame, populations are constructed as pure and as hybrid (admixtures).

And Danger

The genomic production of a Taiwanese population and the derivation of stem cell lines with that population's specific genetics suggest identity to be biologically inscribed.[60] A prominent genomic researcher who returned from the United States to become an important player in Taiwan's biotech progress advocates for a strong and democratic Taiwan that acknowledges its own unique history. She characterizes more clearly the elements of voluntarism and choice in identity making. "I think whichever way you decide, you want to be Chinese, you want to be Taiwanese, you want to be Aboriginal, it's fine. But you have to make that decision or choice based on knowledge, not based on ignorance. And what bothers me is that there is so much ignorance, it's that they weren't given the facts and then allowed to make a choice. That to me is not acceptable."[61]

Her concern, it appears, is not with making a specific Taiwanese identity per se, but with recuperating a valorized identity, rather than accepting an imposed identity and historical narrative. The KMT period of martial law largely took the form of authoritative and sometimes brutal rule by a minority group. In this sense, the new discourse of Taiwanese identity based in genetic uniqueness may be viewed as an insurrectionary recuperation of a subjugated identity.

This same researcher, however, also alludes to what might be the problem with constructing a genetic narrative of Taiwanese identity: "Like Nazis, you raise those Nazi kids. You are very patriotic. You're doing the right thing for the country, right, but do they really know all the facts? Before they were given that choice to say, 'I want to be a Nazi'? That's how I feel, that a real democratic society ought to have that. Be given all the facts, then you decide—not that you only know half-facts—then make a choice."

She refers to the tactics of the KMT during the period of martial law as well as in contemporary politics, in promoting the narrative that all people in Taiwan with roots in mainland China are descendants of Huang Di.[62] As such, they are positioned as either inheritors of the "real" China as claimed by the KMT government, or as subjects of mainland China as claimed by the CCP. Both positions are resisted in these new narratives of Taiwanese identity. In claiming a genetic basis for identity, however, the specter of race thinking is raised, and with it the dangers of biologized identity making that finds an exemplar in Nazi Germany. While the researcher uses the Nazi analogy to vilify the KMT, it nonetheless underscores the danger of constructing biologized identities more generally, including the new genetic Taiwanese identity.

These examples of Taiwanese identity making and Taiwanese stem cell making both rely on the production of a population defined in a biological sense. In the work of Lin's team this population is defined based on a set of genetic markers, counted, and distinguished from other populations, also understood as biological. The goal of making stem cells with Taiwanese genetic characteristics underscores one researcher's project of ensuring that this population is included in the therapeutic promise of regenerative medicine that stem cell research hopes to signal. Both moves can be viewed as parts of a project of nation building, and both rely on fundamental practices of purification and hybridization—discursive and technical—and on the production of a population.

It is this population that Foucault identifies as the object and target of biopower. In his formulation of the emergence of modern European state racism, he traces the fragmentation of a single race (understood as a discursive political construct with multiple shifting meanings and power effects) into plural and hierarchically organized races.[63] This racism functions to create biological distinctions within a population—to subdivide the race into races—and then to place them in evolutionary and civilizational tension. Here, it is the interiority of the other, the corrupting influence of the subrace(s), that comes to be perceived as threatening to the purity and quality of the general population.

Such internal exclusions are heightened in the genetic discourse of Taiwanese identity with its strong divisions between who is and who is not authentically Taiwanese. I do not suggest that Taiwan must follow a twentieth-century European course of nation building, state making, modernization, or racism; clearly it has its unique course to take. And the construction of a Taiwanese identity as genetically hybrid would seem to foreclose the possibility of a purity-based racial politics. Nonetheless, the biological production of categories of people, and medical discourses of regeneration, do appear to call for a biopolitical analysis.

Subjecting the specificities of identity making and stem cell making in Taiwan to critique is, following Foucault, not to suggest that it is bad, but that it is dangerous. The creation of categories of people who qualify, in a biological sense, as authentically Taiwanese necessitates the concomitant creation of those who do not so qualify, providing yet another way to figure difference in an already deeply factionalized Taiwan.

Notes

The research and writing of this essay was supported in part by the California Institute for Regenerative Medicine, the Fulbright Foundation, a Charlotte W. Newcombe fellowship from the Woodrow Wilson National Fellowship Foundation, the Doreen B. Townsend Center for the Humanities, and the U.C. Berkeley Science and Technology Studies Center. I thank the following for their helpful comments on earlier versions of this essay: Aihwa Ong, Charis Thompson, Vincanne Adams, Cori Hayden, Patty Chang, Rosie Poitra-Chalmers, Thurka Sangaramoorthy, and two anonymous reviewers.

1. This statement was made at an internal laboratory lecture given on October 20, 2005, in Taipei. Both anthropological convention and compliance with my human subjects protocol require the maintenance of confidentiality, and therefore I name neither the researcher nor the site.
2. Bruno Latour, *We Have Never Been Modern*, trans. Catherine Porter (Cambridge, Mass.: Harvard University Press, 1993).
3. Michel Foucault, *The History of Sexuality*, vol. 1: *An Introduction* (New York: Vintage Books, 1981), 69.
4. I use the term "Taiwanese" in its most inclusive sense—that is, it might include Minnan, Hakka (*Kejia ren*), Aborigines (*yuanzhumin*—"original inhabitant"), and mainlanders (*waishengren*—"outside the province," although a more inclusive term is also in circulation, *xinzhumin*—"new inhabitants"). I use "Taiwanese" in quotes either when referring to others' usages of the term, or to call attention to its potentially problematic or specific usage. Similarly, "Chinese" is a problematic designation, since it can be used to mean both an ethnic or cultural designation and a national identity. When using the term in its ethnic valence, I often attach the qualifier "Han" for clarity. This is, however, still problematic, since who counts as Han (and by whom) is part of the question addressed here.
5. Paul Brodwin, "Genetics, Identity, and the Anthropology of Essentialism," *Anthropological Quarterly* 75, no. 2 (2002): 323–30. Also, Carl Elliott and Paul Brodwin, "Identity and Genetic Ancestry Tracing," *British Medical Journal* 325 (2002): 21–28.
6. Paul Rabinow, "Artificiality and Enlightenment: From Sociobiology to Biosociality," in *Essays on the Anthropology of Reason* (Princeton, N.J.: Princeton

University Press, 1996). Also, Nikolas Rose and Carlos Novas, "Biological Citizenship," in *Global Assemblages: Technology, Politics, and Ethics as Anthropological Problems*, ed Aihwa Ong and Stephen J. Collier (Malden, Mass.: Blackwell, 2005).

7. Paul Rabinow, *French DNA: Trouble in Purgatory* (Chicago: University of Chicago Press, 1999), 131.
8. Joan H. Fujimura, "Transnational Genomics: Transgressing the Boundary between the 'Modern/West' and the 'Premodern/East,'" in *Doing Science and Culture*, ed. Roddey Reid and Sharon Traweek (New York: Routledge, 2000).
9. The 2003 *Taiwan Yearbook* estimates Taiwan's ethnic composition as follows: Aborigines 2 percent; Minnan and Hakka 85 percent (in a ratio of approximately 3:1); post-1945 Han Chinese 14 percent. Interestingly, they also state that "the Han form the largest ethnic group in Taiwan, making up roughly 98 percent of the population; 15 percent of this group came to Taiwan after 1945," thus giving another example of the flexible naming practices at play in Taiwan that refer to the Minnan and Hakka as Han, Chinese, or Taiwanese, or a combination of these. *Taiwan Yearbook 2003* (Taipei: Government Information Office, 2003), 25.
10. I refer to the DPP and the KMT as the representative parties in Taiwanese politics. It should be noted, however, that other parties are active. The KMT and its affiliated parties are commonly glossed as the "pan-blue" alliance, while the DPP and its affiliates are "pan-green." Here, DPP and KMT can be read as stand-in references for "pan-green" and "pan-blue" respectively. Under President Ma Ying-Jeou (elected to office in 2008), a deliberate rapprochement between China and Taiwan is developing.
11. Daniel C. Lynch, "Taiwan's Self-Conscious Nation-Building Project," *Asian Survey* 44, no. 4 (2004): 513–33.
12. Lowell Dittmer, "Taiwan and the Issue of National Identity," *Asian Survey*, 44, no. 4 (2004): 483, emphases in original. Note that *benshengren* is used to denote the Minnan and Hakka while *waishengren* refers to those who came in the 1940s immigration wave.
13. I hesitate over this usage as it reinscribes Taiwanese as Chinese, which is precisely what is at issue in these narratives.
14. Donald M. Nonini and Aihwa Ong, "Chinese Transnationalism as an Alternative Modernity," in *Ungrounded Empires: The Cultural Politics of Modern Chinese Transnationalism*, ed. Aihwa Ong and Donald M. Nonini (New York: Routledge, 1997), 12.
15. Tai Hung-chao, ed., *Confucianism and Economic Development: An Oriental Alternative?* (Washington, D.C.: Washington Institute for Values in Public Policy, 1989). Also, Gordon S. Redding, *The Spirit of Chinese Capitalism* (Berlin: Walter de Gruyter, 1990).
16. See for instance, Ong and Nonini, *Ungrounded Empire*; Aihwa Ong, *Flexible Citizenship: The Cultural Logics of Transnationality* (Durham: Duke University

Press, 1999); Lisa Rofel, *Other Modernities: Gendered Yearnings in China after Socialism* (Berkeley: University of California Press, 1999).

17. I take a nominalist sensibility to each of these terms—"ethnic," "ancestral," "territorial," "cultural"—and consider them to be indicative of narrative tropes that people invoke in flexible and meaningful ways, and not as stable signifiers.
18. Tu Wei-ming, "Cultural China: The Periphery as Center," *Daedalus* 120, no. 2 (1991): 1–32, quotation at 3.
19. What exactly Huang Di represents is somewhat open to interpretation. One of my colleagues, Wenshan, suggests that while Huang Di can refer to a blood-based ancestral lineage, it can also be interpreted as a symbolic reference constitutive of an inclusive symbolic family.
20. In his fascinating account of Taiwanese identity making during the Japanese colonial period, Ching posits particular emergences of Chinese and Taiwanese consciousness to colonialist situations: "The universalistic assertion of a 'Chinese consciousness' is a response to the real danger posed by the equally universalizing tendency of Western (and to some degree Japanese) imperialism. Likewise, the emergence of a specifically Taiwanese consciousness and its imagined and imaginable Chineseness are overdetermined by the specific status of Chinese nationalism on the one hand and Japanese colonialism on the other." Leo T. S. Ching, *Becoming Japanese* (Berkeley: University of California Press, 2001).
21. Nonini and Ong, "Chinese Transnationalism as an Alternative Modernity," 4. Also, Hsing You-tien, "Building *Guanxi* across the Straits: Taiwanese Capital and Local Chinese Bureaucrats," in Ong and Nonini, *Ungrounded Empires*.
22. Ong and Nonini, *Ungrounded Empires*, 327.
23. As Ong and Nonini saliently articulate *Ungrounded Empires* (esp. 22–25), many, and especially the gendered poor, are absent and silenced in these discourses of Chinese capitalism and entrepreneurialism.
24. Tu, "Cultural China."
25. Melissa Brown, *Is Taiwan Chinese?: The Impact of Culture, Power, and Migration on Changing Identities* (Berkeley: University of California Press, 2004).
26. Chen Ching-chih, "Taiwan, China Share Little Culture," *Taipei Times*, September 16, 2005, 8.
27. Brown, *Is Taiwan Chinese?*; *Taiyu* can be viewed as a problematic way of referring to the language spoken by the Minnan (*Minnan hua*), since it means "Taiwanese language," and therefore creates a categorical exclusion of other kinds of Taiwanese.
28. Marie Lin et al., "The Origin of Minnan and Hakka, the So-called 'Taiwanese,' Inferred by HLA Study," *Tissue Antigens* 57 (2001): 192–99.
29. Of course, some Aborigines also call themselves Taiwanese, and they are arguably the only people who can legitimately claim nativist attachments to the land.

30. Excerpts from fieldnotes, 2005–6.
31. T. Y. Wang and I-Chou Liu, "Contending Identities in Taiwan," *Asian Survey* 44, no. 4 (2004): 568–90.
32. Emerson M. S. Niou, "Understanding Taiwan Independence and Its Policy Implications," *Asian Survey* 44, no. 4 (2004): 555–67.
33. HLA allele counting is a counting of genetic sequences in a region of the human genome thought to be of importance to immune system function.
34. Lin et al., "The Origin of Minnan and Hakka," 192, emphases in original.
35. Ibid., 197, emphasis added.
36. Most notably, see Foucault, *The History of Sexuality*, vol. 1; Ian Hacking, "Making Up People," in *The Science Studies Reader*, ed. Mario Biagioli (1986; New York: Routledge, 1999); Geoffrey C. Bowker and Susan Leigh Star, *Sorting Things Out: Classification and Its Consequences* (Cambridge, Mass.: MIT Press, 1999).
37. Nikolas Rose, *Powers of Freedom: Reframing Political Thought* (Cambridge: Cambridge University Press, 1999).
38. Marie Lin et al., "Heterogeneity of Taiwan's Indigenous Population: Possible Relation to Prehistoric Mongoloid Dispersals," *Tissue Antigens* 55 (2000): 1–9, quotation at 4–5.
39. They are not the first to make such a move. See, for example, T. Imanish, T. Akaza, et al., "Allele and Haplotype Frequencies for HLA and Complement Loci in Various Ethnic Groups," in *HLA 1991: Proceedings of the 11th International Histocompatability Workshop and Conference*, ed. K. Tsuki, M. Aizawa, T. Sasazuki T (Oxford: Oxford University Press, 1992) (cited in Lin et al., "Heterogeneity of Taiwan's Indigenous Population"); Yao Yong-Gang et al., "Phylogeographic Differentiation of Mitochondrial DNA in Han Chinese," *American Journal of Human Genetics* 70 (2002): 635–51.
40. Lin et al., "The Origin of Minnan and Hakka," 194.
41. Though mainly beyond the scope of this essay, this highlights the importance of geography in identity. This geographic element is manifestly visible in the distinction between northern and southern Han made in Lin's papers, as well as in the mainland mobilization of their genetic relationship to respective regional minorities. Furthermore, within Taiwan's independence movement, many have aligned themselves ethnically with a somewhat more southeastern Asia, as is suggested through claimed genetic links to Singapore and Thai populations.
42. Field interview, April 2006.
43. Lin et al., "The Origin of Minnan and Hakka," 193.
44. See, for instance, Tu, "Cultural China"; and Aihwa Ong, *Flexible Citizenship*, 261 n. 64.
45. Brown, *Is Taiwan Chinese?*
46. Margaret Sleebom-Faulkner, "How to Define a Population: Cultural Politics and Population Genetics in the People's Republic of China and the Republic of China," *BioSocieties* 1 (2006): 399–419.

47. Lin et al., "The Origin of Minnan and Hakka"; and Lin et al., "Heterogeneity of Taiwan's Indigenous Population." Differences in individual bases within a chromosomal region (single nucleotide polymorphisms) tend to occur at specific locations and such genetic variants, when located near each other, tend to be inherited together. These regions of single base variants that are inherited together are known as haplotypes.

"A set of polymorphic, linked alleles inherited as a unit is considered a haplotype" (Rick Kittles and Charmaine Royal, "The Genetics of African Americans: Implications for Disease Gene Mapping and Identity," in *Genetic Nature/Culture: Anthropology and Science beyond the Two-Culture Divide*, ed. Alan H. Goodman, Deborah Heath, and M. Susan Lindee [Berkeley: University of California Press, 2003], 223).

48. Lin et al., "Heterogeneity of Taiwan's Indigenous Population," 1.
49. Troy Duster, "Buried Alive: The Concept of Race in Science," in Goodman, Heat, and Lindee, *Genetic Nature/Culture*.
50. Fieldnotes, October 2005.
51. On anticipation and anticipatory practice, especially in relation to biomedicine, see Vincanne Adams, Michelle Murphy, and Adele E. Clarke, "Anticipation: Technoscience, Life, Affect, Temporality," *Subjectivity* 28, (2004): 246–65. On the promissory component of biotechnology and biocapital, see Charis Thompson's lecture, "The Biotech Mode of Reproduction," quoted in Sarah Franklin, "Ethical Biocapital: New Strategies of Cell Culture," in *Remaking Life and Death: Toward an Anthropology of the Biosciences*, Sarah Franklin and Margaret Lock, eds. (Santa Fe, N.M.: School of American Research Press, 2003), 97–128.
52. The science and the practicability of his project are matters of some debate. One researcher suggested that this project would require ten to twenty thousand human embryonic stem cell lines to be therapeutically meaningful, and another suggested that the meaning of the HLA markers may be based on a scientific fallacy.
53. On the concept of race in population genetics, see Jenny Reardon, *Race to the Finish: Identity and Governance in an Age of Genomics* (Princeton, N.J.: Princeton University Press, 2005). For a discussion of how race, as a variable concept, is inscribed in ethnoracial considerations in genetic research, disease incidence, and biomedical practice see Duster, "Buried Alive."
54. Chen Bow-wen, "Current Status of Sun Yat-sen Cord Blood Bank," paper presented at the Asia Pacific Donor Registry Conference, Hualien, Taiwan, April 8–9, 2006.
55. Stefan Sperling, "Managing Potential Selves: Stem Cells, Immigrants, and German Identity," *Science and Public Policy* 31, no. 2 (2004): 139–49.
56. Jackson Laboratory, "Hybrid Mice: Definition and Application," http://jaxmice.jax.org/type/hybrid/index.html (accessed February 12, 2009).
57. This points to the need to interrogate both the technique itself and its underlying assumptions, but that is beyond the scope of this chapter.

58. Templeton, "Human Races in the Context of Recent Human Evolution," 236. On the convergence of allele frequencies, see also Matthew B. Hamilton, *Population Genetics*. (Hoboken, N.J.: Wiley-Blackwell, 2009), esp. 133–35.
59. Bruno Latour, *We Have Never Been Modern*, trans. Catherine Porter (Cambridge, Mass.: Harvard University Press, 1993); Mary Douglas, *Purity and Danger* (1966; London: Routledge, 2002).
60. I play upon Mary Douglas's use of danger as a constitutive outside to purity. I invoke it here not to suggest a reinvigoration of that binary or of structuralism more generally, but to write against them in showing that purity and hybridity are not in static opposition but, rather, in dynamic relations of co-constitution.
61. Interview excerpt, April 10, 2006.
62. This rendition of Chinese/Taiwanese history is still taught in Taiwanese classrooms, although recent changes include a consideration of Taiwan's history in its own right, in addition to a history of China.
63. Michel Foucault, *The History of Sexuality*, vol. 1, and *Society Must Be Defended: Lectures at the Collège de France, 1975–1976*, ed. Mauro Bertani and Alessandro Fontana, trans. David Macey (New York: Picador, 2003).

WEN-CHING SUNG

Chinese DNA | GENOMICS AND BIONATION

The body is a center for the politics of similarity. The boundary of a group is recognized and enhanced by its shared similarities: skin color; diet pattern; one's way of walking, sitting, and squatting; and even vulnerability to certain diseases.

Since science investigates the body, it inevitably entangles with the politics of similarity. In fact, the science of categorizing human beings has been closely related to the nation-building project. Many studies have demonstrated the role of the science of humans in nationalism.[1] In his recent work *The Cultivation of Whiteness*, for instance, historian Warwick Anderson finds that in nineteenth- and twentieth-century Australia, biological and medical research on the Aboriginal as well as immigrating people was loaded with the political agenda of making a Caucasian nation-state. Underlying those investigations were undisguised racial discourses concerning the anxiety of the white people's "racial degeneration"; "whiteness" as a category in public health, medicine, and physical anthropology; and "whitening" the native population. What is notable in Warwick Anderson's work is that he clearly articulates the close relation between science and "imagined communities." To Warwick Anderson, science—especially the biological categorization of peoples—is a crucial component in the building of the "imagined communities"—one that Benedict Anderson did not include in his famous work. Thus, mass media and similar cultural tools are not the only major means to evoke nationalism, the sense of sameness, or the sense of belonging. Warwick Anderson suggests that "the clinic and laboratory should be added to those sites where the nation—any nation—may be imagined."[2]

This chapter explores how genomics, a cutting-edge biological science of category making, is appropriated in an Asian context for constructing arguably one of the most important kinds of imagined communities in modern times. Enlarging Anderson's thesis to include laboratory and clinic as sites of imagining the nation, I examine an emerging trend in China that turns genomic research into vehicles for recapitulating and substantiating the notion of Chinese ethnicity. "Who are Chinese (in blood) and who are not?" is a central question as China engages debates over sovereignty with Taiwan and Tibet, as well as over Uyghurs, Mongols, and other minority groups on the border. In the case of China and Taiwan, both sides mobilize cutting-edge biological science—in Anderson's sense—for the construction of their respective imagined national-ethnical identities. Jennifer Liu's essay in this volume, "Making Taiwanese (Stem Cells)," demonstrates the Taiwanese side of such an imagination and how stem cell research and genetics help define a distinct Taiwanese ethnicity as opposed to a Chinese one. In this essay, I examine the Chinese side of this imagination and the roles of genomics in building a unified "Chineseness."

Bionation in Late Capitalism

In defining "Chineseness" with the aid of genomics, the nation-state comes closer and closer to what anthropologist Paul Rabinow calls "biosociality," a social group that shares the same biological identity.[3] In the original definition of biosociality, Rabinow focuses on the level of individual orientation and practice. Not to distort Rabinow's concept, however, I think the meanings of biosociality do not have to be restricted at the levels of individuals or patient groups. If we consider biosociality as a mode of forming groups and engendering collective actions based on certain biology-laden identification, then the notion can refer to broader social processes. Hence I extend the concept of biosociality to the national level. We may name this biologized nation-state the "bionation." It is a universal emerging form of life not just a particularly Chinese phenomenon: scholars have discovered that in many countries, human genome projects have led to biologization of national identity that is consistent with the current waves of ethnopolitics around the world.[4]

Genomics has not created these deliberations on race, nation, and ethnicity; in China, they have existed for more than a century. At the end of the Qing reign, revolutionaries and reformers proposed the notion of *Zhonghua minzu* (roughly translated as Chinese ethnicity) as a cloak category to include the Han and all the minority peoples within the territory. To modernists such as Sun Yat Sen, the idea of Zhonghua minzu was a constitutive element to turn China into a nation-state in the Western sense, for it unified all the ethnic groups into a single Chinese people. Zhonghua minzu and the related concept of ethnicity were under continual controversies, however. While some scholars, intellectuals, and politicians viewed ethnicity as a biological category, believed that distinct ethnic groups did inhere different bloods, and sought to identify those ethnic groups in terms of their physical attributes, others viewed ethnicity as a cultural category, doubted the precision of the genealogical hypothesis, and chose to identify ethnic groups in terms of languages, customs, and oral tales. When the Chinese Communist Party embarked on a grand ethnic identification project in the 1950s, their criteria were cultural rather than biological. In China's dominant ideology after the 1950s, *minzu*, or ethnicity, is largely a social phenomenon, referring to people using the same language, sharing the same culture, living in the same place, and having the same sense of identity.

The introduction of genomics since the 1990s nonetheless adds another spin to the discourses and practices on China's ethnic categorization. Following their Western colleagues, Chinese molecular biologists and geneticists moved quickly to sequence the genomes of the Chinese people. They seek the distinctiveness of genetic data among China's fifty-six ethnic groups, but also, paradoxically the sameness across all of them; they also look for the groups' evolutionary past and interrelations and attempt to identify disease-causing genes specific to Chinese populations. What emerges from their studies is a notion of "Chinese DNA" that gives new meanings to the Chinese nation and "Chineseness." "Zhonghua minzu" now seems to have a novel biological connotation, owing to the new genetic science; it implies not only the same languages, the same customs, the same sense of identity, and even the same physical appearances, but also the same genes. Following Warwick Anderson, the imagination at genome-sequencing centers, biochemical laboratories, and public health data centers is inevitably a biologized one.

Nevertheless, ethnic politics and solidarity of the state are not the only relevant aspects underlying the notion of the bionation. Not only does the bionation utilize category making among human populations as a means to rally for national identity, it also highlights the biological differences of its citizens as crucial *biological resources*. Contrasting Warwick Anderson's racist state, which exercises the politics of exclusion and separation in the name of medicine, the bionation today engages with a politics of resource making that treats people's bodies as national treasure. This, of course, has been embedded in the biotech-based global political economy since the late twentieth century. Scholars have noted the discourses and practices on transacted tissues, organs, blood, body parts, and embryos in late capitalism.[5] And such value-creating objects from human bodies are not restricted to material substance. The new genomic science goes even further to imply that the information coded in the genes of different human populations also constitutes important resources, which the state does not hesitate to grasp.

Like Rabinow's biosociality, the bionation refracts all the hopes and fears that contemporary bioscience and biotechnology have raised in our public and individual lives. For the building of a minzu identity, the flip side of the Chinese DNA is the utilization of the Chinese peoples' genetic data as *resources* for the country to maintain its economic competence and provide better health care for its citizens, which are exactly the supposed raison d'être of the nation-state. As early as 1977–78, Michel Foucault pointed out two canonical rationales for the development of the modern state—achieving the "competitive state," with regard to the country's economic and military power compared to other members of the international community; and achieving the "*Wohlfahrt* state," with regard to the tranquility, happiness, and wealth of its peoples.[6] The discourses on Chinese DNA, as employed by government, scientists, and the media, point precisely to the centrality of these two rationales in China's emerging bionation. On the one hand, the huge Chinese population is a "genetic reservoir" and thus a valuable asset for the country as it competes with the West and other Asian states for global pharmaceutical, medical, and biotechnological markets. On the other hand, the genetic information associated with the Chinese populations is also important enough for the state to promise institutional measures in promoting the sanitation, health, and general well-being of its citizens. Chinese DNA thus constitutes stakes of nation building, state security, and capitalistic venture at the same time. Like the cases of "French DNA" and "Icelandic DNA" (both of which have been subjects of study), the story of Chinese DNA intertwines national identity and sovereignty with biovalue and biopolitics, as Aihwa Ong highlights in the introduction to this volume. And compared to its Western counterparts, the strong Chinese state leads to an accentuation of the collective and national aspects over the individualistic and private aspects in the story.

In the remainder of this essay I examine, first, a certain "prehistory" of Chinese DNA by tracing the formation and development of the notion of Zhonghua minzu and related biopolitics through the twentieth century. Following this, I discuss the notion of Chinese DNA that emerges from recent human genome projects and the relevant popular imaginations on genomics. Then I will give a brief overview of human genomics and outline various current human genome projects in which Chinese scientists are participating. I conclude the chapter by exploring the roles of Chinese DNA in bionation building. This entails a discussion of Chinese DNA in the international context, in the genomic research cited in sovereignty debates with Taiwan and Tibet, in the question that arises in global scientific communities of whose genomes are the "best representatives" of a particular ethnicity or nationality, and in the concern about foreign appropriation of China's human genetic resource.

Ethnicities, Minzu, and Biopolitics

Similarities and differences among populations lie at the center of discourses on the notion of national DNA. Those ideas about categorization have, however, existed much longer than the human genome projects. In China, genomics does not create new ingredients but adds to centuries-old deliberations of race, nation, and ethnicity. Thus, the concept of Chinese DNA should be considered a representation of the most updated stage of a *longue-durée* process regarding the birth and evolvement of the minzu narratives.

China is a multiethnic country. At present, the Chinese government officially recognizes fifty-six ethnic groups: the Han majority and fifty-five ethnic minorities. According to the fifth nationwide population census in 2000, the "national minority" (*shaoshu minzu*) numbered 104.49 million and constituted 8.41 percent of the total Chinese population.[7] Chinese ethnic minorities are spread all over China but reside mainly in the nation's peripheral areas. In addition to living on the geographical periphery, minorities are also at the cultural and political margins of the society. The relationship between the Han and the minority people has always been a highly sensitive political issue in Chinese society.

In today's China, the fifty-six ethnic groups are known as the fifty-six minzus. It is worth examining how this expression, as well as the number fifty-six, came about. Coined circa 1889, "minzu" is a word deriving from the Japanese term *minzoku*.[8] The word does not have a synonym in English, since it signifies an ambiguous category, often glossed alternatively as "ethnicity" or "nationality."[9] What usually accompanies this word is another term, "Zhonghua" (Chinese). Since the beginning of the republic, Sun Yat Sen and his followers at the Nationalist Guomindang Party (GMD) had used the term "Zhonghua minzu" to refer to all peoples residing in China as a single ethnic group. "Zhonghua minzu" appeared at a turbulent time, when the revolutionaries were trying to save the country from the threat of Western colonial empires while terminating the Manchu monarchy. It was a product of nation building. To Sun Yat Sen, a single and distinct Chinese ethnicity served his cause of making China a unified modern national state; the rhetoric of a unified single nationality promised to accommodate the fact that the Republic of China, a Han-dominated political regime, inherited the Qing Empire's myriad non-Han subjects and the vast peripheral lands where they resided. Before and during the Sino-Japanese War (1937–45), the GMD government further stressed the country's ethnic unity to promote the sense of national solidarity.[10]

Although Sun Yat Sen's slogan of Zhonghua minzu was "a union of five ethnic communities [Han, Manchu, Mongol, Muslin, and Tibetan]," the term nonetheless carried some culturalist bias. "Zhonghua" refers to Chinese; it has been used since ancient China (circa 2000 BCE) to distinguish those who lived in the Central Plains region (Zhongyuan) from those who did not. From the perspective of the people who considered themselves part of Zhonghua, all those residing outside the Central Plains—Yi in the East, Rong in the West, Di in the North, and Man in the South—were barbarians. Although that geographical charting of barbarity gradually faded into history as China expanded its territory beyond the Central Plains, "Zhonghua" has still referred dominantly to the Han civilization, even to this date. In this sense, "Zhonghua minzu" is part of a Han-centered discourse.[11]

The connotation of Zhonghua minzu and the views about China's ethnicities that it implies and draws on were by no means monolithic, however. According to the historian Thomas Shawn Mullaney, there were at least four distinct perspectives, falling into two competing camps, on Chinese ethnic groups in the early twentieth century. They were held respectively by physical anthropologists, ethnologists, the GMD, and the Chinese Communist Party (CCP). In academic circles, physical anthropologists contended that all Chinese belong to a single *race*, having the same physical appearance, body figure, skeleton dimensions, and skin color. Their opponents were the ethnologists, who argued that Chinese are constituted of diverse *ethnicities* with different cultures, customs, living styles, and social structures. This dichotomy between singularity and diversity had a parallel in the political domain. Siding with the physical anthropologists, the GMD stuck to the notion of a singular Chinese *nation*—Zhonghua minzu, in Sun's original sense. In contrast, the CCP was more sympathetic with the ethnologists' view and adopted a Soviet-style discourse on the multiethnic union: that is, that China consists of multiple *nationalities* whose differences cannot be dismissed.[12]

As the CCP was winning the civil war against the GMD, the ethnologists' perspective about Chinese ethnic groups was also gaining upper hand over the physical anthropologists'. Soon after the establishment of the People's Republic of China in 1949, the Chinese Communist Party launched surveys of the minorities. From 1954 to 1990, the Chinese government embarked on an "Ethnic Classification Project" (*minzu shibie jihua*) to identify all the minority groups within the territory. The project was a political and scientific program. It reflected a convergence of the communists' and ethnologists' views about ethnicity and nationality. "Experts"—mainly ethnologists and other social scientists—were responsible for its execution. Their aim was to find the "correct" categorization of ethnic groups in China. In the first stage of the project, names of ethnic groups were collected. More than four hundred names of ethnicities were reported to the CCP. But these names did not necessarily represent the "real" ethnicities. The next stage was therefore to identify "authentic ethnic groups" among the reported populations, based on four criteria proposed by Joseph Stalin in his 1912 essay on nationalism—common language, common territory, common culture with a similar psychological base, and common economic approach.[13]

As a result, the recognition of minzu in China has a strong historical relationship with the Soviet (especially Stalinist) theory of nationality.[14] In 1990, the Ethnic Classification Project officially recognized fifty-six Chinese ethnicities in total. The government soon initiated programs to manage these ethnicities. In this process, knowledge of culture and languages has been a central component of governance.

Two points about China's ethnopolitics are worth noting here. First, although the CCP has been more supportive than the GMD to the position of ethnic diversity, it can by no means get away from the discourse of Zhonghua minzu. The Chinese government does not identify its state as a multiracial "melting pot" in the U.S. fashion, and not even a U.S.S.R.-style multiethnic federation in the strict sense. Rather, the CCP has made it clear that China is "a unified nation-state comprising a number of ethnicities" (*tongyi de duo minzu guojia*).[15] The aim of the Ethnic Classification Project was to substantiate this ambivalent duality. On the one hand, China is composed of multiple ethnicities (minzu). On the other hand, all these ethnicities are parts of the same nation. This paradoxical "unity in diversity" would crop up again and again in China's biotech discourses and its sovereignty contention with other lands.

Second, the Ethnic Classification Project and the associated ethnic policies should be considered as part of modern China's exercise of biopolitics and biopower. The project exemplified how the state governed its populations with scientific knowledge. The systematic ethnological investigation sponsored by the Chinese Communist Party aimed at mapping China's ethnic demography and identifying the true ethnic categories, which served as a basis for the administration to form policies and measures on the minorities. This rational control of population is comprehensive, and ethnicity is only one of its several aspects. In addition to the ethnic policies that concerned the *categories* of population, the Chinese government is also active in administering the *quantity* of population. Like the Ethnic Classification Project, the famous "One Child Policy"—each couple is allowed to have only one child, with few exceptions—launched in the 1970s was also a product of scientific governmentality. The anthropologist Susan Greenhalgh and Edwin Winckler, a political scientist, have demonstrated how a group of systems engineers responsible for the missile and rocket programs played a key role in forming this policy as they produced a daunting calculation result from demographic statistics showing that China's population, if not checked, would undergo a Malthusian explosion.[16]

Note that China's population policies (and minority policies) have been measures of Leninist, centralized state control, and hence are somehow distinct from Foucault's canonical cases of biopolitics that involve the construction of discourses, promotion of forms of life, and noncoercive exercise of power in Western liberal democracies. This does not mean that Foucault's notion of biopolitics is irrelevant here, however. As Greenhalgh and Winckler point out, "Although China's modern political trajectory takes a distinctively Chinese form, far from being outside modern power relations . . . China has become ever more enmeshed in them."[17] In China's minority administration and population control projects, the stress on the "scientific basis" of policy making, the close connections between the government's exercise of power and the state sponsorship of the pursuit of knowledge about humans, and its supposedly noble aim of improving citizens' quality of life, are all clear characteristics of the modern biopolitics that concerned Foucault.

From this angle, the ongoing human genome projects and the ethnopolitical implications associated with them can be viewed as a continuation of biopower and biopolitics in the PRC. Genomics adds to China's rational "state-crafting" and population control, in terms of both categories and quantity. But of course, the mode of this new biopower is different. While the Ethnic Classification Project involved a Stalinist ethnological worldview and the One Child Policy presupposed a Leninist cybernetic mentality, the novel biopolitics is connected with the hypes and hopes of genomic science and the neoliberal, knowledge-based biocapitalism it promises.

Chinese DNA

In China, the outbreak of severe acute respiratory syndrome (SARS) and the suffering it caused provided an opportunity to form discourses on a physical component of Chineseness. In late 2003, when SARS still cast shadows upon global health, a book titled *The Last Line of De-*

fense [*Zuihou yidao fangxian*] proposed a conspiracy theory for the epidemic.[18] Based on the impression that SARS infected mostly Chinese (within China and abroad), the author Ceng Tong conjectured that SARS has an unusual ability to recognize *Chinese genes* (*Zhongquoren jiyin*). Hence, he proposed that the virus was neither natural nor from wild animals but was actually a genetically engineered bioweapon (*jiyin wuqi*) invented by the United States to target the *Chinese ethnicity* (*Zhongguo renzhong*). His book, with its hysterically nationalistic tone, soon captured public attention in China. Chinese scientists immediately argued against this conspiracy theory; they held that there is no such thing as a *Chinese gene* that distinguishes Chinese from non-Chinese.[19]

What draws my attention to this book is the entangled multiple layers of political imaginations it propagates. First, the story portrays the United States as a strong world power armed with advanced technologies to intervene in the international order; SARS, a seemingly natural disaster occurring in China, is, according to the book, the product of this global empire. Second, China was attacked by a Western power; SARS reminds Chinese of the European, Russian, American, and Japanese invasions that occurred after the Opium Wars. Finally, Tong's conjecture about a disease targeted to the nation reveals a politics of similarity. In other words, he asserts a homogeneous Chinese body, which is more prone to infection by the SARS virus. Here, nationalistic anxiety and anti-West feeling weave together with a biologized identity politic.

At the commonsense level, the extreme view in *The Last Line of Defense* seems absurd and easy to refute. Although connections between specific diseases and populations have been identified from time to time, the reasons behind such connections have been proven complicated. Humans' inherited biological traits constitute only one aspect in a group's susceptibility; geography, lifestyle, nutrition, climate, and even social relations all play parts in the persistence and spread of diseases. Nevertheless, Tong's contention implies an emerging social conviction—or at least the discourses about it—that we cannot easily dismiss. "Scientifically" or not, what underlies the panic over the "Chinese-targeted" SARS is the belief that the biological distinctiveness of a specific population is real, and that such distinctiveness becomes most explicit in the selection of a disease. In other words, who contracts the disease and who does not may constitute the most dramatic markers of racial or ethnic identities. And the biological distinctiveness of the Chinese population consists of a specific genetic makeup more prone to the attack of the SARS virus. Here this pathology-based identity serves as a crucial component in the politics of similarity and the imagination of homogeneity. No doubt such discourses are facilitated by the rising genomic science and new perspectives on the body, disease, medication, race, ethnicity, and human species that it brings about.

Although Chinese lay people and scientists do not use the term "Chinese genes" (*Zhongquoren jiyin*) as Ceng Tong does, Tong is not alone in believing that there are significant genetic differences between Chinese and other populations. Before Tong published his book, some Chinese had argued on the World Wide Web about whether SARS was a genetic weapon targeted at Chinese populations. The Chinese government also called for a meeting of biologists to discuss whether the SARS virus might be a genetic weapon. Therefore, Tong's book *The Last Line of Defense* is reflective of thinking about the physical uniqueness of the Chinese body. Such thinking also influenced the implementation of scientific projects. When I was conducting fieldwork at scientific research establishments in Beijing and Shanghai, a few informants told me that a major reason for China's initial hesitation to participate in the U.S.-led Human Genome Project in the early 1990s was that the genome sequenced in that project was collected from the blood of about two hundred Caucasian employees at the U.S. National Institutes of Health. To the Chinese scientists criticizing the Human Genome Project, these samples simply did not represent the genome of the Chinese population, and thus the project was of little practical use to China. Needless to say, the subsequent Chinese Human Genome Project and Genographic Project are both built upon the premise that Chinese people have genetic traits different enough—in the evolutionary sense—from other populations to justify the separate, national projects.

We may use the term "Chinese DNA" to reflect an emic concept that connotes the discourses, imaginations, practices, and politics of the population categorization associated with the new genomic science. (I prefer the term "Chinese DNA" to "Chinese genes," because it highlights the roles of the new genomic science in this discourse. Like "French DNA," Chinese DNA represents a novel phenomenon that—

despite its longstanding root in racial narratives—becomes prominent only after the introduction of molecular-biology-based genetic engineering.) Chinese DNA is a cultural concept shared by some laypeople as well as professionals, that Chinese have certain biologically distinct features inherited in their ancestral blood, and these features are different in nontrivial ways from those of non-Chinese. Simply put: the Chinese comprise one nation, and that nation has a genetic basis. Chinese DNA as a cultural belief is also connected to certain social, institutional, and political phenomena: the employment of genomic research in the sovereignty debates with China's neighboring lands, readdressing the issues of ethnic identification, the reification of human population genes as national resources, the mobilization of the nationalistic ethos to turn scientific research into a competition with the West and the rest of Asia for entering the center of the world stage, and so on.

Although the concept somehow does carry a racist tone, Chinese DNA is not necessarily a racist discourse by nature. One reason is that traditional racist rhetoric emphasizes the "purity" of blood, the supremacy of a race over others, the fear of "racial degradation," the biological foundation for different peoples' distinct intellect, behaviors, and life styles, and hence the legitimacy of apartheid measures of one kind or another. It is an *exclusive* rhetoric. By contrast, a large portion of the notion of Chinese DNA stresses more the uniformity and homogeneity of different ethnicities across and sometimes even outside the country: Taiwanese, Tibetans, Mongols, Uyghurs, and Muslins are all Chinese in blood. This is an *inclusive* rhetoric. Even for the more exclusive part of the notion that highlights the differences between Chinese and the rest (most conspicuously Caucasians), the goal is not to argue for a system exclusively tailored for Chinese and essentially different from that of the West. Rather, it is to call for the effective participation of the universal system—biotech, bioscience, knowledge-based economy, biomedicine-based health care—by focusing on projects that take better care of needs related to the biological features of Chinese people.

The concept of Chinese DNA has parallels in other places. Scholars have shown that the human genome projects led to multiple forms of biologization of identity in many countries and an emerging wave of ethnopolitics around the world.[20] Rabinow's study of French DNA—a story of how blood and belonging are turned into national resources in public deliberations—is the most salient example. In recent media, the debates over Icelandic DNA and Jewish DNA illustrate tangential but equally interesting points on the implications of geneticizing the nation: in the Icelandic case, the genealogical constituency of the population is simple. What is controversial is who owns the right to possess and use the genetic data of this population. In the Jewish case, the discourse of genes as resources has yet to be developed. What is under the spotlight today is whether this diasporaic people, which has migrated to all corners of the world for thousands of years, share some common genetic identity. In Asia, the notion of national DNA becomes more and more visible, too. Not only Chinese but also many Japanese scientists and laypeople believe that drugs act differently in different populations.[21] As a result, Japan's government and the public have issued a pressing demand to the international pharmaceutical community that new medications should have separate clinical trials with different standards using Japanese subjects.[22]

Chinese DNA (and other national DNA as well) is a biocultural-geographical concept with genomic underpinnings. This view of the human body constitutes a knowledge core underlying the political actions and rhetoric of a bionation; the politics of similarities and differences—no matter if it concerns national identity, territory claim, minority relations, or resource making—exercised by the state and society is more and more contingent upon assumptions about the genetic makeup of Chinese populations. In other words, Chinese DNA is an epistemic presupposition in China's building of a bionation.

The notion of national DNA is made possible by the rise of genomics and the various human genome projects that have occupied the center stage of world science since the 1990s. In the next section, I will briefly review the human genome projects in which Chinese scientists have participated and discuss their implications to China's bionation building.

Human Genome Projects in China

The various human genome projects all study the complete set of human genetic material. The first project of this kind was launched in the United States in 1990.[23] Before that, investigation into the whole genome had been deemed unrealistic, since it would take an inordinate amount of time and effort to isolate and identify all the single genes of any vertebrate. Finding the complete set of human genes—which, as we now know, comprise three billion pairs of nucleotide bases—was simply beyond the capacity of any laboratory. The human genome projects were made possible by the invention of several critical technologies, such as the polymerase chain reaction (PCR) and automatic sequencing machines. These technologies have transformed the scientific practice for finding the DNA sequences of genes and identifying their order, taking it from manual work to industrial large-scale production. These technological breakthroughs have resulted in the high-throughput machinery of genetic data generation. The considerable compression of data-producing time in turn makes genome sequencing and analysis much more tractable. As PCR and sequencing technologies disseminate into laboratories around the world, genomic projects proliferate. Gradually, the genome sequencing technologies are turned from the subject of cutting-edge scientific research into common and routine practice at a set of genomic research centers that are emerging swiftly among the international scientific communities. More and more human genome projects have been launched in North America, Europe, and Asia.

The global endeavors of the genomic projects accompany a profound social transformation.[24] One aspect of this is the rise of the new research area of genomics.[25] It is a brand new way of conducting research in life sciences that emphasizes genes as the ultimate cause of biological phenomena and the interplay of different genes in such causal functionality.[26] Related to the establishment of genomics is a shift of pharmaceutical paradigms, which turns the search for new drugs into the identification of gene-targeted chemicals.[27] This inevitably changes the general public's concepts about diseases.[28] It also leads to the state's appropriation of genes as a valuable national resource.[29]

As a rising economic power eager to return to the center of the world stage, China does not stay outside the global game of genomics. In 1994, the Chinese state launched its first national human genome project. Soon afterward, a group of Chinese scientists in Beijing and Seattle joined the U.S.-led Human Genome Project on behalf of their country. Since then, the Chinese government has actively sponsored human genomic research at its state scientific institutions.

All of China's human genome projects are part of the transnational research initiatives. They fall into two types, reflecting two different goals, as well as two different underlying assumptions about human biology. The first type emphasizes variations across different populations, and the aim is to study human diversity in order to construct the evolutionary history of the human species. The international endeavor best representing this type of inquiry is the Human Genome Diversity Project (HGDP), at Stanford University. In China, investigations along this line also include the Chinese Human Genome Project (CHGP), the Surname Project, and the Genographic Project.

THE CHINESE HUMAN GENOME PROJECT

In 1994, China started its first national project on the human genome with an attempt to acquire the necessary research infrastructure and core sequencing technology, as well as to construct a Chinese genetic database of the fifty-six ethnicities.[30] Under the title of the Chinese Human Genome Project (CHGP), the program was led by Chen Zhu and Qiang Boqin at the Chinese Academy of Sciences. Some scientists involved in this project were also members of the Human Genome Organisation (HUGO), and they collaborated with the HGDP to study genetic variants among global populations. A goal of the Chinese Human Genome Project was to "collect and preserve diverse cells and genetic materials of the 55 minority groups before they vanish genetically" due to the "increasing miscegenation of different ethnic groups."[31]

As with the Human Genome Diversity Project, the CHGP's research focus was human evolution. In 1998, Chinese scientists participating in both the CHGP and the Human Genome Diversity Project used microsatellites (a technique of pinpointing the locations of short but repetitive nucleotide base pairs in DNA) to study the genetic relationship among twenty-eight sampled populations in China.[32] From their study, the scientists reported a clear genetic distinction between southern and northern Chinese populations. They also confirmed that "modern humans [who] originated in Africa constitute the majority of the current gene pool in East Asia."[33] This finding adds new information to the longstanding debate in the Chinese paleontological community regarding the origin of the human beings residing in China today: whether the Chinese came from the species *Homo sapiens* of African origin (as the mainstream view holds), or whether they evolved independently into intelligent primates on Chinese land (as some scholars still insist). Yet, how the new evidence affects such a debate is still under study.

THE SURNAME PROJECT

Ethnicity is not the only useful category for genomic research. Since Chinese surnames are much older than those in many other parts of the world (hence perhaps old enough to map genetic diversity), a group of scientists have used surnames as a grouping guide to construct genetic relationships among Chinese populations. Specifically, they have compared the genetic similarities and differences of people with the same surnames, and made cross-surname comparisons, too. The results of these studies indicate that China's South is genetically more heterogeneous than its North. In other words, while northern people sharing the same family names are more uniform in their genetic makeup, southern people with the same family names have more diverse genetic constitutions.[34]

Using surnames as a categorical reference in genomic research risks a cultural bias, however. Since Chinese families are patrilineal, scientists analyzing the DNA of those with the same surnames trace only the genetic features of patrilineal descent. Yet, chances are that individuals with different family names may have equally similar genetic makeup because of their genealogical relationship on the maternal side. Why not a human genome project based on, for instance, mitochondrial DNA (a maternally inherited genetic material)? The point here is not to debunk scientific research of this kind, but to make explicit the underlying cultural assumption built into the Surname Project. Like the CHGP that reflected China's ethnic imagination, the Surname Project also embodied a Chinese (or more specifically, a Han) cultural order that stresses a blood-based patrilineal family tie.

The Genographic Project

A major international research program is being developed along the lines of the Human Genome Diversity Project and CHGP, and China is part of it. In April 2005, China announced its participation in the Genographic Project initiated by IBM and the National Geographic Society. The Genographic Project shares the same goal as the Human Genome Diversity Project in studying genetic variants among populations. The project's manifesto goes even further to claim that the "ultimate human history is written in human genes."[35] Luca Cavalli-Sforza, the leader of the Human Genome Diversity Project, chairs the advisory board of the Genographic Project. Li Jin in the School of Life Sciences at Fudan University, Shanghai, is in charge of sample collections and analysis in East and Southeast Asia.

The aim of the Genographic Project is to map human migration patterns from prehistoric times to the present. It is an evolutionary inquiry on when humans came to different parts of the world, when they became (genetically) different, what the exact family tree of the entire human species is, and how the (racial and ethnic) categorization of human beings is associated with place. The presuppositions underlying such questions fit the standard theory of evolution. Since Darwin, geographical separation has been considered a key factor for organisms to evolve into different species. Note that this place-oriented view is also consistent with a conception about ethnicity in China: that is, that ethnicities have strong ties with geography. With a few exceptions (such as Han, Manchu, Muslin, and Hakka within Han), most Chinese ethnic or subethnic groups aggregate in definite geographical regions and are known by their location.[36]

The CHGP, the Surname Project, and the Genographic Project all seek to uncover humans' evolutionary history and path of subdivision. They are exactly the kind of category-making biology that has preoccupied scholars from Linnaeus and Darwin to evolutionary biologists today. Parallel to this "anthropological" pursuit, however, there is another type of human genome project in which China has actively participated. This second type of genomic research is much more medically oriented. It aims to discover the genetic makeup of diseases, boost private biotechnology in the diagnosis and treatments of illnesses, and ultimately provide applications to clinical practices. The (first) Human Genome Project epitomizes this type of program. Other projects along this line of investigation include the HapMap Project and the Cancer Genome Project.

THE HUMAN GENOME PROJECT, HAPMAP PROJECT, AND CANCER GENOME PROJECT

The Human Genome Project, HapMap Project, and Cancer Genome Project were all initiated by the National Institutes of Health of the

United States. This series of projects ultimately aims to decode the relationship between diseases and genes. Previous genetic research on diseases studied specific genes in relation to a single disease, and the research design often relied on hypotheses presupposing the causal connections between the disease and certain genes. By contrast, the Human Genome Project, HapMap, and Cancer Genome Project are not hypothesis-driven. They adopt a blanket coverage approach to study the *whole* genome in an attempt to sort out the complicated correlation between multiple genes and diseases simultaneously. Accordingly, the nature of this new type of genetic research is data production, not hypothesis testing. These U.S.-initiated projects have evolved into programs of international collaboration. In the Human Genome Project, multiple teams in different countries sequence different parts of the human genome in parallel to reduce cost and shorten time. In this sense, the project is built upon a global division of labor that is similar to David Harvey's notion of "flexible production" in manufacturing.[37] The HapMap Project has one more practical need for international cooperation, as it involves a comparative study of different populations around the world: the participation of international scientists facilitates the collection of genetic samples in different countries. At present, the most extensive international collaboration on cancer genome research is the International Cancer Genome Consortium (ICGC). Current ICGC members include scientific institutions in Australia, Canada, China, European Union, France, India, Japan, Singapore, United Kingdom, and United States.[38] The ICGC was launched comparatively recently, so it is premature to assess the productiveness of this international collaboration.

Through the coordination of Henry Yang, Chinese scientists are participating in the Human Genome Project, HapMap Project, and the International Cancer Genome Consortium. China's entrance to the Human Genome Project was not a plan guided by the state. Instead, a group of Chinese scientists including Henry Yang utilized their academic connections with American scientists involved in the Human Genome Project to join the consortium without informing the Chinese government in advance. (The government and funding agencies were later mobilized to support the project.) As mentioned earlier, some Chinese scientists hesitated to join the Human Genome Project because the sequenced genome was not taken from the blood of Chinese.

Another reason for such hesitation was that the end product of the Human Genome Project was still too far from medical applications. The Chinese funding agencies' attitude toward the HapMap Project and Cancer Genome Project has been more positive since these two projects are closer to disease research and medical applications.

So, there are two types of genome projects—CHGP and its like, and the Human Genome Project and its like. In the early phase of genomic research, a major distinction between these two types of projects was their respective assumptions about human genes. When the Human Genome Project was founded in 1990, its purpose was to "sequence" the entire human genome (i.e., to determine the exact sequence of the three billion DNA subunits)[39] and identify universal human genes in the sequence. By contrast, the Human Genome Diversity Project, launched in 1993, aimed to study the global diversity of human genomes and examine the genetic differences between distinct races and populations living in separate regions. Put in a somewhat simplified but not distorted way, the Human Genome Project assumes that the human genome is a "common thread," a static and monolithic entity unchanging across time and space and invariant from population to population. By contrast, the Human Genome Diversity Project not only acknowledges genetic variants among populations but also reveals the history of human migration and evolution.

In the field of biology, these two projects have their respective supporters. Molecular biologists in general view a species as a single entity sharply defined by a set of genes and a set of associated forms and functions. The major question for molecular biologists is thus what makes us, as humans, different biologically from other animals. But while molecular biologists emphasize the essential features that define a species, population geneticists emphasize the variations that evolution has worked upon the species. Thus, population geneticists emphasize diversity over uniformity. Their question is about variations of humans across the species; in other words, how we differ from one another.[40]

Such a clear-cut distinction has, however, faded in recent years. The follow-up programs of the Human Genome Project have started to examine population differences in disease profiles. And molecular biologists no longer promulgate the simplistic hypothesis that the human genome is singular, uniform, and homogeneous across populations, especially in the clinical context—the popular discourses on "patient-tailored" "gene therapy" is just one conspicuous example of this shift of emphasis. Now, the distinction between the two types of human genome projects is much more about the scope and aim of study. As a director of the U.S. National Institutes of Health pointed out to me, the Human Genome Diversity Project, CHGP, Surname Project, and Genographic Project are "anthropological inquiries," whereas the Human Genome Project, HapMap, and Cancer Genome Project are health research.[41]

In China, two different groups of scientists are involved in these two types of human genome projects. Jin Li in the School of Life Sciences at Fudan University is the coordinator of various human genome diversity projects (Human Genome Diversity Project, Genographic Project, etc.) in China. Henry Yang (Yang Hungming) at the Bejing Genomics Institute is the head of the Chinese constituencies for the Human Genome Project, HapMap, and the Cancer Genome Project. The constituency of these groups indicates that the distinction is more about the research aim than about the disciplinary boundary: both teams consist of population geneticists and molecular biologists. Jin and Yang are geneticists by training, but some of their important collaborators are molecular biologists.

Although we can no longer hold the simple view that the two types of projects are governed by two different assumptions on singularity and diversity, this apparent dichotomy nonetheless does play a part—though with a twist—in the Chinese context. The questions now for Chinese scientists as well as laypeople are: Are the *Chinese* (rather than human beings in general) the same or different? Do the Chinese belong to a single biological category? Or are they actually a collection of diverse categories? Their cutting-edge genomic research resonates with the popular imagination of Chinese DNA in the biological constituency of the Chinese nation; those human genome projects also mediate the country's vague but mighty hope to turn the genes of its populations into valuable national resources.

Chinese DNA and Bionation Building

Biology has involved category making since early in its history. A significant part of Aristotle's natural history consisted of identifying and naming flora and fauna. In the eighteenth century, Carl Linnaeus developed a binomial taxonomical system to name, classify, and rank organisms based on morphology. The ambition of Linnaeus and the systematists after him was to find the "natural kinds" of the living creatures of God. Their paradigms came and went. Their methods changed from time to time. But their dream of getting down the essential categories of animals and plants remains.[42]

Since the late twentieth century, the most fashionable means of fulfilling the dream of finding the "natural system of classification" has been the new science of genomics. Based as it is on the study of the complete genetic makeup (i.e., the genome) rather than physical appearances of organisms, genomics promises a more precise taxonomy of living beings. It offers not only a more "scientific" definition of species and a measure of how close distinct species are, but also a means to reconstruct their evolutionary relationships.

The genomic implications for category making apply to human beings, too. Today, the various human genome projects championed in popular media and academic journals claim that they will decode the secret of *Homo sapiens*: what our origin was, how ethnic populations formed, how different or similar we are. Moreover, genomics is not only providing keys to those central questions about where we came from and who we are. The new science also promises a leap in medicine, by explaining why certain people are more vulnerable to specific diseases, and by offering a faster way to develop new drugs. Thus human genome projects have proliferated in countries in both hemispheres.

Classifying human beings is never just a scholarly enterprise. By establishing evolutionary, genetic, biochemical, and bioinformational criteria to group or distinguish people living in heterogeneous societies and cultures, the various human genome projects—like their predecessors in physical anthropology—invite all kinds of politics. Here the endeavors of parsing the "natural kinds" among human populations become the boundary-setting work that inevitably tangles with complex social issues ranging from state construction and identity politics to governmentality and capitalism. In short, the biological science of category making constitutes what Donna Haraway calls "situated knowledge," whose efficacy and implications depend on the social situations in which the knowledge is produced and embedded. While

Haraway does not deny the existence of nature or the possibility of knowledge about it, she contends that both have to be contextualized and appraised in terms of their political and cultural circumstances.[43]

Embedded in China's century-long minzu discourses, the emerging genetic view of the body, and the neocapitalistic logic of biovalue, Chinese DNA plays an increasingly important role in the building of a bionation. Such a role becomes most explicit when China encounters international communities in the political and scientific domains related to genomics. There are three important areas where Chinese DNA plays an important role in the building of China as a bionation—territory, ethnicity, and resources—and we will examine each in more detail.

TERRITORIAL CLAIMS

Today, the sovereignty disputes over claims by the Taiwanese, Tibetans, and to a lesser extent Uyghurs and Mongols are perhaps one of the most sensitive political issues for China. For Chinese, a standard way to engage such debates is to appeal to the idea of Zhonghua minzu: all of these people, in this view, belong to the unified Chinese nationality. As I mentioned earlier, Zhonghua minzu is an ideology of shared languages, cultures, and histories—our languages and cultures are highly correlated to one another, and we share a strongly overlapped past. The introduction of genomics since the 1990s adds a biological component to the minzu narratives surrounding the sovereignty disputes—we share not only the same culture and history but also a common blood. With this new shared feature, minzu takes on the characteristics of a Rabinowian biosocial unit.

Such political implications are explicit in the recent research on the genetic makeup of Taiwanese and Tibetans. Scientists in Mainland China and Taiwan continue to debate the degree of genetic similarity between the Chinese and the Taiwanese, and each group has conducted scientific research to support its arguments.[44] Similarly, in 2007, several Chinese scientists at Fudan University who had been studying the genetic makeup of Han and Tibetans announced that their studies showed that the two peoples had a common origin.[45] The answer to the question "Who are genetically Chinese, and who are not?" is still pending as more research, politics, and discourses are being developed. Nevertheless, this debate shows that in China, blood ties are crucial in legitimizing and imagining nationality. To all the parties involved in these debates, genes are becoming a biological marker for claiming or rejecting an imagined boundary around the "One China."

Does this highly politicized genomics mean the Chinese genomic scientists are driven by the government to distort deliberately their research results? I doubt it. The exact relationship between the Chinese scientists and the state in the human genome research needs to be further investigated, but in any case, the interaction between politics and science is more complex than naïve assumptions like "Politics drives science" or (conversely) "Science is independent of politics" suggest.The influence of politics on science often takes subtler forms than direct government control. As Jenny Reardon demonstrates in her analysis of the Human Genome Diversity Project in the United States, it is impossible for scientists to retreat to a neutral or apolitical ground to conduct their research.[46] According to Foucault, "there is no knowledge on one side and society on the other, or science and the state, but the basic form of power-knowledge."[47] Knowledge is not the servant of power, neither is power the servant of knowledge; they exist in symbiosis.

ETHNIC REPRESENTATIVENESS

The issues of ethnic representativeness challenge the norm of genomic science. Should minorities be included in clinical studies? As soon as the National Institutes of Health initiated the HapMap Project, which aims to study human genetic variants, Chinese scientists joined the consortium. However, when NIH asked whether Chinese scientists could provide blood samples of minorities in China, the Chinese scientist in charge of sample collection replied: "No, we only plan to provide samples of Han, because Han is the majority in China." This incident reveals the nature of the duality of Chineseness—while ethnic diversity is espoused by the contemporary Chinese state, it is really a backhanded acceptance of diversity, which attempts to assert homogeneity within heterogeneity. The NIH coordinator who asked for the samples further strengthened this Han-centered perspective by stating that the project only aims to study diseases of major populations of the world.[48]

Another clash that occurred in the HapMap Project was over the question whether Chinese and Japanese are biologically similar. While their Western colleagues did not give too much thought to this question, both the Chinese and Japanese scientists participating in the project believed that there was a *scientific* need to include genetic samples from their respective ethnicities.

These small episodes actually point to a greater issue underlying all the human genome projects: how to select the (ethnic) blood samples, and whose genome is the better representation of that ethnicity? The Human Genome Project had been criticized for its exclusive reliance on Caucasian blood samples. But broadening the sampling space into different races did not seem to be sufficient. After the Human Genome Diversity Project encountered difficulty in the United States and came to a standstill, its organizers urged that scientists of different racial and ethnic groups should study their own genes. "Asians working on Asia, for instance—not only Indians, but also Chinese and so on."[49]

The result is a proliferation of national genome projects around the world. The Pan-Asian SNP Initiatives established in 2004 by the Human Genome Organization, which looked at SNPs (single nucleotide polymorphisms) is an example. This consortium was established by scientists from China, India, Indonesia, Japan, South Korea, Malaysia, Nepal, the Philippines, Singapore, Thailand, and Taiwan. One of its goals is to construct a genetic map of human history in Asia, for these scientists believe that the regional Asian populations share unique genetic variations that go back thousands of years. This initiative also aims "to uncover the breadth of genetic diversity and the extent of genetic similarity in Asia. This information will form the basis for future studies in genomic medicine for the Asian populations."[50] Among the consortium's member states, South Korea did not join the international HapMap Project but launched its own genome project, since the government considered that HapMap put too much focus on the Chinese and Japanese in the East Asian category and thus excluded the Korean population.

The appearance of the myriad national human genome projects around the world witnesses the working of ethnic representative politics. The underlying discourse is: We, people of a national state, are different from those of other nation-states; and thus we deserve our own representative genome. (The flip side of this narrative is, as the Han-majority talk at the HapMap Project indicates, that your differences are not significant enough to deserve a representative.) Rhetoric like this certainly carries a strong nationalistic tone. But what is at stake under such disputes about representativeness is not the right of participatory democracy or independence of nationality but the health and health care of the nation's populations. In the context of genomic research and its clinical connotations, the nation becomes more and more a biological category. And the issues of ethnic representativeness are also issues of biopolitics.

RESOURCE MAKING

The numerous human genome projects can also be viewed as explorations of genetic resources. Since the early 1990s, China, in collaboration with a few other countries, initiated a series of genetics projects to study its ethnicities. The purpose of these projects is not solely for governance or academic interests, but also for the development of biotechnology.

There has been a global gold rush of genes since the Human Genome Project began in 1990. In 2000, the *Washington Post* reported that some American scientists went to a remote village in China's Anhui Province to collect blood samples for DNA analysis. This and other previous large-scale collections of Chinese blood samples in studies by foreign scientists irritated the scientific community in China. The Chinese scientists considered this imperial science, that is, the West came to China to rob its biological resources for its own pharmaceutical industry. China, in this view of global research, was solely a provider of raw materials. Chinese scientists therefore united together to argue for the need to protect the country's genetic resources and develop their own genome research.[51]

In 1997, the Chinese government set regulations to protect their "genetic heritage." Thereafter, Chinese scientists become the gatekeepers of these genetic materials. Any foreign scientist who wants to obtain blood samples of genes from China has to collaborate with Chinese scientists. By voicing the need to protect China's human genetic resources from foreign exploitations, the Chinese scientists obtained a monopoly of Chinese DNA.[52]

Now, ethnic diversity has become not only China's national pride but also its national heritage in the popular imagination. It is widely believed that China's ethnic diversity is the country's key to winning the international competition in science and economy in the twenty-first century.

In the age of genomics, we are seeing an increasing biologization of identity. The sociologist Nikolas Rose points out that "the nature of the classification schema shape our forms of life, our ways of governing others, and our ways of relating to and governing ourselves."[53] The complex story of national DNA is about the classification scheme shaped by the new genomic science. The implications of this emerging cultural code are still being developed, and scholars have different perspectives about how it will go. Some see the biologization of identity as a liberating force, since it represents a capacity to manipulate the body that serves as a strategy for individuals to plan their lives. Others fear that the manipulation may lead to eugenics and pose discrimination to certain groups. In any case, the novel social phenomena associated with the cutting-edge biotech are so important and conspicuous that we cannot ignore them.

What we have seen in China is the emergence of Chinese DNA as a crucial discursive ingredient for the building of a bionation. It marks a convergence of the longstanding discourses about peoplehood/nationality/minzu with the increasingly dominant genetic view of the body and hence a pull of existing ethnic categories toward a more biologized one. This rhetoric of Chinese DNA plays a role in the country's ethnopolitics, and in its sovereignty debates with the neighboring lands. Moreover, it entails certain biopower and biovalue narratives that view the genes of domestic populations as objects for national health, as well as valuable national resources for the country's competency in a knowledge-based global economy. Chinese DNA constitutes a significant part of the social, cultural, political, and economic landscapes of the Asian biotech today.

Notes

1. A lot has been written on the part that eugenics played in the nationalistic project, especially in twentieth-century Europe. Recent works on Nazi Germany's eugenics include Götz Aly, Peter Chroust, and Christian Pross, *Cleansing the Fatherland: Nazi Medicine and Racial Hygiene* (Baltimore, Md.: Johns Hopkins University Press, 1994); and Dieter Kuntz, ed., *Deadly Medicine: Creating the Master Race* (Chapel Hill: University of North Carolina Press, 2004). The classic work on American eugenics is Daniel Kevles, *In the Name of Eugenics: Genetics and the Uses of Human Heredity* (Cambridge, Mass.: Harvard University Press, 1985).

2. Warwick Anderson, *The Cultivation of Whiteness: Science, Health and Racial Destiny in Australia* (New York: Basic Books, 2003), 2; Benedict Anderson, *Imagined Communities: Reflections on the Origin and Spread of Nationalism* (London: Verso, 2006).
3. Paul Rabinow, "Artificiality and Enlightenment: From Sociobiology to Biosociality," in *The Science Studies Reader*, ed. Mario Biagioli (New York: Routledge, 1999).
4. Nikolas Rose, *The Politics of Life Itself: Biomedicine, Power, and Subjectivity in the Twenty-first Century* (Princeton, N.J.: Princeton University Press, 2007).
5. Catherine Waldby and Robert Mitchell, *Tissue Economies: Blood, Organs, and Cell Lines in Late Capitalism* (Durham: Duke University Press, 2006).
6. Michel Foucault, "Security, Territory, and Population," in *Ethics: Subjectivity and Truth*, vol. 1 of *Essential Works of Foucault, 1954–1984*, ed. Paul Rabinow, trans. Robert Hurley and others (New York: New Press, 1997), 70.
7. See the announcement that appeared on the official Web site of the China Population and Development Research Center, "Major Figures of the 2000 Population Census, by National Bureau of Statistics People's Republic of China," March 28, 2001, http://www.cpirc.org.cn/en/e5cendata1.htm (accessed February 12, 2010).
8. Quangxue Huang and Lianzhu Shi, *Recognition of Ethnicities in China* (Beijing: Minzu Publisher, 1995).
9. Stevan Harrell, *Cultural Encounters on China's Ethnic Frontiers* (Seattle: University of Washington Press, 1995).
10. Before the Human Genome Project, one salient biological feature of Chineseness, which Chinese themselves recognize, is their "yellow" skin. Interestingly, Chinese used to call their own complexion "white" in ancient times. But when the discourse of Zhonghua minzu was being formulated, Chinese started to see themselves as "yellow." See Frank Dikotter, *The Construction of Racial Identities in China and Japan: Historical and Contemporary Perspectives* (Honolulu: University of Hawaii Press, 1997). In this discourse of Chineseness, the yellow skin of Zhonghua minzu is tied to the Yellow River in space, and to the Yellow Emperor in temporality. In China's recognition of human populations, Asians such as the Japanese and Koreans are also yellow-skinned populations.
11. Chinese claim that Zhonghua minzu has five thousand years of history. Myths also indicate that Chinese are descendents of the Yellow Emperor, and even more symbolically, *Long de chuanren* (descendants of the dragon). In other words, for Chinese nationalists and ordinary people in China, their country is an ancient body that has evolved up to the present time.
12. Thomas Shawn Mullaney, "Coming to Terms with the Nation: Ethnic Classification and Scientific Stratecraft in Modern China, 1928–1954," Ph.D. dissertation, Columbia University, 2006.
13. Harrell, *Cultural Encounters on China's Ethnic Frontiers.*

14. Ibid.
15. Xiao-Tong Fei, *The Pattern of Diversity in Unity of the Chinese Nation* (Beijing: Zhongyang Minzu University, 1999).
16. Susan Greenhalgh and Edwin Winckler, *Governing China's Population: From Leninist to Neoliberal Biopolitics* (Stanford, Calif.: Stanford University Press, 2005).
17. Ibid., 32.
18. The book *The Last Line of Defense* was published by the Social Science Academy Press, one of the prestigious publishers for social sciences in China. The author, Ceng Tong, earned his master's degree in international law from Beijing University; he did not receive formal training in biology.
19. Fang Zhouzi, a well-known expatriate Chinese social critic, who used to hold a postdoctoral position in the Salk Institute for Biological Studies, argued against Ceng Tong's conspiracy theory because there are no genes for a "Chinese DNA" that could distinguish Chinese from non-Chinese. The Chinese population is mainly defined by history and culture, he explained; it was never a biologically distinct category, that is, a race. See Fang's article on his Web site "Xin Yu Si," October 20, 2003, http://www.xys.org/xys/netters/Fang-Zhouzi/science/sars_gene3.txt (in Chinese) (last accessed on February 12, 2010).
20. Paul Rabinow, *French DNA: Trouble in Purgatory* (Chicago: University of Chicago Press, 1999); Jenny Reardon, *Race to the Finish: Identity and Governance in an Age of Genomics* (Princeton, N.J.: Princeton University Press, 2005); Rose, *The Politics of Life Itself.*
21. Rose, *The Politics of Life Itself.*
22. Wen-Hua Kuo, "Japan and Taiwan in the Wake of Bio-globalization: Drugs, Race, and Standards," Ph.D. dissertation, Massachusetts Institute of Technology, 2005.
23. The Human Genome Project was coordinated by the Department of Energy and the National Institutes of Health for thirteen years after its founding in 1990. It aims to identify all the genes in human DNA, determine the sequences of the three billion chemical base pairs that make up human DNA, store this information in databases, improve tools for data analysis, and transfer related technologies to the private sector. The estimated number of genes in the human genome has varied at different stages of the project. Before 2000, scientists believed the number to be about 100,000. In 2001, the number became 30,000–40,000. By 2004, it decreased further to 20,000–25,000. See http://www.ornl.gov/sci/techresources/Human_Genome/faq/genenumber.shtml (accessed February 12, 2010).
24. Joan Fujimura, "Transnational Genomics: Transgressing the Boundary between the 'Modern/West' and the 'Premodern/East,'" in *Doing Science and Culture*, ed. Roddey Reid and Sharon Traweek (New York: Routledge, 2000); Rabinow, "Artificiality and Enlightenment."

25. "Genomics" refers to the scientific discipline of mapping, sequencing, and analyzing genomes.
26. James Anderson, Valerie A. Luzadis, Barry D. Solomon, Paul Baer, and Richard B. Norgaard, "Interdisciplinary Research at NIH," *Science* 283, no. 5410 (1979): 2017d; Sydney Brenner, "Genomics: Hunting the Metaphor," *Science* 291, no. 5507 (2001): 1265–66; Joel Hagen, "Timeline: The Origins of Bioinformatics," *Nature Review Genetics* 1 (2000): 231–36; Elizabeth Pennisi, "Human Genome Project: Funders Reassure Genome Sequencers," *Science* 280, no. 5367 (1998): 1185.
27. William Haseltine, "The Power of Genomics to Transform the Biotechnology Industry," *Nature Biotechnology* 16 (1998 Supplement): 25–27; Patrick Kleyn and Elliot Vesell, "Pharmacogenomics: Genetic Variation as a Guide to Drug Development," *Science* 281, no. 5384 (1998): 1820–21; Eliot Marshall, "Genomics: Drug Firms to Create Public Database of Genetic Mutations," *Science* 284, no. 5413 (1999): 406–7.
28. Fujimura, "Transnational Genomics"; Jocelyn Kaiser, "Biobanks: Population Databases Boom, from Iceland to the U.S.," *Science* 298, no. 5596 (2002): 1158–61; Gisli Palsson and Paul Rabinow, "Iceland: The Case of a National Human Genome Project," *Anthropology Today* 15, no. 5 (1999): 14–18; Larissa K. F. Temple, Robin S. McLeod, Steven Gallinger, and James G. Wright, "Defining Disease in the Genomics Era," *Science* 293 (2001): 807–8.
29. Rabinow, *French DNA*.
30. Boqin Qiang, "Human Genome Research in China," *Journal of Molecular Medicine* 82, no. 4 (2004): 214–22. The funding for the Human Genome Project in China came from diverse sources: the National Natural Science Foundation of China sponsored the first phrase of the project; the State Commission of Education, the Ministry of Public Health, and local governments funded the nineteen laboratories involved in the project.
31. Human Genome Organisation, http://www.hugo-pacific.genome.ad.jp/2contents/project.html (no longer available).
32. The twenty-eight sampled populations included four Taiwanese Aboriginal groups.
33. Luigi Luca Cavalli-Sforza, "The Chinese Human Genome Diversity Project," *Proceedings of the National Academy of Sciences of the United States of America* 95, no. 20 (1998): 11501–3; J. Y. Chu, W. Huang, S. Q. Kuang, J. M. Wang, J. J. Xu, Z. T. Chu, Z. Q. Yang, K. Q. Lin, P. Li, M. Wu, Z. C. Geng, C. C. Tan, R. F. Du, and L. Jin, "Genetic Relationship of Populations in China," *Proceedings of the National Academy of Sciences of the United States of America* 95, no. 20 (1998): 11763–68.
34. Cavalli-Sforza, "The Chinese Human Genome Diversity Project."
35. Genographic Project, http://www3.nationalgeographic.com/genographic/index.html.
36. Sow-Theng Leong, *Migration and Ethnicity in Chinese History: Hakkas, Pengmin, and Their Neighbors* (Stanford, Calif.: Stanford University Press, 1997).

37. David Harvey, *The Condition of Postmodernity* (Oxford: Basil Blackwell, 1989).
38. See the announcement that appeared on the official Web site of the Cancer Genome Consortium, "Scientists Form International Cancer Genome Consortium," April 29, 2008, http://www.icgc.org/.
39. Nucleotides form the basic double-helix structure of the DNA molecule. A nucleotide consists of three molecules—a sugar, a phosphate group, and a molecule called a base. There are four different bases, abbreviated as A, C, G, and T for adenine, cytosine, guanine, and thymine. To sequence a genome is to find out the exact order of bases in DNA.
40. Walter Gilbert, "A Vision of the Grail," in *The Code of Codes: Scientific and Social Issues in the Human Genome Project*, ed. Daniel Kelves and Leroy Hood (Cambridge, Mass.: Harvard University Press, 1992), 84–85.
41. Interview with Mark S. Guyer, director for Extramural Research at National Human Genome Research Institute (NHGRI), NIH, August 27, 2007.
42. See University of California Museum of Paleontology, "Carl Linnaeus (1707–1778)," n.d., http://www.ucmp.berkeley.edu/history/linnaeus.html.
43. Donna Haraway, "Situated Knowledge: The Science Question in Feminism and the Privilege of Partial Perspective," in Biagioli, *The Science Studies Reader*.
44. For the controversy on the genetic similarities and differences between Chinese and Taiwanese, see Jennifer Liu's essay in this volume.
45. Feng Zhang, Bing Su, Ya-ping Zhang, and Li Jin, "Genetic Studies of Human Diversity in East Asia," *Philosophical Transactions of the Royal Society of London*, ser. B, Biological Sciences, 362, no. 1482 (2007): 987–95.
46. Reardon, *Race to the Finish*.
47. Michel Foucault, "Penal Theories," in *Ethics: Subjectivity and Truth*, 17.
48. Field observation, the First Strategy Meeting of the International HapMap Project, Washington, D.C., October 28, 2002.
49. Reardon, *Race to the Finish*, 134.
50. See the press releases that appeared on the official Web site of the Genome Institute of Singapore, "HUGO Pacific Pan-Asian SNP Initiative to Explore Genetic Diversity for Pan-Asian Populations," November 19, 2004, http://www.gis.a-star.edu.sg (accessed May 16, 2005).
51. Hui Li and Jue Wang, "Backlash Disrupts China Exchanges," *Science* 278, no. 5337 (1997): 376–77.
52. General Office of the State Council (of the PRC), "Interim Measures for the Administration of Human Genetic Resource," June 10, 1998, Ministry of Science and Technology and Ministry of Public Health, People's Republic of China.
53. Rose, *The Politics of Life Itself*, 167.

AFTERWORD **NANCY N. CHEN**

Asia's Biotech Bloom

The expansion of biotechnology industries across Asia in the twenty-first century has been described by media and scientific journals as a biotech bloom.[1] The rise of this region goes beyond being a genomic assembly line for sequencing, lab research, or drug trials. Rather, as contributors to this volume have documented, the production of knowledge in Asia reflects the formation of an increasingly global technoscientific culture in which researchers, private firms, and state investors are forging a distinctive biotech industry.[2] Scientists trained in the United States and Europe have been drawn to national and private industry labs in the region for many reasons, which include professional enhancement based on financial incentives such as bonuses, capital earmarked for lab infrastructure and personnel, and generous cost-of-living expenses. More than a site of return for Asian citizens trained abroad, the centers for biotechnology and genomic research are emerging as lively arenas of collaboration and diversity where scientists from a range of backgrounds can visit and participate. Research and development in the biosciences are celebrated and deemed significant to national progress and sense of modernity. In the aftermath of the Asian financial crises of the 1990s, such assemblages offer timely and significant investment in the economic and social landscape through the life sciences.

The rush of biotech firms to this region is also shaped by incentives provided by nation-states, which include vast research centers, indigenous populations to develop genomic products, and projections of a vast market. Asia is deemed the site where new products can be tested through clinical trials in biopharmaceuticals, as Sunder Rajan illustrates in his chapter on the changing experimental landscape in India.[3]

Extensive state investment on the part of many Asian governments has formed a biotech bubble in which scientific programs with an R & D focus on stem cell research, genetically modified agricultural products, and genomic sequencing can be developed in synch with the market economy. Asia is on the cusp of technical and economic innovations precisely because of its investments and focus on biotech. The anthropologists in this volume trace the effects of these new technologies in this expansive and all-encompassing field, and, more specifically, examine the claims of progress being made for ordinary citizens on the part of governing institutions. The chapters on blood by Vincanne Adams, Kathleen Erwin, and Phuoc Van Le in China, as well as the chapter by Aihwa Ong in Singapore, voice some of the concerns raised for both individuals as well as nation-states.

The biotech bloom is a critical site of inquiry as market speculators and media have focused attention on the new economy. The combination of blurred public and private funding for such projects indicates the ways in which life and the biosciences are being reconfigured for nation making under the rubric of market consumption. In the present moment of global financial downturn, compounded by ongoing concerns of contagion and pandemics, it is useful to consider how biotechnologies in the Asian context are situated: against a precipice of recession and, yet, full of hopes of opportunity in the midst of crisis.[4]

Biotechnology in an Age of Crisis

The Asian financial crisis of 1997–98 was a formative experience for the region. Though the economies of Thailand, South Korea, and Indonesia were the most devastated, the impact was felt throughout the region. Sharp devaluations of currencies and assets across Asian markets became dubbed by media as the "Asian flu." When the International Monetary Fund responded by raising interest rates, critics of the move, including many in the region, renamed the economic crisis the "IMF crisis."[5]

Little more than a decade later, the global financial recession, sparked by the failure of subprime real estate loans in the United States, has accompanied continuing rises in fuel and food costs worldwide. As this volume goes to press, the broader context of credit crises, devaluations of assets, and global recession prompts the question of how these might impact the biotechnology industry across Asia. By the end of

2008, it was clear that start-up biotech firms in financial markets that depend upon infusions of capital to assemble products were experiencing the squeeze. Smaller biotech firms both in Asia and worldwide with higher ratios of research and development costs have faced restructuring, even buyouts by larger firms, mostly Big Pharma seeking to develop its pipeline of products.[6] As patents for blockbuster drugs expire, pharmaceutical giants sweep the globe to acquire smaller biotech firms with promising new products.[7] The wave of fiscal tightening is expected to slow down the Asian biotech industry during 2009–10, but the biotechnology sector seemed to be less exposed than the pharmaceutical sector in the early period of the recession.

Financial crises, whether local, regional, or global, have a clear impact on biotechnology research and development. Yet, while the downturn may prove to be another check on the growing influence of Asian biotech, it could emerge that the financial crisis of the late 1990s inoculated the industry in Asia, since it gave rise to resilient networks and structures: public financing, diversified sectors, and, most significantly, key participants in labs, corporations, and governing entities. The presence of state investors as primary stakeholders in the advancement of techniques, labs, and markets suggests a different formation of the postgenomic industry in this region. As the ethnographic studies in this volume reflect, the region is quite diverse, with distinct histories and industrial foci that have led to a diversified industry overall. The region's bioeconomies of DNA range from genomic sequencing to stem cell research, tissue collection, and seed and drug development, with new techniques and practices such as xenotransplantation and biopharming in the making.[8] The assemblage of products would not be possible without human capital, the skilled workers who engage in genomic research, development, and production in the industry. This volume has addressed key sites across India, China, South Korea, Singapore, Thailand, Japan, and Taiwan, where the biotech industry has taken on specific formations of nation making and biocapital. The biotech industry has also grown in other parts of Asia and Australasia, such as Malaysia, Indonesia, the Philippines, Australia, and New Zealand. While it may seem that densely urbanized sectors have an advantage in the concentration of capital and knowledge, regions in Asia with a greater degree of biodiversity also have the potential to shape new sectors in the industry. The assemblages of bioprospecting, state-funded laboratories engaged in genomic knowledge production, and second-generation biotech firms have been hailed as the next step in developing the health biotech sector, which focuses on personalized medicine and the consumption of new drugs.[9]

Genomic Pipelines: Knowledge, Property, and Consumption

In her comparative study of biotechnology endeavors in the United Kingdom, Europe, and the United States, Sheila Jasanoff found very distinct state approaches to the biological scientific industry, based on their national politics.[10] Such findings are instructive as we consider the development of biotechnology across Asia, not always as a unified entity, but each national context with its distinct history, assemblages of knowledge, materiality, and ultimately market share. While personalized medicine is hailed as the next generation of biotechnology, the findings of the volume's contributors suggest that market frameworks are not sufficient to understand biotech in Asian countries; biotech in this region is also shaped by historical notions of medicine, the body, and food. Other factors are discussed by Charis Thompson, in her comparative analysis of "nationalist" and "internationalist" strategies of regenerative medicine or stem cell research, which suggests that differences in the region are defined by specific articulations of biocapital geared toward innovation and staking claims on scientific futures. The political adage "Follow the money" suggests another important strategy to illustrate the flows of biocapital and the ways in which biocitizens have emerged, concerned with care of the self through consumption and health practices. Such cultivation of self-care takes place not just for patients, but also for medical practitioners, who are inculcated into pharmaceutical corporate citizenship, as witnessed by Stefan Ecks in this volume. The widespread rise in drug consumption across Asia dovetails with long traditions of self-management of health care. Ara Wilson's analysis of medical tourism as the intersection of state and corporate shared interests also reflects how the region's focus on health biotechnology will continue to shape domestic health services in addition to the consumption of pharmaceuticals. New consumers are raised in an environment of the market and biotech conjoined. Thus the work of biotech can be seen as a means to cultivate biocitizens in regimes of order that are simultaneously private and public.[11] Pharmaceutical firms and the pipeline economics of bringing drugs to market currently play a great role in developing the emerging health biotech sector. The ethnographers in this volume suggest additional sites to trace biocapital and its effects beyond health care settings and laboratories. Careful attention to consortial collaborations between labs that lead to patents such as agricultural biotechnology on key crops in Asia is another intersection to track, as I show in my chapter on the analysis of the rice genome. Developing markets for biotech products, whether of genetically modified seeds or state-of-the-art medicine, hinge upon maintaining standards of intellectual property. In this regard, both China and India have increasingly called for enforcement of intellectual property particularly as part of their engagement with the World Trade Organization.

Redefining property not solely in terms of intellectual property, but from the framework of biosovereignity has been a critical interest of this volume and its contributors. Blood, stem cells, DNA, even large populations, are not simply material entities but also deeply symbolic of vitality and belonging to nation-states. The race to determine Chinese and Taiwanese DNA, traced by Wen-Ching Sung and Jennifer Liu, or the regulation of stem cell research in terms of protecting reproductive futures by Margaret Sleeboom-Faulker, reflect how genomic pipelines are used not only by corporations to stake claims but also by knowledge makers funded by public and private entities. These intersections of sovereignity and property suggest already differential formations of biotechnology that may also lead to distinct practices of owning and, perhaps, consuming biotechnology.

Bioinsecurity and Governance

The vision of biotechnology as a generative force in Asian markets and society is inextricably linked with ongoing concerns of population growth, unpredictable market economies, and epidemiological and ecological disaster. These states of exception underscore the risks and hopes in which formations of Asian biotechnology are situated. Ensuring the collective good in terms of adequate material resources has facilitated assemblages of biotechnology as distinctively made in Asia. Conventional meanings of nature and ethics are displaced to allow for new practices and forms that suggest collective technoscience for shared livelihoods and futures. In a moment of deepening environmental concerns and financial market volatility, perhaps the directions taken by governments in the region foreground the difficult choices that nation-states elsewhere may likely face. In this context of limited goods, the anthropologists in this volume present the dramatic extremes of life and cosmopolitan transformation that have been wrought by market expansion in this region.

The development of biopharmaceutical and genomic products is overshadowed by repeated incidents of exposure to contaminated foods and fake medicines that underscore deep concerns about life and death. Bioinsecurity in such contexts reflects the need to develop extensive frameworks of governance that can address food and drug safety or containment of pandemics. By attending to the formations of nationalism and ethical considerations that are built on the promise of biotech, this volume offers ways to track notions of governance that emerge not only in the face of new pandemics but also in everyday contexts, when parents provide for children, care for the elderly, or consume new food and drugs. A steady focus on people, plants, and animals, as well as the pathogens that endanger sources of livelihood are anthropological interventions that can inform new directions in the study of biotechnology. In sum, the collective analyses of Asian biotechnology formations in this volume suggest the contingent and yet extensive formations of knowledge, ideologies, and practices that frame the biopolitical elements of this industry.

Notes

1. The term "boom" is often used in business media to describe biotech startups and reflects the generous infusion of venture capital during a period flush with funding. The similar term "bloom" tends to be used more frequently for Asian biotech. "Let a hundred flowers bloom" was a Maoist slogan, but Michael M. J. Fischer has pointed out a metaphorical association with algae blooms and other microbial formations that grow quickly in response to the right conditions (comments in the "Socio-technical Imaginary Workshop," November 14, 2008). See also Nancy N. Chen, "China's Biotech Bloom," *Genewatch* 17, no. 1 (January–February 2004).
2. Sarah Franklin's work on global stem cell collaboration introduces the concept of the global biological which engages with Margaret Lock's notion of local biological. See "Stem Cells R Us: Emergent Life Forms and the Global Biological," in *Global Assemblage: Technology, Politics and Ethics as Anthropological Problems*, ed. Aihwa Ong and Stephen J. Collier (Malden, Mass.: Blackwell, 2005).
3. See also Adriana Petryna, *When Experiments Travel: Clinical Trials and the*

Global Search for Human Subjects (Princeton, N.J.: Princeton University Press, 2009), which tracks the clinical trial industry across the United States, Poland, and Brazil.

4. The interlinked terms of "crisis" and "opportunity" are almost a cliché in recent media. In Mandarin, the pinyin for "crisis" combines the terms for danger and opportunity.
5. For a comparative assessment of the Asian financial crisis, see T. J. Pempel's edited volume *The Politics of the Asian Economic Crisis* (Ithaca, N.Y.: Cornell University Press, 1999).
6. Glen Giovannetti and Gautam Jaggi, eds., *Beyond Borders: Global Technology Report 2008*, Ernst & Young Global Ltd., http://www.ey.com (accessed April 3, 2009).
7. Joe Dumit addresses this practice in his research on blockbuster drugs, "Pharmaceutical Witnessing: Drugs for Life in an Era of Direct-to-Consumer Advertising," in *Technologized Images, Technologized Bodies*, ed. Jeanette Edwards, Penny Harvey, Peter Wade (Oxford: Berghahn Books, forthcoming).
8. Catherine Waldby and Robert Mitchell address the different forms and politics of tissue collection and circulation in *Tissue Economies: Blood, Organs, and Cell Lines in Late Capitalism* (Durham: Duke University Press, 2006).
9. Sarah E. Frew et al. have written extensively on the China and India health biotechnology markets. See "Chinese Health Biotech and the Billion-Patient Market," *Nature Biotechnology* 26 (2008): 37–53; and "India's Health Biotech Sector at a Crossroads," *Nature Biotechnology* 25 (2007): 403–17.
10. Sheila Jasanoff, *Designs on Nature: Science and Democracy in Europe and the United States* (Princeton, N.J.: Princeton University Press, 2005).
11. Nikolas Rose has written on biological citizens in *The Politics of Life Itself: Biomedicine, Power, and Subjectivity in the Twenty-first Century* (Princeton, N.J.: Princeton University Press, 2006). See also Adriana Petryna, *Life Exposed: Biological Citizens after Chernobyl* (Princeton, N.J.: Princeton University Press, 2002).

Bibliography

Abraham, John, and Graham Lewis. "Citizenship, Medical Expertise and the Capitalist Regulatory State in Europe." *Sociology* 36 (2002): 67–88.

Adams, Vincanne. *Doctors for Democracy: Health Professionals in the Nepali Revolution*. Cambridge: Cambridge University Press, 1998.

Adams, Vincanne, Michelle Murphy, and Adele E. Clarke. "Anticipation: Technoscience, Life, Affect, Temporality." *Subjectivity* 28 (2009): 246–65.

Ahern, Emily M. "The Power and Pollution of Chinese Women." In *Women in Chinese Society*, edited by M. Wolf and R. Witke. Stanford, Calif.: Stanford University Press, 1975.

Aizura, Aren Z. "The Romance of the Amazing Scalpel: 'Race,' Labour and Affect in Thai Gender Reassignment Clinics." Manuscript, 2008.

Aly, Götz, Peter Chroust, and Christian Pross. *Cleansing the Fatherland: Nazi Medicine and Racial Hygiene*. Baltimore, Md.: Johns Hopkins University Press, 1994.

Anagnost, Ann. "The Corporeal Politics of Quality (Suzhi)." *Public Culture* 16, no. 2 (spring 2004): 189–208.

——. *National Past-Times: Narrative, Representation and Power in Modern China*. Durham: Duke University Press, 1997.

Anderson, Benedict. *Imagined Communities: Reflections on the Origin and Spread of Nationalism*. 1983. 2nd ed., London: Verso, 1991; rev. ed. 2006.

Anderson, James, Valerie A. Luzadis, Barry D. Solomon, Paul Baer, and Richard B. Norgaard. "Interdisciplinary Research at NIH." *Science* 283, no. 5410 (1979): 2017d.

Anderson, Warwick. *The Cultivation of Whiteness: Science, Health and Racial Destiny in Australia*. New York: Basic Books, 2003.

——. "Re-Orienting STS: Emergent Studies of Science, Technology, and Medicine in Southeast Asia." *East Asian Science Technology, and Society: An International Journal* 2 and 3 (2009).

Applebaum, Kalman. *The Marketing Era: From Professional Practice to Global Provisioning*. New York: Routledge, 2004.

Archard, David "Selling Yourself: Titmuss's Argument against a Market in Blood." *Journal of Ethics* 6 (2002): 87–103.

Arradau, Claudia. "Beyond Good and Evil: Ethics and Securitization/Desecuritization Techniques." *E-Journal Rubicon*, December 2001.

Bai, Jingyu. "China Moves to Reform Biotech Policies." *Nature Biotechnology* 22, no. 10 (October 204): 1197.

Balibar, Etienne, and Immanuel Wallerstein. *Race, Nation, Class: Ambiguous Identities*. New York: Verso, 1992.

Barlow, Tani. *Formations of Colonial Modernity in East Asia*. Durham: Duke University Press, 1997.

Barry, Andrew. "Ethical Capitalism." In *Global Governmentality*, edited by Wendy Larner and William Walters. London: Routledge, 2004.

Beck, Ulrich. "The Reinvention of Politics: Towards a Theory of Reflexive Modernization." In *Reflexive Modernization*, edited by U. Beck, A. Giddens, and S. Lash. Stanford, Calif.: Stanford University Press, 1994.

Beech, Hannah. "Asia's Great Science Experiment." *Time* magazine, October 23, 2006.

Benjamin, Ruha. "Culturing Consent: Science and Democracy in the Stem Cell State." Ph.D. dissertation, University of California, Berkeley, 2008.

Bioworld and General Biologic. *China Biotech 2008*. Atlanta, Ga.: Bioworld and General Biologic, 2008.

Birch, Kean. "The Neoliberal Underpinnings of the Bioeconomy: The Ideological Discourses and Practices of Economic Competitiveness." *Genomics, Society, and Policy* 2, no. 3 (2006): 1–15.

Bourdieu, Pierre. "Utopia of Endless Exploitation: The Essence of Neoliberalism." *Le Monde Diplomatique*, December 1998, http://mondediplo.com/1998/12/08bourdieu.

Bowker, Geoffrey C., and Susan Leigh Star. *Sorting Things Out: Classification and Its Consequences*. Cambridge, Mass.: MIT Press, 1999.

Brenner, Sydney. "Genomics: Hunting the Metaphor." *Science* 291, no. 5507 (2001): 1265–66.

Brodwin, Paul E. "Genetics, Identity, and the Anthropology of Essentialism." *Anthropological Quarterly* 75, no. 2 (2002): 323–30.

Brown, Melissa. *Is Taiwan Chinese?: The Impact of Culture, Power, and Migration on Changing Identities*. Berkeley: University of California Press, 2004.

"Bt30 Health Fee May Be Scrapped." *The Nation* (Thailand), October 13, 2006, http://www.nationmultimedia.com/2006/10/13/national/national_30016065.php.

Buckley, Sandra. *Broken Science. Voices of Japanese Feminism*. Berkeley: University of California Press, 1997.

Cavalli-Sforza, Luigi Luca. "The Chinese Human Genome Diversity Project." *Proceedings of the National Academy of Sciences of the United States of America* 95, no. 20 (1998): 11501–3.

Chanasongkram, Kanokporn. "Siriraj Hospital Continues to Lead the Way in Healthcare." *Bangkok Post*, September 21, 2007.

Chang Ai-lien. "Parents Save Son by Having Another Baby." *Straits Times* (Singapore), August 6, 2004.

Chen, Bow-wen. "Current Status of Sun Yat-sen Cord Blood Bank." Paper presented at the Asia Pacific Donor Registry Conference, Hualien, Taiwan, 2006.

Chen, Ching-chih. "Taiwan, China Share Little Culture." *Taipei Times* (Taiwan), September 16, 2005.

Chen, Nancy N. "China's Biotech Bloom." *Genewatch* 17, no. 1 (January–February 2004): 10–12.

——. "Consuming Medicine and Biotechnology in China." In *Privatizing China, Socialism from Afar*, edited by Li Zhang and Aihwa Ong. Ithaca, N.Y.: Cornell University Press, 2008.

Ching, Leo T. S. *Becoming "Japanese": Colonial Taiwan and the Politics of Identity Formation.* Berkeley: University of California Press, 2001.

Chiu, Yu-tzu. "Taiwanese Scientists Find Genetic Links to SARS." *Nature Medicine* 9, no. 1335 (November 2003).

Cho, Hae-joang. "Constructing and Deconstructing Koreanness." In *Making Majorities: Constituting the Nation in Japan, Korea, China, Malaysia, Fiji, Turkey, and the United States*, edited by Dru Gladney. Stanford, Calif.: Stanford University Press, 1998.

Choe, Sang-Hun, "Korean Lab Roiled by Egg Donor Disclosures." *International Herald Tribune*, November 23, 2005.

Choy, Tim. "Articulated Knowledges: Environmental Forms after Universality's Demise." *American Anthropologist* 107, no. 1 (2005): 5–18.

Chu, J. Y., W. Huang, S. Q. Kuang, J. M. Wang, J. J. Xu, Z. T. Chu, Z. Q. Yang, K. Q. Lin, P. Li, M. Wu, Z. C. Geng, C. C. Tan, R. F. Du, and L. Jin. "Genetic Relationship of Populations in China." *Proceedings of the National Academy of Sciences of the United States of America* 95, no. 20 (1998): 11763–68.

Clarke, Adele E., Janet K. Shim, Laura Mamo, Jennifer R. Fosket, Jennifer R. Fishman. "Biomedicalization: Technoscientific Transformations of Health, Illness, and U.S. Medicine." *American Sociological Review* 68 (2003): 161–94.

Cohen, Lawrence. "Operability, Bioavailability, and Exception." In *Global Assemblages: Technology, Politics, and Ethics as Anthropological Problems*, edited by Aihwa Ong and Stephen J. Collier. Malden, Mass.: Blackwell, 2005.

——. "Where It Hurts: Indian Material for an Ethics of Organ Transplantation." *Daedelus* 128, no. 4 (1999): 135–65.

Collier, Stephen J., and Andrew Lakoff. "Distributed Preparedness: The Spatial Logic of Domestic Security in the United States." *Environment and Planning D: Society and Space* 26, no. 1 (2008): 7–28.

——. "On Regimes of Living." In *Global Assemblages: Technology, Politics, and Ethics as Anthropological Problems*, edited by Aihwa Ong and Stephen J. Collier. Malden, Mass.: Blackwell, 2005.

——. "The Vulnerability of Vital Systems: How 'Critical Infrastructure' Became a Security Problem." In *Securing "the Homeland,"* edited by Myriam Anna Dunn and Kristian Søby Kristensen. New York: Routledge, 2007.

Collier, Stephen J., and Aihwa Ong. "Global Assemblages, Anthropological Problems." In *Global Assemblages: Technology, Politics, and Ethics as Anthropological Problems*, edited by Aihwa Ong and Stephen J. Collier. Malden, Mass.: Blackwell, 2005.

Coonan, Clifford, and David McNeill. "Japan's Rich Buy Organs from Executed Chinese Prisoners." *Independent* (United Kingdom), March 21, 2006.

Cooper, Melinda, Brian Salter, and Amanda Dickins. "China and the Global Stem Cell Bioeconomy: An Emerging Political Strategy?" *Regenerative Medicine* 1, no. 5 (2006): 671–83.

Cyranoski, David. "Japan Sets Rules for Stem Cell Research." *Nature Medicine* 10, no. 8 (2004): 763.

——. "Chinese Bioscience: The Sequence Factory." *Naturenews* online edition, March 3, 2010, http://www.nature.com.

Daar, Abdallah S. "Rewarded Giving." *Transplantation Proceedings* 24 (1992): 2207–11.

Davis, Joseph E. "An Interview with Francis Fukuyama." *[Paleopsych] Hedgehog*, October 19, 2004, http://lists.extropy.org/pipermail/paleopsych/2004-October/000710.html.

Dean, Mitchell. *Governing Societies*. Maidenhead, United Kingdom: Open University Press, 2007.

Dikotter, Frank. *The Construction of Racial Identities in China and Japan: Historical and Contemporary Perspectives*. Honolulu: University of Hawaii Press, 1997.

——. *Imperfect Conceptions: Medical Knowledge, Birth Defects, and Eugenics in China*. New York: Columbia University Press, 1998.

Dillon, Michael, and Luis Lobo-Guerrero. "Biopolitics of Security in the 21st Century: An Introduction." *Review of International Studies* 34, no. 2 (2008): 265–92.

Dittmer, Lowell. "Taiwan and the Issue of National Identity." *Asian Survey* 44, no. 4 (2004): 475–83.

Donaldson, Thomas. "Decompacting the Global Compact." Paper presented at the All-Academy Symposium, "The Global Compact: Building Corporate Citizenship in a World of Networks," at the 2002 Academy of Management Conference, Denver, Colo., August 12, 2002.

Donzelot, Jacques. *The Policing of Families*. New York: Random House, 1997.

Douglas, Mary. *Purity and Danger*. 1966; London: Routledge, 2002.

Dumit, Joseph. *Drugs for Life*. Durham: Duke University Press, forthcoming.

——. *Technologized Images, Technologized Bodies*, ed. Jeanette Edwards, Penny Harvey, Peter Wade. Oxford: Berghahn Books, forthcoming.

Duster, Troy. "Buried Alive: The Concept of Race in Science." In *Genetic Nature/Culture: Anthropology and Science beyond the Two-Culture Divide*, edited by Alan H. Goodman, Deborah Heath, and M. Susan Lindee. Berkeley: University of California Press, 2003.

Ecks, Stefan. "Global Pharmaceutical Markets and Corporate Citizenship: The Case of Novartis' Anti-cancer Drug Glivec." *BioSocieties* 3, no. 2 (2008): 165–81.

——. "Three Propositions for an Evidence-based Medical Anthropology." In "Objects of Evidence," edited by Matthew Engelke, special issue of *Journal of the Royal Anthropological Institute* (2008): S77–S92.

Elliott, Carl, and Paul Brodwin. "Identity and Genetic Ancestry Tracing." *British Medical Journal* 325 (2002): 21–28.

Elmore, Mick. "Thailand's Plastic Surgeons Cut a Niche for Themselves." International News, Deutsche Press-Agentur, February 7, 1997.

Enloe, Cynthia H. *Bananas, Beaches, and Bases: Making Feminist Sense of International Politics*. Berkeley: University of California Press, 1990.

Epstein, Steven. *Impure Science: AIDS, Activism, and the Politics of Knowledge*. Berkeley: University of California Press, 1996.

Ernst & Young [Ernst & Young Global Ltd. (EYG)]. "Unveiling India's Pharmaceutical Future." *Health Sciences Industry Report 2005*. London: EYG, 2005.

Erwin, Kathleen. "The Circulatory System: Blood Procurement, AIDS, and the Social Body in China." *Medical Anthropology Quarterly* 20, no. 2 (2006): 139–59.

Fackler, Martin. "Scientist at Work: Shinya Tamanaka, Risk Taking Is in His Genes." *New York Times*, December 11, 2007, Science section, 1, 4.

Faiola, Anthony. "Koreans 'Blinded' to Truth about Claims on Stem Cells." *Washington Post Foreign Service*, January 13, 2006, A10.

Farquhar, Judith. *Appetites: Food and Sex in Post-Socialist China*. Durham: Duke University Press, 2002.

Fei, Xiao-Tong. *The Pattern of Diversity in Unity of the Chinese Nation*. Beijing: Zhongyang Minzu University, 1999.

Ferguson, James, and Akhil Gupta. "Spatializing States: Towards a Study of Transnational Governmentality." *American Ethnologist* 24 (2002): 981–1002.

Fernandez, Elizabeth. "Legislators Touched by Leukemia Push to Save Umbilical Cord Blood." *San Francisco Chronicle*, August 13, 2007, A1, A10.

Fischer, Michael M. J. *Emergent Forms of Life and the Anthropological Voice*. Durham: Duke University Press, 2003.

——. "Four Genealogies for a Recombinant Anthropology of Science and Technology." *Cultural Anthropology* 22, no. 4 (November 2007): 539–615.

Fisher, Jill. "Human Subjects in Medical Experiments." In *Science, Technology, and Society*, edited by Sal Restivo. Oxford: Oxford University Press, 2005.

Foucault, Michel. *Ethics: Subjectivity and Truth*. Vol. 1 of *Essential Works of Foucault, 1954–1984*, edited by Paul Rabinow, translated by Robert Hurley et al. New York: New Press, 1997.

——. "Governmentality." In *Power*, vol. 3 of *Essential Works of Foucault, 1954–1984*, edited by James Faubion, series editor Paul Rabinow. New York: New Press, 2000.

——. *History of Sexuality*, vol. 1, *An Introduction*. New York: Vintage Books, 1981.

——. *Naissance de la biopolitique: Cours au Collège de France, 1978–1979*. Paris: Gallimard/Seuil, 2004.

——. "Penal Theories." In *Ethics: Subjectivity and Truth*, edited by Paul Rabinow. New York: New Press, 1997.

——. "Security, Territory, and Population." In *Ethics: Subjectivity and Truth*, edited by Paul Rabinow. New York: New Press, 1997.

——. *Security, Territory, Population: Lectures at the Collège de France, 1997–1978*. Edited by Michel Senellart, English series editor Arnold I. Davidson, translated by Graham Burchell. New York: Palgrave Macmillan, 2007.

——. *"Society Must Be Defended": Lectures at the Collège de France, 1975–1976*. Edited by Mauro Bertani and Alessandro Fontana, translated by David Macey. New York: Picador, 1997.

Franklin, Sarah. "Ethical Biocapital: New Strategies of Cell Culture." In *Remaking Life and Death: Toward an Anthropology of the Biosciences*, edited by Sarah Franklin and Margaret Lock. Santa Fe, N.M.: School of American Research Press, 2003.

——. "Life Itself: Global Nature and the Genetic Imaginary." In *Global Nature, Global Culture*, edited by Sarah Franklin, Celia Lury, and Jackie Stacey. London: Sage, 2000.

——. "Rethinking Nature-Culture: Anthropology and the New Genetics." *Anthropological Theory* 3, no. 1 (2003): 65–85.

——. "Stem Cells R Us: Emergent Life Forms and the Global Biological," in *Global Assemblages: Technology, Politics and Ethics as Anthropological Problems*, ed. Aihwa Ong and Stephen J. Collier. Malden, Mass.: Blackwell, 2005.

Franklin, Sarah, and Susan McKinnon, "Introduction: Relative Values: Reconfiguring Kinship Studies." In *Relative Values: Reconfiguring Kinship Studies*, ed. Sarah Franklin and Susan McKinnon. Durham: Duke University Press, 2001.

Frew, Sarah E., et al. "Chinese Health Biotech and the Billion-Patient Market." *Nature Biotechnology* 26 (2008): 37–53.

——. "India's Health Biotech Sector at a Crossroads." *Nature Biotechnology* 25 (2007): 403–17.

Fujimura, Joan. "Transnational Genomics: Transgressing the Boundary between the 'Modern/West' and the 'Premodern/East.'" In *Doing Science and Culture*, edited by Roddey Reid and Sharon Traweek. New York: Routledge, 2000.

Fukuyama, Francis. *Our Posthuman Future: Consequences of the Biotechnology Revolution*. New York: Farrar, Straus, and Giroux, 2002.

Gentzler, J. Mason. *Changing China*. New York: Praeger Publishers, 1977.

Gilbert, Walter. "A Vision of the Grail." In *The Code of Codes: Scientific and Social Issues in the Human Genome Project*, edited by Daniel Kelves and Leroy Hood. Cambridge, Mass.: Harvard University Press, 1992.

Goodale, Mark. "Ethics, Human Rights, and Anthropology." *American Anthropologist* 108, no. 1 (2006): 25–37.

Gottweis, Herbert, and Robert Triendl. "South Korean Policy Failure and the Hwang Debacle." *Nature Biotechnology* 24, no. 2 (February 2006): 141–43.

Grace, Patricia. *Baby No-Eyes*. Honolulu: University of Hawaii Press, 1998.

Greenhalgh, Susan. *Just One Child: Science and Policy in Deng's China*. Berkeley: University of California Press, 2008.

Greenhalgh, Susan, and Edwin Winckler. *Governing China's Population: From Leninist to Neoliberal Biopolitics*. Stanford, Calif.: Stanford University Press, 2005.

Hacking, Ian. "Making Up People." In *The Science Studies Reader*, edited by Mario Biagioli. 1986; New York: Routledge, 1999.

Hagen, Joel. "Timeline: The Origins of Bioinformatics." *Nature Review Genetics* 1 (2000): 231–36.

Hamilton, Matthew B. *Population Genetics*. Hoboken, N.J.: Wiley-Blackwell, 2009.

Haraway, Donna. "A Cyborg Manifesto." In *Simians, Cyborgs, and Women: The Reinvention of Nature*. New York: Routledge, 1991.

——. "Situated Knowledge: The Science Question in Feminism and the Privilege of Partial Perspective." In *The Science Studies Reader*, edited by Mario Biagioli. New York: Routledge, 1999.

Harrell, Stevan. *Cultural Encounters on China's Ethnic Frontiers*. Seattle: University of Washington Press, 1995.

Harris, Sara. "Asian Pragmatism." *EMBO Reports* 3, no. 9 (2002): 816–17, http://www.nature.com/embor/.

Harvey, David. *A Brief History of Neoliberalism*. Oxford: Oxford University Press, 2005.

——. *The Condition of Postmodernity*. Oxford: Basil Blackwell, 1989.

——. *The New Imperialism*. Oxford: Oxford University Press, 2003.

Haseltine, William. "The Power of Genomics to Transform the Biotechnology Industry." *Nature Biotechnology* 16 (1998 Supplement): 25–27.

Hayden, Cori. "Benefit-sharing: Experiments in Governance." Paper presented at the Social Science Research Council Workshop "Intellectual Property, Markets, and Cultural Flows," New York, October 24–25, 2003.

——. "Taking as Giving: Bioscience, Exchange, and the Politics of Benefit-Sharing." *Social Studies of Science* 37, no. 5 (2007): 729–58.

——. *When Nature Goes Public: The Making and Unmaking of Bioprospecting in Mexico*. Princeton, N.J.: Princeton University Press, 2003.

Held, David, Anthony McGrew, David Goldblatt, and Jonathan Perraton. *Global Transformation: Politics, Economics, Culture*. London: Routledge, 1999.

Hennig, Wolfgang. "Bioethics in China: Although National Guidelines Are in Place, Their Implementation Remains Difficult." *European Molecular Biology Organization (EMBO) Reports* 7 (2006): 850–54.

Hepeng, Jia. "GM Rice May Soon be Commercialized." *China Business Weekly*, January 26, 2005.

Hewison, Kevin. *Pathways to Recovery: Bankers, Business and Nationalism in Thailand*. Working Paper Series no. 1. Hongkong: Southeast Asia Research Centre, City University of Hong Kong, April 2001.

High Flyers Think Tank. "Emerging Diseases—Ready and Waiting?" Paper presented at the Shine Dome, Australian Academy of Science, Canberra, October 19, 2004.

Hochschild, Arlie Russell. *The Managed Heart: Commercialization of Human Feeling*. Berkeley: University of California Press, 1983.

Holland, Suzanne, Karen Lebacqz, and Laurie Zoloth. *The Human Embryonic Stem Cell Debate.* Cambridge, Mass.: MIT Press, 2001.

Hong, Sungook. "The Hwang Scandal That Shook the World of Science." *East Asian Science, Technology and Society* 2 (2008): 1–7.

Honig, Emily, and Gail Herschatter. *Personal Voices: Chinese Women in the 1980's.* Stanford, Calif.: Stanford University Press, 1988.

Hsing, You-tien. "Building *Guanxi* Across the Straits: Taiwanese Capital and Local Chinese Bureaucrats." In *Ungrounded Empires: The Cultural Politics of Modern Chinese Transnationalism*, edited by Aihwa Ong and Donald Nonini. New York: Routledge, 1997.

Huang, Jikun, Scott Rozelle, Carl Pray, and Qinfang Wang. "Plant Biotechnology in China." *Science* 295 (2002): 674–76.

Huang, Quangxue, and Lianzhu Shi. *Recognition of Ethnicities in China.* Beijing: Minzu Publisher, 1995.

ICFAI Center for Management Research. *Bumrungrad's Global Services Marketing Strategy.* ICFAI Case Collection. Hyderabad, India: Institute of Chartered Financial Analysts of India Center for Management Research, 2003.

Ida, Ryuuichi. "Ethical Questions of the Human Embryonic Stem Cells Research." *Rinsho Shinkeigaku* [Clinical Neurology] 42, no. 11 (November 2002): 1147–48.

Imanish, T., T. Akaza, et al. "Allele and Haplotype Frequencies for HLA and Complement Loci in Various Ethnic Groups." In *HLA 1991: Proceedings of the 11th International Histocompatability Workshop and Conference*, edited by K. Tsuki, M. Aizawa, and T. Sasazuki. Oxford: Oxford University Press, 1992.

Jacques, Martin. *China Rules the World: The End of the Western World and the Birth of a New Global Order.* New York: The Penguin Press, 2009.

"Japanese Scientist Says Regulations Needed for Non-embryo Stem Cells to Avoid Abuse." *International Herald Tribune*, January 9, 2008.

Jasanoff, Sheila. *Designs on Nature: Science and Democracy in Europe and the United States.* Princeton, N.J.: Princeton University Press, 2005.

Jing, Jun. *Feeding China's Little Emperors: Food, Children, and Social Change.* Stanford, Calif.: Stanford University Press, 2000.

Kafatos, Fotis. "A Revolutionary Landscape: The Restructuring of Biology and Its Convergence with Medicine" *Journal of Molecular Biology* 319, no. 4 (2002): 861–67.

Kaiser, Jocelyn. "Biobanks: Population Databases Boom, from Iceland to the U.S." *Science* 298, no. 5596 (2002): 1158–61.

Kaptchuk, Ted. *The Web That Has No Weaver: Understanding Chinese Medicine.* 2nd ed. New York: McGraw-Hill, 2000.

Kato, Kazuto. "The Ethical and Political Discussions on Stem Cell Research in Japan." In *Grenzüberschreitungen* [Crossing Borders], edited by W. Bender et al. Münster: Agenda Verlag, 2005.

Kay, Lily E. *The Molecular Vision of Life: Caltech, the Rockefeller Foundation, and the Rise of New Biology.* Oxford: Oxford University Press, 1996.

Kayukawa, Junji. *Kuroun Ningen* [Human Cloning]. Tokyo: Koubunsha Shinsho, 2003.

Kevles, Daniel. *In the Name of Eugenics: Genetics and the Uses of Human Heredity*. Cambridge, Mass.: Harvard University Press, 1985.

Khwankhom, Arthit. "Bt30 Health Scheme Still Lacks Funds, Says Official." *The Nation* (Thailand), http://www.nationmultimedia.com/2006/07/14/national/national_30008668.php.

Kittikanya, Charoen. "Dual-Track System." *Bangkok Post*, "Mid-Year Economic Review 2004," http://www.bangkokpost.com/.

——. "Foreigners Still Flock to Thai Hospitals, Attracted by Highly Skilled Doctors and Lower Bills." *Bangkok Post*, "Economic Year-End Review, 2007," http://www.bangkokpost.com/.

——. "Health." *Bangkok Post*, "Economic Year-End Review, 2004," http://www.bangkokpost.com/.

Kittles, Rick, and Charmaine Royal. "The Genetics of African Americans: Implications for Disease Gene Mapping and Identity." In *Genetic Nature/Culture: Anthropology and Science beyond the Two-Culture Divide*, edited by Alan H. Goodman, Deborah Heath, and M. Susan Lindee. Berkeley: University of California Press, 2003.

Kleinman, Arthur. *The Illness Narratives: Suffering, Healing, and the Human Condition*. New York: Basic Books, 1988.

——. *Patients and Healers in the Context of Culture*. Berkeley: University of California Press, 1981.

Kleyn, Patrick, and Elliot Vesell. "Pharmacogenomics: Genetic Variation as a Guide to Drug Development." *Science* 281, no. 5384 (1998): 1820–21.

Koh Buck Song. "Perfect People's Fears." *Today* (Singapore), April 14, 2004.

Kohrman, Matthew. *Bodies of Difference: Experiences of Disability and Institutional Advocacy in the Making of Modern China*. Berkeley: University of California Press, 2005.

——. "Should I Quit? Tobacco, Fraught Identity, and the Risks of Governmentality." In *Privatizing China, Socialism from Afar*, edited by Li Zhang and Aihwa Ong. Ithaca, N.Y.: Cornell University Press, 2008.

Kornberg, Arthur. "Whither Biotechnology in Japan: Why Biotechnology Hasn't Taken Off." *Harvard Asia Pacific Review* 106, no. 2 (fall 2002): 6–9.

Kumra, Gautam. "One Business's Commitment to Society: An Interview with the President of the Novartis Foundation for Sustainable Development." *McKinsey Quarterly* 3 (2006), http://www.mckinseyquarterly.com/.

Kuntz, Dieter, ed. *Deadly Medicine: Creating the Master Race*. Chapel Hill: University of North Carolina Press, 2004.

Kuriyama, Shigehisa. *The Expressiveness of the Body and the Divergence of Greek and Chinese Medicine*. New York: Zone Books, 2002.

Kuo, Wen-Hua. "Japan and Taiwan in the Wake of Bio-Globalization: Drugs, Race, and Standards." Ph.D. dissertation, Massachusetts Institute of Technology, 2005.

Lakoff, Andrew. "The Private Life of Numbers: Audit Firms and the Government of Expertise in Post-Welfare Argentina." In *Global Assemblages: Technology, Politics, and Ethics as Anthropological Problems*, edited by Aihwa Ong and Stephen J. Collier. Malden, Mass.: Blackwell, 2005.

Latour, Bruno. *We Have Never Been Modern*. Translated by Catherine Porter. Cambridge, Mass.: Harvard University Press, 1993.

Leadbeater, Charles, and James Wilsdon. "South-East Asia Economies Herald a New Dawn of Technological Innovation," *Times* (London), January 17, 2007, 51.

Leem, So Yeon, and Jin Hee Park. "Rethinking Women and Their Bodies in the Age of Biotechnology: Feminist Commentaries on the Hwang Affair." *East Asian Science, Technology and Society* 2 (2008): 9–26.

Lemke, Thomas. "The Birth of Bio-Politics: Michael Foucault's Lectures at the Collège de France on Neo-Liberal Governmentality." *Economy and Society* 30 (2001): 1–17.

Leong Chin, "A Life-Saving Gift." *Straits Times* (Singapore), September 25, 2005.

Leong, Sow-Theng. *Migration and Ethnicity in Chinese History: Hakkas, Pengmin, and Their Neighbors*. Stanford, Calif.: Stanford University Press, 1997.

Lewis, Tracy, Jerome Reichman, and Anthony So. "The Case for Public Funding and Public Oversight of Clinical Trials." *Economists' Voice* 4, no. 1, art. 3 (2007).

Li, Hui, and Jue Wang. "Backlash Disrupts China Exchanges." *Science* 278, no. 5337 (1997): 376–77.

Li Zhang and Aihwa Ong, eds. *Privatizing China: Socialism from Afar*. Ithaca, N.Y.: Cornell University Press, 2008.

"Life Line." *Business Times* (Singapore), September 24, 2005.

Lim Say Boon. "Economics and Science at Stake over Stem-Cell Research Debate." *South China Morning Post*, September 8, 2002, 4.

Lim, Sylvia, and Calvin Ho. "The Ethical Position of Singapore on Embryonic Stem Cell Research." *SMA News* (Singapore Medical Association) 35, no. 6 (June 2003): 22–23.

Lin, Marie, et al. "Heterogeneity of Taiwan's Indigenous Population: Possible Relation to Prehistoric Mongoloid Dispersals." *Tissue Antigens* 55 (2000): 1–9.

———. "The Origin of Minnan and Hakka, the So-called 'Taiwanese,' Inferred by HLA Study." *Tissue Antigens* 57 (2001): 192–99.

Liu, Edison. "Asia's Biotech Tiger." *New Scientist* 175, no. 2360 (September 14, 2002): 54–57.

Liu, Jennifer. "Biomedtech Nation: Taiwan, Ethics, Stem Cells and Other Biologicals." Ph.D. dissertation, University of California, Berkeley, 2008.

Liu, Lydia. *The Clash of Empires: The Invention of China in Modern World Making*. Cambridge, Mass.: Harvard University Press, 2004.

Lock, Margaret. "The Alienation of Body Tissue and the Biopolitics of Immortalized Cell Lines." *Body and Society* 7, nos. 2–3 (2001): 63–91.

——. *Twice Dead: Organ Transplants and the Reinvention of Death*. Berkeley: University of California Press, 2002.

Lynch, Daniel C. "Taiwan's Self-Conscious Nation-Building Project." *Asian Survey* 44, no. 4 (2004): 513–33.

Macklin, Ruth. *Mortal Choices: Bioethics in Today's World*. New York: Pantheon, 1987.

Marshall, Eliot. "Genomics: Drug Firms to Create Public Database of Genetic Mutations." *Science* 284, no. 5413 (1999): 406–7.

Marshall, Patricia A., and Abdallah S. Daar. "Cultural and Psychological Dimensions of Organ Transplantation." *Annals of Transplantation* 3, no. 2 (1998): 7–11.

Marshall, Thomas H. "Citizenship and Social Class." In *Citizenship and Social Class*, edited by Thomas H. Marshall and Tom Bottomore. 1949; London: Pluto, 1991.

Martin, Emily. *Bipolar Expeditions: Mania and Depression in American Culture*. Princeton, N.J.: Princeton University Press, 2007.

——. *The Woman in the Body: A Cultural Analysis of Reproduction*. Boston, Mass.: Beacon Press, 1987.

Marx, Karl. *Capital: A Critique of Political Economy*, vol. 1. Edited by Frederick Engels, translated by Samuel Moore and Edward Aveling. 1867; New York: International Publishers, 1967. Penguin edition, translated by B. Fowkes, London: Penguin, 1976.

Marx, Karl, and Friedrich Engels. *Manifesto of the Communist Party*. 1848; Chicago: Encyclopedia Britannica, 1952.

Masahiro, Morioka. "The Ethics of Human Cloning and the Sprout of Human Life." In *Cross-Cultural Issues in Bioethics: The Example of Human Cloning*, edited by Heiner Roetz. Amsterdam: Rodopi, 2006.

Mastro, Timothy D., and Ray Yip. "The Legacy of Unhygienic Plasma Collection in China." *AIDS* 20, no. 10 (2006): 1451–52.

Masui, Tohru. "Cultivating Trust and Motivation in Human Experiments: The Process of Creating Biobanks." In *Human Genetic Biobanks in Asia*, edited by Margaret Sleeboom-Faulkner. London: Routledge, 2008.

Matten, Dirk, and Andrew Crane. "Corporate Citizenship: Towards an Extended Theoretical Conceptualization." Research Paper Series 4. Nottingham: Nottingham University Business School, International Centre for Corporate Social Responsibility, 2003.

McGoey, Linsey. "On the Will to Ignorance in Bureaucracy." *Economy and Society* 36 (2007): 212–35.

McVeigh, Brian. *The Nature of the Japanese State*. London: Routledge, 1998.

McVey, Ruth, ed. *Southeast Asian Capitalists*. Ithaca, N.Y.: Cornell University Press, 1992.

Meyer, Christopher, and Stan Davis. *It's Alive: The Coming Convergence of Information, Biology, and Business*. New York: Crown Business, 2003.

Meyerowitz, Joanne J. *How Sex Changed: A History of Transsexuality in the United States*. Cambridge, Mass.: Harvard University Press, 2002.

Morishima, Michio. *Why Has Japan "Succeeded": Western Technology and the Japanese Ethos*. Cambridge: Cambridge University Press, 1984.

Mullaney, Thomas Shawn. "Coming to Terms with the Nation: Ethnic Classification and Scientific Stratecraft in Modern China, 1928–1954." Ph.D. dissertation, Columbia University, 2006.

Muller, Jessica H. "Anthropology, Bioethics, and Medicine: A Provocative Trilogy." *Medical Anthropology Quarterly*, new ser. 8, no. 4 (December 1994): 448–67.

Murphy, Rachel. "Turning Peasants into Modern Chinese Citizens: 'Population Quality,' Discourse, Demographic Transition and Primary Education." *China Quarterly* 177 (2004): 1–20.

Nakajo, Yukiko, et al. "Physical and Mental Development of Children after *in vitro* Fertilization and Embryo Transfer." *Reproductive Medicine and Biology* 3, no. 2 (June 2004): 63.

Nakanishi, Nao. "China Seen a Crouching Dragon in Biotechnology," Reuters, December 20, 2002.

Nie, Jing-Bao. *Behind the Silence: Chinese Voices on Abortion.* Lanham, United Kingdom: Rowman and Littlefield, 2005.

Niou, Emerson M. S. "Understanding Taiwan Independence and Its Policy Implications." *Asian Survey* 44, no. 4 (2004): 555–67.

Nonini, Donald M., and Aihwa Ong. "Chinese Transnationalism as an Alternative Modernity." In *Ungrounded Empires: The Cultural Politics of Modern Chinese Transnationalism*, edited by Aihwa Ong and Donald Nonini. New York: Routledge, 1997.

Norgren, Tiana. *Abortion before Birth Control: The Politics of Reproduction in Postwar Japan*. Princeton, N.J.: Princeton University Press, 2001.

Normile, Dennis. "SNP Study Supports Southern Migration Route to Asia," *Science Magazine*, vol. 326, December 11, 2009, 1470.

Nudeshima, Jiro. "Human Cloning Legislation in Japan." *Eubios Journal of Asian and International Bioethics* 11, no. 1 (2001): 101–2.

Nundy, Samiran, and Chandra Gulhati. "A New Colonialism?—Conducting Clinical Trials in India." *New England Journal of Medicine* 352, no. 16 (2005): 1633–36.

Olds, Kris, and Nigel Thrift. "Cultures on the Brink: Reengineering the Soul of Capitalism—On a Global Scale." In *Global Assemblages: Technology, Politics, and Ethics as Anthropological Problems*, edited by Aihwa Ong and Stephen J. Collier. Malden, Mass.: Blackwell, 2005.

Ong, Aihwa. "Assembling around SARS: Technology, Body Heat, and Political Fever in Risk Society." In *Ulrich Beck: Kosmopolitisches Projekt*, edited by Angelika Pferl and Natan Szaider. Badan-Baden: Nomos Verlagsgesellschaft, 2004.

——. "Ecologies of Expertise: Assembling Flows, Managing Citizenship." In *Global*

Assemblages: Technology, Politics, and Ethics as Anthropological Problems, edited by Aihwa Ong and Stephen J. Collier. Malden, Mass.: Blackwell, 2005.

——. *Flexible Citizenship: The Cultural Politics of Transnationality*. Durham: Duke University Press, 1998.

——. *Neoliberalism as Exception: Mutations in Citizenship and Sovereignty*. Durham: Duke University Press, 2006.

——. "Scales of Exception: Experiments with Knowledge and Sheer Life in Tropical Southeast Asia." *Singapore Journal of Tropical Geography* 29, no. 2 (July 2008): 1–13.

——. "Zoning Technologies in East Asia." In *Neoliberalism as Exception: Mutations in Citizenship and Sovereignty*. Durham: Duke University Press, 2006.

Ong, Aihwa, and Stephen J. Collier, eds. *Global Assemblage: Technology, Politics and Ethics as Anthropological Problems*. Malden, Mass.: Blackwell, 2005.

Ong, Aihwa, and Li Zhang, "Privatizing China: Powers of the Self, Socialism from Afar." In *Privatizing China, Socialism from Afar*, edited by Li Zhang and Aihwa Ong. Ithaca, N.Y.: Cornell University Press, 2008.

Ong, Aihwa, and Donald Nonini, eds. *Ungrounded Empires: The Cultural Politics of Modern Chinese Transnationalism*. New York: Routledge, 1997.

Ossorio, Pilar, and Troy Duster. "Race and Genetics: Controversies in Biomedical, Behavioral and Forensic Medicine." *American Psychologist* 60, no. 1 (2005): 116–27.

Padmanabhan, Manjula. *Harvest*. London: Aurora Metro Press, 2003.

Palsson, Gisli, and Paul Rabinow. "Iceland: The Case of a National Human Genome Project." *Anthropology Today* 15, no. 5 (1999): 14–18.

——. "The Icelandic Controversy: Reflections on the Transnational Market of Civic Virtue." In *Global Assemblages: Technology, Politics, and Ethics as Anthropological Problems*, edited by Aihwa Ong and Stephen J. Collier. Malden, Mass.: Blackwell, 2005.

Pempel, T. J. *The Politics of the Asian Economic Crisis*. Ithaca, N.Y.: Cornell University Press, 1999.

Pennisi, Elizabeth. "Human Genome Project: Funders Reassure Genome Sequencers." *Science* 280, no. 5367 (1998): 1185.

Petryna, Adriana. "Drug Development and the Ethics of the Globalized Clinical Trial." Working paper. Princeton, N.J.: Princeton Institute of Advanced Studies, 2005.

——. "Ethical Variability: Drug Development and Globalizing Clinical Trials." *American Ethnologist* 32, no. 2 (May 2005): 183–97.

——. *Life Exposed: Biological Citizens after Chernobyl*. Princeton, N.J.: Princeton University Press, 2002.

Petryna, Adryna, Andrew Lakoff, and Arthur Kleinman, eds. *Global Pharmaceuticals: Ethics, Markets, Practices*. Durham: Duke University Press, 2006.

Phongpaichit, Pasuk. "Thailand under Thaksin: Another Malaysia?" Perth, Australia: Asia Research Centre at Murdoch University, 2004, http://wwwarc.murdoch.edu.au/wp/wp109.pdf.

Phongpaichit, Pasuk, and Chris Baker. *Thailand: Economy and Politics*. Oxford: Oxford University Press, 1995.

Pollack, Andrew. "Scientific and Ethical Questions Cloud Plans to Clone for Therapy." *New York Times*, February 13, 2004, A1, A13.

Powell, Colin L. "Nonimmigrant Visas for Medical Treatment." U.S. Department of State, November 1 (no year), http://travel.state.gov/visa/laws/telegrams/telegrams_1533.html.

Pratruangkrai, Petchanet. "Saudi Health Scheme Inked." *The Nation* (Thailand), May 20, 2006, http://www.nationmultimedia.com/.

Pritchard, Chris. "Want to Fix Thailand's Ailing Economy? More Sex Change Operations!" *Medical Post* (Canada) 34, no. 5 (February 3, 1998): 59.

Qiang, Boqin. "Human Genome Research in China." *Journal of Molecular Medicine* 82, no. 4 (2004): 214–22.

Qiu, J. "Is China Ready for GM Rice?" *Nature* 455 (2008): 850–52.

Rabinow, Paul. "Artificiality and Enlightenment: From Sociobiology to Biosociality." In *Essays on the Anthropology of Reason*. Princeton, N.J.: Princeton University Press, 1996. Reprinted in *The Science Studies Reader*, edited by Mario Biagioli. New York: Routledge, 1999.

——. *Essays on the Anthropology of Reason*. Princeton, N.J.: Princeton University Press, 1996.

——, ed. *The Foucault Reader*. New York: Pantheon Books, 1984.

——. *French DNA: Trouble in Purgatory*. Chicago: Chicago University Press, 1999.

Rabinow, Paul, and Nikolas Rose. "Thoughts on the Concept of Biopower Today." *BioSocieties* 1 (2006): 195–217.

Rajagopal, Arvind. "The Menace of Hawkers." In *Property in Question: Value Transformation in the Global Economy*, edited by Katherine Verdery and Caroline Humphrey. New York: Berg, 2004.

Rapp, Rayna. *Testing Women, Testing the Fetus: Amniocentesis in America*. New York: Routledge, 1999.

Rawls, John. *A Theory of Justice*. 1971; Cambridge, Mass.: Belknap, 2005.

Reardon, Jenny. *Race to the Finish: Identity and Governance in an Age of Genomics*. Princeton, N.J.: Princeton University Press, 2005.

Redding, Gordon S. *The Spirit of Chinese Capitalism*. Berlin: Walter de Gruyter, 1990.

Rofel, Lisa. *Desiring China: Experiments in Neoliberalism, Sexuality and Public Culture*. Durham: Duke University Press, 2007.

——. *Other Modernities: Gendered Yearnings in China after Socialism*. Berkeley: University of California Press, 1999.

Rose, Nikolas. *The Politics of Life Itself: Biomedicine, Power, and Subjectivity in the Twenty-first Century*. Princeton, N.J.: Princeton University Press, 2007.

——. *Powers of Freedom: Reframing Political Thought*. Cambridge: Cambridge University Press, 1999.

Rose, Nikolas, and Carlos Novas. "Biological Citizenship." In *Global Assemblages Technology, Politics, and Ethics as Anthropological Problems*, edited by Aihwa Ong and Stephen J. Collier. Malden, Mass.: Blackwell, 2005.

Rundle, Rhonda L. "A Daisy Chain of Kidney Donations." *Wall Street Journal*, September 23, 2008, D1, D2.

Salter, Brian, Melinda Cooper, and Amanda Dickens. "China and the Global Stem Cell Bioeconomy: An Emerging Political Strategy?" *Regenerative Medicine* 1, no. 5 (2006): 671–83.

Sassen, Saskia. *Globalization and Its Discontents: Essays on the New Mobility of People and Money*. New York: New Press, 1998.

——. *Territory, Authority, Rights: From Medieval to Global Assemblages*. Princeton: Princeton University Press, 2006.

Scheper Hughes, Nancy. "The Last Commodity: Post-human Ethics and the Global Traffic in 'Fresh' Organs." In *Global Assemblages: Technology, Politics, and Ethics as Anthropological Problems*, edited by Aihwa Ong and Stephen J. Collier. Malden, Mass.: Blackwell, 2005.

Scott, Christopher Thomas. *Stem Cell Now: A Brief Introduction to the Coming Medical Revolution*. London: Plume Printing, 2006.

Shan, Hua, Jing-Xing Wang, Fu-Rong Ren, Yuan-Zhi Zhang, Hai-Yan Zhao, Guo-Jing Gao, Yang Ji, and Paul M. Ness "Blood Banking in China." *Lancet* 360 (2002): 1770–75.

Shao Jing. "Fluid Labor and Blood Money: The Economy of HIV/AIDS in Rural Central China." *Cultural Anthropology* 21, no. 4 (2006): 535–69.

Shapiro, Peter J. "The New Sovereignists: American Exceptionalism and Its False Prophets." *Foreign Affairs*, November–December 2001, http://foreignaffairs.com.

Shmulewitz, Ascher, Robert Langer, and John Patton. "Convergence in Biomedical Technology." *Nature Biotechnology* 24 (2006): 277.

Silver, Lee. "The God Effect: America's Religious Conservatives Aren't the Only Ones Who Object to Science on Spiritual Grounds—So Do Europe's Greens. The Big Winner Is Asia." *Newsweek International*, April 2004.

"Singapore: The Biopolis of Asia." *Science*, April–May 2003, D1.

Sleebom-Faulkner, Margaret. "How to Define a Population: Cultural Politics and Population Genetics in the People's Republic of China and the Republic of China." *BioSocieties* 1 (2006): 399–419.

Slingby, Brian T., Noriko Nagao, and Akira Akabayashi. "Administrative Legislation in Japan: Guidelines on Scientific and Ethical Standards." *Cambridge Quarterly of Healthcare Ethics* 13 (2004): 245–53.

Smaglik, Paul. "Filling Biopolis." *Nature* 425 (2003): 746–47.

Soleri, D., D. A. Cleveland, G. E. Glasgow, S. H. Sweeney, F. Aragón Cuevas, H. Ríos Labrada, and M. R. Fuentes Lopez. "Testing Assumptions Underlying Economic Research on Transgenic Food Crops for Third World Farmers: Evidence from Cuba, Guatemala and Mexico." *Ecological Economics* 67, no. 4 (2008): 667–82.

Sperling, Stefan. "Managing Potential Selves: Stem Cells, Immigrants, and German Identity." *Science and Public Policy* 31, no. 2 (2004): 139–49.

"S'pore Relaxes Jail Penalty for Human Cloning." *International Herald Tribune*, May 12, 2004.

Star, Susan Leigh. "The Ethnography of Infrastructure." *American Behavioral Scientist* 43, no. 3 (1999): 377–91.

Strange, Susan. *Casino Capitalism*. Manchester: Manchester University Press, 1997.

Strathern, Marilyn. "Emergent Properties." In *Kinship, Law, and the Unexpected*. Cambridge: Cambridge University Press, 2005.

Suehiro, Akira. "Capitalist Development in Postwar Thailand: Commercial Bankers, Industrial Elite, and Agribusiness Groups." In *Southeast Asian Capitalists*, edited by Ruth McVey. Ithaca, N.Y.: Cornell University, Southeast Asian Program, 1992.

Sunder Rajan, Kaushik. *Biocapital: The Constitution of Postgenomic Life*. Durham: Duke University Press, 2006.

——. "Experimental Values: Indian Clinical Trials and Surplus Health." *New Left Review* 45 (2007): 67–88.

——. "Subjects of Speculation: Emergent Life Sciences and Market Logics in the US and India." *American Anthropologist* 107, no. 1 (2005): 19–30.

Sun-Wei Guo, Chang-Jiang Zheng, and C. C. Li. "The Gene War of the Century." *Science* 278. no. 5344 (December 5, 1997): 1693–97.

Susumu, Shimazono. "Why Must We Be Prudent in Research Using Human Embryos?: Differing Views of Human Dignity." In *Dark Medicine*, edited by William R. La Fleur, Gernot Boehme, and Shimazono Susumu. Bloomington: Indiana University Press, 2008.

Tai, Hung-chao, ed. *Confucianism and Economic Development: An Oriental Alternative?* Washington, D.C.: Washington Institute for Values in Public Policy, 1989.

Tay, Michelle. "S'pore Is Easiest City in the World to Do Business; It Is Also Top in Region for Economic Stability and Legal/Political Framework: Survey." *Straits Times* (Singapore), June 10, 2008.

Temple, Larissa K. F., Robin S. McLeod, Steven Gallinger, and James G. Wright. "Defining Disease in the Genomics Era." *Science* 293 (2001): 807–8.

Templeton, Alan R. "Human Races in the Context of Recent Human Evolution: A Molecular Genetic Perspective." In *Genetic Nature/Culture: Anthropology and Science beyond the Two-Culture Divide*, edited by Alan H. Goodman, Deborah Heath, and M. Susan Lindee. Berkeley: University of California Press, 2003.

Terry, Jennifer. *An American Obsession: Science, Medicine, and Homosexuality in Modern Society*. Chicago: University of Chicago Press, 1999.

Thompson, Charis. *Making Parents: The Ontological Choreography of Reproductive Technologies*. Cambridge, Mass.: MIT Press, 2005.

——. "Why We Should, in Fact, Pay for Egg Donation." *Regenerative Medicine* 2, no. 2 (2007): 203–9.

Thompson, Grahame F. "Global Corporate Citizenship: What Does It Mean?" *Competition and Change* 9 (2005): 131–52.

Tierney, John, "Are Scientists Playing God? It Depends on Your Religion." *New York Times*, November 20, 2007.

Titmuss, Richard M. The Gift Relationship: From Human Blood to Social Policy. Edited by Anne Oakley and John Ashton. 1970; New York: Free Press, 1987.

Tourism Investigation and Monitoring Team. "Opinion Divided over Benefits of Medical Tourism." *new frontiers* 12, no. 3 (2006). Third World Network Web site, http://www.twnside.org.sg/title2/nf123.doc.

Traweek, Sharon. *Beamtimes and Lifetimes: The World of High Energy Physicists*. Cambridge, Mass.: Harvard University Press, 1988.

Tsing, Anna. "The Global Situation." *Cultural Anthropology* 15, no. 3 (2000): 327–60.

Tsuge, Azumi. "How Japanese Women Describe Their Experience of Prenatal Testing." In *Predictive and Genetic Testing in Asia*, edited by Margaret Sleeboom-Faulkner, 109–24. Amsterdam: Amsterdam University Press, 2010.

Tu, Wei-ming. "Cultural China: The Periphery as Center." *Daedalus* 120, no. 2 (Spring 1991): 1–32.

Tu, Wei-ming, Milan Hejtmanek, and Alan Wachman, eds. *The Confucian World Observed: A Contemporary Discussion of Confucian Humanism in East Asia*. Honolulu: East West Center, 1992.

UNESCO [United Nations Educational, Scientific and Cultural Organization]. *Towards Knowledge Societies*. Paris: UNESCO, 2005.

Usher, Pat. "Feminist Approaches to a Situated Ethics." In *Situated Ethics in Educational Research*, edited by Helen Simons and Robin Usher. London: Routledge, 2000.

Waldby, Catherine, and Robert Mitchell. *Tissue Economies: Blood, Organs, and Cell Lines in Late Capitalism*. Durham: Duke University Press, 2006.

Wallace, Alfred Russell. "Remarks at the British Association and to 'The Spectator' on the Degeneracy Theory." *Anthropology Review*, October 1869, 420–21. Reprint at http://www.wku.edu/smithch/wallace/S150152.htm.

Wang, T. Y., and Liu I-Chou. "Contending Identities in Taiwan." *Asian Survey* 44, no. 4 (2004): 568–90.

Washington, Harriet A. *Medical Apartheid: The Dark History of Medical Experimentation on Black Americans from Colonial Times to the Present*. New York: Random House, 2008.

Webster's New Collegiate Dictionary. Springfield, Mass.: G. and C. Merriam, 1956.

Whittaker, Andrea. "Pleasure and Pain: Medical Travel in Asia." *Global Public Health* 3, no. 3 (2008): 271–90.

Whyte, G. "Ethical Aspects of Blood and Organ Donation." *Internal Medical Journal* 33 (2003): 362–64.

Wibulpolparsert, Suwit. "International Trade and Migration of Health Workforce: Experienced from Thailand." Paper presented at the Joint WTO-World Bank Symposium on the Movement of Persons (Mode 4) under GATS. World Trade Organization, Geneva, April 11–12, 2008, http://www.wto.org/english/tratop_e/serv_e/symp_apr_02_suwit_e.doc.

Wilsdon, James, and James Keeley. *China: The Next Science Superpower? The Atlas of Ideas: Mapping the New Geography of Science*. London: Demos, 2007

Wilson, Ara. *The Intimate Economies of Bangkok: Tomboys, Tycoons, and Avon Ladies in the Global City*. Berkeley: University of California Press, 2004.

Wipatayotin, Preeyanat Phanayanggoor Apinya. "PM 'Failed to Consult the Public.'" *Bangkok Post*, January 9, 2006.

World Bank. *World Bank Development Report 1998–1999: Knowledge for Development*. Washington D.C.: World Bank, 1999, http://www.worldbank.org/wdr/wdr98.

World Mental Health Survey Consortium. "Prevalence, Severity, and Unmet Need for Treatment of Mental Disorders in the World Health Organization World Mental Health Surveys." *Journal of the American Medical Association* 291 (2004): 2581–90.

Yamanaka, Shinya. "Scientists at Work." *New York Times*, December 11, 2007.

Yan Xuetong. "The Rise of China in Chinese Eyes." *Journal of Contemporary China* 10 no. 26 (2001): 33–39.

Yang, Mayfair Mei-Hui. *Gifts, Favors and Banquets: The Art of Social Relationships in China*. Ithaca, N.Y.: Cornell University Press, 1994.

Yao, Yong-Gang, et al. "Phylogeographic Differentiation of Mitochondrial DNA in Han Chinese." *American Journal of Human Genetics* 70 (2002): 635–51.

Yoshida, Masayuki. "Reconsidering the Japanese Negative Attitude toward Brain Death and Organ Transplantation." *Eubios Journal of Asian and International Bioethics* 14 (2004): 91–95.

You, May-Su, and Vladimir Korzh. "Zebrafish in the Tropical One-North." *Zebrafish* 1, no. 4 (March 1, 2005): 327–34.

Yu, Jun, et al. "A Draft Sequence of the Rice Genome (*Oryza sativa* L. ssp. *indica*)." *Science* 296, no. 5565 (April 5, 2002): 79–92.

Zaller, Nickolas, Konrad E. Nelson, Paul Ness, Guoxing Wen, Turgun Dewir, Xuhua Bai, and Hua Shan. "Demographic Characteristics and Risks for Transfusion-transmissible Infection among Blood Donors in Xinjiang Autonomous Region, People's Republic of China." *Transfusion* 46 (2006): 265–71.

——. "Knowledge, Attitude and Practice Survey Regarding Blood Donation in a Northwestern Chinese City." *Transfusion Medicine* 15 (2005): 277–86.

Zhan, Mei. "Wild Consumptions: Relocating Responsibilities in the Time of SARS." In *Privatizing China, Socialism from Afar*, edited by Li Zhang and Aihwa Ong. Ithaca, N.Y.: Cornell University Press, 2008.

Zhang, Feng, Bing Su, Ya-ping Zhang, and Li Jin. "Genetic Studies of Human Diversity in East Asia." *Philosophical Transactions of the Royal Society of London*, ser. B, Biological Sciences, 362, no. 1482 (2007): 987–95.

Zhang, Qifa. "China: Agricultural Biotechnology Opportunities to Meet the Challenges of Food Production." In *Agricultural Biotechnology and the Poor*, edited by G. J. Persley and M. M. Lantin. Report of the International Conference on Biotechnology, convened by the Consultative Group on International Agricultural Research of the World Bank and the U.S. National Academy of Sciences, in Washington, D.C., October 21–22, 1999.

Contributors

VINCANNE ADAMS is director of the Medical Anthropology Program at the University of California, San Francisco (joint program with University of California, Berkeley) and a professor of medical anthropology. She is the author of three books and numerous articles on medical anthropology, women's health, and the politics of modernity in Inner Asia.

NANCY N. CHEN is professor of anthropology at the University of California, Santa Cruz (on leave from Scripps College). A medical anthropologist, she is author of *Food, Medicine, and the Quest for Good Health* (2009) and *Breathing Spaces: Qigong, Psychiatry, and Healing in China* (2003), and coeditor of *China Urban: Ethnographies of Contemporary Culture* (2001) and *Bodies in the Making: Transgression and Transformation* (2006).

STEFAN ECKS is codirector of the Anthropology of Health and Illness Program and a senior lecturer in social anthropology at the University of Edinburgh. Ecks has conducted fieldwork in South Asia since 1999. His current work looks at emerging forms of pharmaceutical uses, evidence-based medicine, and global corporate citizenship. He recently completed a collaborative project that traced how three key pharmaceuticals (fluoxetine, oxytocin, rifampicin) are regulated, produced, distributed, and prescribed in India and Nepal.

KATHLEEN ERWIN is director of the Research Program Application and Review Center at the University of California Office of the President. She received her Ph.D. in anthropology from the University of California, Berkeley, and completed a postdoc in AIDS prevention studies at UCSF. Dr. Erwin first lived in Shanghai in 1984, and has conducted research in China since 1993 on topics ranging from gender and sexual culture to her more recent work on blood donation and HIV.

PHUOC V. LE has a master's of public health degree from the University of California, Berkeley, and a medical degree from Stanford. He is currently a resident in the Harvard Affiliated Residency in Internal Medicine and Pediatrics, and a Global Health Equity resident at Brigham and Women's Hospital in Boston, Massachusetts.

JENNIFER LIU is a graduate of the University of California, Berkeley–University of California, San Francisco, Joint Program in Medical Anthropology and a CEAPS Freeman Postdoctoral Fellow in Chinese science and technology at the Department of History at University of Illinois, Urbana-Champaign. She has conducted field research in Taiwan and California on stem cell research and bioethics. Her current research focuses on biomedical technologies, biobanks, and ethics, with a specific interest in how biological collections articulate with notions of identity and ethnicity.

AIHWA ONG is professor of anthropology at the University of California, Berkeley. Her research focuses on questions of modernity, citizenship, neoliberalism, and biosciences in Asia-Pacific contexts. She is the author of many books, including *Flexible Citizenship* (1999), *Buddha is Hiding* (2003), and *Neoliberalism as Exception* (2006); and co-editor of *Global Assemblages* (2005) and *Privatizing China, Socialism from Afar* (2008). Her writings have been translated into many languages, including Chinese. She serves as the chair of the U.S. National Committee on the Pacific Science Association.

MARGARET SLEEBOOM-FAULKNER is senior lecturer in anthropology at the University of Sussex. Her work focuses on nationalism and processes of nation-state building in China and Japan and on biotechnology and society in East Asia. She currently directs the Socio-genetic Marginalization in Asia Programme (SMAP) institutionally located in the International Institute for Asian Studies (IIAS), Leiden (2004–09), and conducts comparative research into the social, political, and international aspects of stem cell research in East Asia.

KAUSHIK SUNDER RAJAN is associate professor of anthropology at the University of Chicago. He is the author of *Biocapital: The Constitution of Post-Genomic Life* (2006), which is an ethnographic study of genomics-driven marketplaces in the United States and India. He is currently studying the globalization of clinical trials, with a focus on the United States and India.

WEN-CHING SUNG is an assistant professor in the Department of Anthropology at the University of Toronto. She is a social cultural anthropologist with training in both medical anthropology and anthropology of science. She conducts field research in China, Taiwan, and North America. Her overall intellectual interests are in the production and social implications of medical knowledge and technologies. She is working on a book, an ethnographic investigation of the scientific, political, and social circumstances under which biotechnology has developed in contemporary China.

CHARIS THOMPSON is associate professor of rhetoric and gender and women's studies at the University of California, Berkeley, and codirector of the University of California, Berkeley, Science, Technology, and Society Center. She is author of *Making Parents: The Ontological Choreography of Reproductive Technologies* (2005), which won the 2007 Rachel Carson Prize from the Society for the Social Study of

Science. She serves on two embryonic stem cell research oversight ethics committees, and runs a gender, race, nation, and science initiative.

ARA WILSON is director of the program in the study of sexualities and associate professor of women's studies and cultural anthropology at Duke University. She is the author of *The Intimate Economies of Bangkok: Tomboys, Tycoons and Avon Ladies in the Global City* and a book in progress titled *Sexual Latitudes: The Erotic Life of Globalization*, which analyzes globalization as a stage for sexual politics. Medical tourism in Southeast Asia is the subject of her next ethnographic research project.

Index

Page numbers in italics refer to illustrations.

Aihwa Ong is professor of anthropology at the University of California, Berkeley.

Nancy N. Chen is professor of anthropology at the University of California, Santa Cruz.

Library of Congress Cataloging-in-Publication Data
Asian biotech : ethics and communities of fate /
edited by Aihwa Ong and Nancy N. Chen.
p. cm.—(Experimental futures : technological lives, scientific arts, anthropological voices)
Includes bibliographical references and index.
ISBN 978-0-8223-4793-4 (cloth : alk. paper)
ISBN 978-0-8223-4809-2 (pbk. : alk. paper)
1. Biotechnology—Asia. 2. Biotechnology—Moral and ethical aspects—Asia. I. Ong, Aihwa. II. Chen, Nancy N. III. Series: Experimental futures.
HD9999.B443A7815 2010
338.4′76606095—dc22   2010017239